The Complete Book
of Cosmetic Surgery

THE COMPLETE BOOK OF
Cosmetic Surgery

A CANDID GUIDE FOR MEN, WOMEN, & TEENS

Elizabeth Morgan, M.D., F.A.C.S.

WARNER BOOKS

A Warner Communications Company

Copyright © 1988 by Elizabeth Morgan
All rights reserved.
Warner Books, Inc., 666 Fifth Avenue, New York, NY 10103

Ⓦ A Warner Communications Company

Printed in the United States of America
First Printing: February 1988
10 9 8 7 6 5 4 3 2 1

Library of Congress Cataloging-in-Publication Data
Morgan, Elizabeth, 1947–
    The complete book of cosmetic surgery.
    1. Surgery, Plastic—Popular works. I. Title.
[DNLM: 1. Esthetics—popular works. 2. Surgery,
Plastic—popular works. WO 600 M8472c]
RD118.M68   1988   617′.95   87-40178
ISBN 0-446-51370-9

Book design: H. Roberts

This book is dedicated to my patients, past, present and future, and to my office staff who help me and my patients so much.

Contents

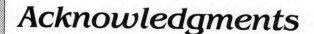

Acknowledgments

It is a great pleasure to thank my editor, Jamie Rothstein, for her astute criticism, hard work, encouragement, and perseverance. She is a wonderful editor.

I would also like to thank Molly Friedrich, my agent and dear friend, who encouraged the idea of this book and worked hard to bring it to life.

Praise also goes to Joyce Hurwitz, the artist whose illustrations appear in this book. Besides being an excellent artist, she had wonderful suggestions of her own and worked long and hard to make her work artistic as well as accurate.

I would like to thank Antonia, Paul, and Meg for their critical readings of various chapters, and Lillian Rodberg for her very diligent and creative copyediting.

A very special thanks goes to Dr. Robert Goldwyn for his critical reading and excellent advice on certain chapters as well.

Finally, I am grateful to my daughter, Hilary, for her enthusiasm and her company during my many hours of writing and typing.

Preface

I decided to become a *plastic* surgeon the morning that, as a resident, I helped Dr. Irving Polayes at Yale correct a child's cleft lip. He told me I had "good hands," and I thought I had just seen the closest thing to a miracle. However, I was sure I would never countenance doing *cosmetic* surgery: It wasn't "real" medicine, it wasn't "serious" surgery, and the surgeons who did cosmetic work always felt a need to justify doing "unnecessary" procedures. I was wrong about cosmetic surgery. It is not only technically difficult, but every year has seen new ways of getting better results. And it is overwhelmingly important—cosmetic surgery changes not only your body but your psyche as well. Even so, other doctors still ask cosmetic surgeons why they are "wasting" their talents—*until the questioner or someone in that doctor's family decides to turn to cosmetic surgery.* Then they come to learn what this unique specialty is all about.

Does "Cosmetic" Mean Unnecessary?

As a patient, you may find some of the same prejudice. People tend to be opposed to something new which they don't understand. You may feel, or may be made to feel, that a cosmetic operation is something that you ought to be embarrassed or guilty about having. I hope to persuade you *not* to feel that way.

Cosmetic surgery is like much of modern surgery: Cataract surgery, hip replacement surgery, bunion surgery as well as facelift surgery are all life-*improving*, not life-*saving* operations. If someone labels your cosmetic operation "unnecessary," don't bother to feel guilty. You're in good company.

And cosmetic surgery isn't insignificant "just" because it makes you look better. Almost every patient I have tells me, "I know I'm only doing this for my looks." True, perhaps, but it makes "looks" sound of little importance. In fact, like it or not, your looks are very important because they affect how you feel about yourself and how others feel about you. Surgery that's "just" for looks includes everything from cosmetic breast enlargement to reconstructing a badly burned face—any kind of operation that changes your body *visibly*.

Pauline was a slightly discouraged teenager who had had a series of operations for a stomach disorder. Her upper lids were heavy and drooped over her lashes; this ran in her family. When Pauline needed another stomach operation, she pleaded to have her eyelids cosmetically improved at the same time. She couldn't explain why. She desperately wanted it done. Reluctantly, her parents agreed, though they clearly felt that they were encouraging vanity and frivolity. After all, Pauline needed the stomach surgery. The eyelid surgery was "totally useless."

The two operations were done together. For the first time, Pauline was not seriously depressed after an operation. In fact, her therapist found her in bed with a palette of eyeshadows and a book on makeup. Ten days after surgery, when she was discharged home, she was allowed to wear her eye makeup. "Needing my stomach operated on always makes me feel like something defective that ought to be thrown away," said Pauline. "But now that my eyes are fixed and the eye shadow shows, I feel pretty good." Her cosmetic surgery had done what nothing else could do: It made her feel that she was attractive, not a reject.

What Makes Surgery "Cosmetic"?

Insurance companies think that the distinction between cosmetic and reconstructive surgery is easy. Reconstructive surgery is what they pay for. Cosmetic surgery is what makes your insurance company laugh when you send in a claim form. But much as your insurance company wants you to think that it has all the answers, these companies change their definition of "cosmetic" all the time. There are no fixed rules. Insurance companies once argued strenuously that reconstructing a breast after a mastectomy was cosmetic. After a while, they changed their minds and agreed that it was cancer reconstruction. Insurance payment problems also abound around correcting "Dumbo" ears in little children, dermabrasion of acne scars, and making enlarged breasts smaller. All of these operations were once written off by insurance companies as cosmetic. Patients who had them were not reimbursed. Doctors and patients who didn't think that was fair convinced most insurance companies to change their minds.

Insurance companies are *not* the last word. I consider surgery to be cosmetic if you have the operation because you don't like the way your looks make you *feel*. If your biggest benefit is psychological, then I call the surgery cosmetic. Not everyone agrees with me, but I think it is the best practical definition.

Edward had a bump on his nose, and everyone told him he was "dumb" to have it fixed. He was a good-looking athlete and had lots of friends. They all agreed he should not waste his time and money.

Edward had cosmetic nose surgery when he finished college. He was not only happy to get rid of the bump, but he felt more sure of himself and less intimidated by going into sales, which was what he wanted to do. "People tell me I look fine," he said afterwards, "but I don't feel it inside me. Changing my nose makes me feel inside as though I can go out and sell, and people will be listening to me, not wondering why I don't get my nose fixed."

Rita had heavy hips, no matter how much she exercised and dieted. She was successful in her career as an account executive. She was married. She was happy. She just wanted to stop thinking of herself as "the girl with the hips." She had a liposuction done to take out her hip bulges. "I love it," she said afterwards. "No one notices. My husband loved me before. People at work couldn't care less. I always felt fat as a teenager. I couldn't forget as long as I had hips. A thousand people would think it was silly, but it finally let me grow up and be the me I am now, not what I was back then."

Why I've Written This Book the Way I Have

I've been a doctor for almost 20 years, and in plastic surgery for 12. I've always been struck by how little time surgeons have to explain surgery to their patients and how much people want to know about the operation before they have it done. Like a lot of surgeons, I spend a lot of time answering my patients' questions. And, at the end of the consultation *I* know, and *they* know, that there is so much to know that they can't possibly remember it all when they go home to think about it. Time and time again I have been asked, "Is there something I can read before I come in to see you or before I have the surgery?" There *are* books, but none that seemed right to me. Some were too glorified (plastic surgery is *not* for everyone). Some were out of date. Some were interesting but incomplete. So, since no one else had done it, I decided that I had to do it, for you, so that you could know as much as you want to know about your surgery—and go back and study the information—before your operation.

This book will also see you through your recovery period. No one really believes the surgeon when he tells them that *time* is necessary after cosmetic surgery to let swelling diminish, scars fade, and final results appear. This book takes you through your healing period so that you can know when you are healing like everyone else and when you may not be, and what to do about it.

You Need to Know the Facts

This book is as honest and candid as I can possibly make it. Doctors don't like to alarm patients—especially not about something like cosmetic surgery, when chances are you'll do fine, be pleased, and should almost enjoy the surgery. But the overwhelming tendency in anything you read about cosmetic surgery is to portray it as nothing more serious than getting a permanent or a workout at a health spa. As a result, doctors know the truth—that this is *surgery*—but you have a misconception about what is involved and what surgery can do. You might not want all the details. Fine—you can skip those parts of my book. But at least you'll know they are here. And you'll know that when your cosmetic surgeon tells you "no one ever has a problem with this operation," what he really means is that most people are pleased with the result, not that this is risk-free surgery with guaranteed results. That is why the examples in this book reflect what *really* happens, including complications, side effects, and comments from patients—most of whom are pleased, but not all.

For the same reason, the illustrations in this book are more graphic, and the "before and after" photographs less spectacular, than in other cosmetic surgery books. During the consultation, I like to show my patients surgical textbook illustrations of their operation to help them understand what will be done to their bodies. Because you are entitled to know this too, I wanted the illustrations in my book to reveal more than just the end results of your operation. So to the extent that I could (without making you uncomfortable) I have chosen illustrations that show you at least some of what a surgical textbook might.

As for the "before and after" photos in this book, they were chosen to show *average* results. My intention is really to give you more of an idea of why photos *aren't* reliable indicators of your surgical result, rather than to demonstrate the "miracle of cosmetic surgery." I want you to understand that "blah," unflattering medical photographs such as these are for your doctor's record—and that even with a spectacular result you may not be "wowed" by a medical photo.

Some Last Thoughts

There are a few other things I'd like you to know before you go on to the rest of the book. First, I am a woman, and yet I refer to your cosmetic surgeon, throughout this book, as "he." I've done this because our language has no pronoun that means "he or she." "Heesh" won't do and he/she is tedious to read over and over again. We live in a democracy, and I decided that I had to represent the majority—and the majority of plastic surgeons, so far, are men.

Every good surgeon has his own way of doing things. If your

surgeon tells you *not* to get your stitches wet, and my book says you can get them wet—listen to *him*. He knows what kind of stitches he put in you. But most surgeons don't have the time or organization to tell you all the details. This book has the hundred or so things he didn't mention and that you wanted, or perhaps needed, to know.

The prices I quote for various operations in Part II are the current range as of June 1987. Inflation is always with us. These prices may soon be out of date, but they should help you to compare the relative costs of cosmetic operations. Please don't be surprised if your surgeon charges more than I say he "ought" to charge—or, if he uses a new drug or equipment not mentioned here, because of new discoveries.

In Part II, I also tell you about insurance—when it might or should pay for your surgery. However, do keep in mind that you will pay *in advance* for cosmetic surgery. Insurance reimburses you *afterwards*, if at all.

Then, there's that difficult question: Who is a "cosmetic surgeon"? I am a Board Certified plastic surgeon. There are not quite 4000 of us in the United States. When I refer to a "good" or qualified surgeon in this book, I am thinking of my colleagues in plastic surgery. However, Board Certified plastic surgeons are not the only ones who do cosmetic surgery. Cosmetic surgery is not a recognized medical specialty, and there is no medical board certification in it. Before you have a cosmetic operation, I want you to know who your cosmetic surgeon is and what his qualifications are—which I discuss in Chapter 2.

Finally, I wrote this book to help you. I didn't write it to convince you that I should operate on you. There are lots of good plastic surgeons doing cosmetic surgery, but not all of them like to write as well as operate. I have many friends and family members who have had or want to have cosmetic surgery. This book consists of what I would tell them if we had all weekend to sit down and talk.

I have been asked at times to name my "ghostwriter." It is *me*. I wrote it—not "with" or "as told to" or "by" someone else, but as though you were sitting in my office with a list of things you wanted to know.

If you want something glossy in three seconds that tells you "don't worry, there's nothing to it," well, this book isn't for you. But if you want the most complete information you can get, without going to medical school and doing a seven-year residency . . . this is it!

P A R T

What No One Has Told You Before

ONE

CHAPTER   1

"Why Am I Doing This?"— Examining Your Motives

Nancy bred St. Bernard dogs. Her face developed jowls around her jawline. "I know people who end up looking like the animals they keep," she explained to me, laughing. "I'm damned if I'm going to let myself look as jowly as a St. Bernard!"

Almost everyone is physically imperfect. Perfection in a face is so rare that I have seen only one woman—Ingrid Bergman in her youth— whose face *I* considered perfect. Other people see perfection in Tom Selleck, Brooke Shields, Vanessa Williams, and other celebrities who seem to be naturally sculpted beyond criticism. Only a fraction of the population does *not* have a physical flaw that surgery could improve.

I'm certainly not one of them. My nose is broad with a twist at the tip. My upper lids sag. My ears stick out at the top . . . I could go on. Most people think I look fine. But *I* know my imperfections better than anyone else. When a big change occurred in my personal life, I wanted a cosmetic operation, and it probably would have helped me psychologically. But I didn't have the time.

YOUR MOTIVES: RIGHT, WRONG, OR IN BETWEEN?

There is a difference between using cosmetic surgery as a crutch—having unreasonable expectations—and using it to help you through a transition in your life. Most people have cosmetic surgery when their lives are changing for better or worse: at times of marriage, divorce, birth, or deaths, or after a child is grown and gone. Other popular "surgery times" are when you change or lose a job, graduate from high school or college, or have a birthday—especially one that marks the decade!

Such changes shake your confidence because they force you to see yourself in a new way. You can worry as much about your ability when you are promoted as when you are fired. Your new marriage may make you as fearful about *possible* failure as a divorce can make you feel a failure. You wonder how you will manage. You know there has to be a "you" that you haven't been before. Cosmetic surgery is a powerful psychological aid to being that *new you*, to start fresh. It's *never* too late.

Debby was an attractive woman, married, with a family of three. Her breasts sagged after her pregnancies. She wanted a breast enlargement to correct this. I did the surgery. Debby healed with a perfect surgical result. When she came back for a routine checkup, I could tell that she had something important to say.

"Do you want to know the real *reason I had this surgery?" she asked me.*

"Yes, I would," I said. I knew there was one.

Debby took a big breath. "It is hard for me to say. My father used me sexually for years. I hated myself. After I left home, I was raped. All this complete stranger said while he attacked me was 'Your breasts are shrunken like prunes.' I hated my body. I knew that if I could have this breast surgery, somehow it would put those things all behind me. My mind could rest."

That was part of her reason. There was more. Debby's husband abused her, physically. Her cosmetic surgery was also her preparation for the impending divorce. Having the surgery gave her the confidence to face the change.

Cosmetic surgery can give you the confidence and the psychic boost to surmount a hurdle in life. The need for such a boost can arise

from something as bad as Debby's abuse, or from something as seem-
ingly insignificant as being teased about your appearance, even years
before.

*Ed was a young man who graduated from high school with good
grades after lots of hard work. He was accepted in college but felt he could
not face the challenge. He was intimidated by college and wanted to drop
out—before he'd begun. Ed had scars from acne five years before. He had
been called "Goober" in eighth grade. He saw his face as grotesque. I did
a dermabrasion (skin sanding) of Ed's face and injected some of the deeper
scars with collagen (a liquid skin protein). Ed's treatment improved his
skin noticeably, but it improved his psyche dramatically. After surgery, at
the end of the summer, he went off to college optimistic and secure.*

Such renewed confidence may come from cosmetic surgery at any
time in your life.

*Franceen was an older woman, widowed for a year. She had disliked
her nose since her sisters called her "Parrot" at the age of fifteen. Franceen's
nose had become coarser and more bulbous with time. She was moving to
Florida to live with her sister, but she felt depressed at the prospect. She
did not think she could face strangers. Franceen had nose surgery before
she moved. She left for her new life happy and hopeful because she felt
better about herself and was not so afraid of rejection by strangers.*

When people use cosmetic surgery for the wrong reasons, the
surgery may not help.

*George was a middle-aged businessman who remarried after his di-
vorce. George's new wife was young, willowy, and athletic. He was per-
petually anxious that she would feel embarrassed by the difference in their
ages, so he had cosmetic eye surgery, to look and feel younger. It made
him look less tired, but it didn't make him feel more secure. Actually his
wife thought George looked fine, but George's self-doubts about his energy
and ability to keep up with her and fit in with her friends had nothing to
do with his looks, and were not "fixed" with plastic surgery.*

Another person who had cosmetic surgery for the wrong reasons
was a very glamorous airline stewardess. She said that she wanted
surgery to keep up with the younger women she worked with. In fact,

not only was her job secure, but she looked great. She had cosmetic face and eye surgery and had a perfectly good surgical result. However, it didn't change what she wanted to change. Her real reason for surgery was that her marriage was in trouble. Her husband was dating other women. It was *his* personality and not *her* looks that were the root of the trouble. Cosmetic surgery couldn't cure that.

YOUR "KNOWING-YOUR-MOTIVATIONS" CHECKLIST

Why do *you* want cosmetic surgery? Below are 35 of the most common reasons. Choose ones closest to yours by marking "True" or "False" next to each statement.

1. I want my face (nose, breasts, etc.) to look better so I can feel better about my looks. ☐ **True** ☐ **False**

2. I don't like my nose (thighs, ears, etc.) and want to see the improvement when I look in the mirror. ☐ **True** ☐ **False**

3. My makeup can do just so much. It needs help. ☐ **True** ☐ **False**

4. I'm tired of putting everyone else first. It's *my* turn. ☐ **True** ☐ **False**

5. I've *always* wanted to do this. I can see what I don't like and I know how to change it. ☐ **True** ☐ **False**

6. I want to erase or change what grief has etched in my face. ☐ **True** ☐ **False**

7. I want to forget about ever having been teased. ☐ **True** ☐ **False**

8. I can see the changes in my face and I don't like them. I want them improved. ☐ **True** ☐ **False**

9. I do everything I can to make the best of myself, and this is just one of those ways. ☐ **True** ☐ **False**

10. I can see what the physical problem is, and it bothers me enough to make surgery worthwhile. ☐ **True** ☐ **False**

11. My family *owes* me this surgery. ☐ **True** ☐ **False**

12. I *hate* having the "family resemblance." ☐ True ☐ False
13. It never bothered me until _____ ☐ True ☐ False
    happened.
14. I'm so boring! I've *got* to make a change ☐ True ☐ False
    in my life.
15. I *refuse* to grow old. ☐ True ☐ False
16. I want to be happier. ☐ True ☐ False
17. I look older than I want to feel inside. ☐ True ☐ False
18. I hate myself and I want to change. ☐ True ☐ False
19. I want to show him/her that I *don't care* ☐ True ☐ False
    about being rejected.
20. My mom/dad/husband/wife/lover will hate ☐ True ☐ False
    my having surgery, and it serves them
    right.
21. I'm exhausted and I *look* it. ☐ True ☐ False
22. If I get rid of the flaw, I just know I'll ☐ True ☐ False
    have a better chance of attracting a new
    boyfriend/girlfriend.
23. So-and-so had the surgery and six months ☐ True ☐ False
    later he/she was engaged.
24. My looks are all that are standing between ☐ True ☐ False
    me and that promotion.
25. I want my clothes to *fit* right for a change. ☐ True ☐ False
    (Applies only to body surgery.)
26. I want to look *great* for the reunion/mar- ☐ True ☐ False
    riage/party.
27. The surgery will make me a successful ☐ True ☐ False
    model.
28. I just know surgery will help me look more ☐ True ☐ False
    like Bo Derek/Tom Selleck/whomever.
29. I'm determined to: be a 34B bra/have a ☐ True ☐ False
    28-inch waist/be able to go without
    makeup/be able to wear my hair long/
    not to be bald anymore/etc.
30. Everyone else is doing it. I can afford it, ☐ True ☐ False
    so why not?
31. My parents offered to get me a nose job ☐ True ☐ False
    for graduation. I may not get another chance
    to have one, if I don't have it now.

32. My doctor said I should have it done and   ☐ **True**   ☐ **False**
he's the expert.
33. I know my husband/wife/children want   ☐ **True**   ☐ **False**
me to have the surgery. If it means that
much to them . . . why not?
34. Anything's got to be better than the way   ☐ **True**   ☐ **False**
I look now.
35. I'm not sure I know why I want to have   ☐ **True**   ☐ **False**
cosmetic surgery. I just do.

Understanding Your Answers

Common Simple Reasons. Those of you who answered "True" only to reasons from 1 to 10 will be happiest with your cosmetic surgery result. Your reasons for surgery are realistic. Your desire is not an impulse. Your expectations are in line with what surgery can do.

Complex Reasons. If most of your reasons are similar to those from 11 to 20, you might reconsider your motivations. These reasons suggest that one or more important events or people in your life make you feel confused, angry, or unhappy. Surgery may be helpful, but it won't resolve these conflicts. You'll be *much* happier with your surgery if you *also* arrange some kind of therapy to help you rid yourself of your inner turmoil. For instance, can you resign yourself to aging, instead of attempting the impossible by *refusing* to age? Who *made* you feel old or boring? For your best surgical result, *resolve complex inner feelings in addition to having cosmetic surgery.*

Overly Specific Reasons. Reasons similar to those between 21 and 29 suggest that you *may* be asking surgery to do something beyond its power. I have *often* seen surgery being followed promptly by a promotion, a marriage, or a new relationship, but the surgery itself cannot predictably lead to these changes. If you are counting on surgery to deliver great or rested looks, you may be disappointed. Surgery can only *help*. Successful surgery may not deliver such specific goals as looking good in certain clothes or hairstyles. And, since no surgery could make Tom Selleck look like Paul Newman, how can it make you look like Tom Selleck? To want to be able to "see the change in the mirror" is realistic; to have exactly a 28-inch waist may not be. Can you modify your hopes to be more compatible with what surgery can deliver? If so, you greatly increase your chances of happiness with the result!

Inadequate Reasons. For those of you who answered "True" to reasons 30 to 35, you must understand that cosmetic surgery is not like buying a loaf of bread. This is an *operation*! So what if everyone else is doing it—is it right for *you*? As for showing you have the money—won't a mink, a Mercedes, or a monster diamond do a better job? If a doctor recommended an operation, such as a breast reduction, you should consider his opinion—but you shouldn't follow it blindly. The same goes for the opinions of friends and relatives. It's *your body*. Do *you* want the surgery? Having an inadequate reason, especially if it is your *only* reason, suggests either that you are much too blasé about surgery or that you aren't aware of why you're doing it. I strongly recommend that you wait until you do know. You won't regret it.

CHAPTER   2

Choosing a Cosmetic Surgeon

So, you are serious about having a cosmetic operation. At least, you want to talk to a surgeon to find out what is involved. You don't have any referrals, so you reach for the Yellow Pages to check the "Cosmetic Surgeon" listing. *Not yet, please!* The terms *cosmetic* and *plastic* are *not* registered trademarks. In fact, you're probably wondering what the difference is between "plastic" and "cosmetic" surgery. There is no difference now. Doctors as well as patients tend to use the words interchangeably.

We've Come a Long Way

A century ago, shady self-styled cosmetic surgeons moved from city to city in America doing cosmetic operations. These operations only cut out a little skin. The results were poor. The scars were bad. The traveling surgeon left his patients and their complications behind him as he moved on. Surprisingly there were still such itinerant surgeons in the 1930s. Not surprisingly, they gave cosmetic surgery a bad reputation. Yet, at about the same time, pioneering work was being done by surgeons such as Dr. Jacques Joseph.

Dr. Joseph, working in Berlin, developed the first cosmetic nose operation, did it properly, and reported it in a scientific journal in 1898. Today, Dr. Joseph would be called an orthopedic surgeon, one who specializes in operations on the bones and joints. At that time, no surgical specialities had been officially established. Any surgeon who worked on reshaping the human body could have been called a plastic surgeon, since "plastic" in this sense derives from the Latin *plasticere*, which means "to mold." During World War I many military surgeons put their talents to work repairing the faces and bodies of wounded soldiers. After the war these surgeons went into private practice. Patients came to these plastic surgeons for treatment of cosmetic problems because they were known to have developed operations to mold the human body in ways that seemed almost miraculous in the 1920s. Plastic surgery became a recognized specialty in the United States in 1937, when the American Board of Plastic and Reconstructive Surgery was founded. It established exams and qualifications for surgeons doing plastic surgery, which included cosmetic surgery as well as reconstructive surgery. The term *plastic surgeon* became synonymous with *cosmetic surgeon*.

What Qualifications Should I Look For?

Today, any doctor can call himself a cosmetic plastic surgeon. All he needs is his medical degree and a state license to practice medicine. He need not have seen, done, or read about a single cosmetic operation. He can have a sign saying "Cosmetic Plastic Surgeon." He can have fancy "Cosmetic Surgery" business cards, and he can operate on you in his own fully equipped office operating room. This is completely legal. And office operating rooms are *fine* so long as the surgeons operating in them are qualified to do your operation.

It's easy for me to tell you that you must never take your surgeon's training or ability on faith. (Once you have facts to back it up, faith in your surgeon is super. Studies show it can actually promote healing.) But how can you judge his competence? Don't panic. Once you understand the qualifications needed to perform cosmetic surgery, you'll be able to make an informed decision yourself.

Doctors from several surgical specialties do cosmetic operations: plastic and reconstructive surgeons; ear, nose, and throat (ENT) surgeons; and eye surgeons. What about me? I am board certified in general surgery and also in plastic and reconstructive surgery. This is called "double boarded." I had one of the longest possible trainings for cosmetic surgery: four years of college, four years of medical school, five years of general surgery training, and two years of plastic surgery training. This was a total of 15 years after high school.

A much shorter road to being a cosmetic surgeon would be, for instance, combining college and medical school in six years, then doing three years in general surgery and two in plastic surgery: an 11-year training period. Such a surgeon could be trained in all plastic surgery operations, just as I am. Or, if such a surgeon wanted to do only cosmetic surgery of the face, he could limit his training to ENT surgery, which would be a total of nine or ten years after high school. Many ENT surgeons are trained these days in cosmetic surgery of the face but not in other areas of plastic surgery.

Understanding Professional Feuds

These three specialties compete—and I mean *compete*—in cosmetic surgery. Why does professional jealousy exist? My field, plastic and reconstructive surgery, invented and developed virtually all cosmetic operations as well as such major reconstructive operations as microsurgery and kidney transplants. We feel as though the cosmetic procedures belong to us, and that we do them *better* than anyone else. Our entire training is devoted to learning how to make the body look and work as perfectly as possible. Still, in medicine, what one specialty discovers and perfects, other specialties will also learn. (For instance, the first kidney transplant was done by a plastic surgeon in 1953 in Boston. Now there are surgeons who limit their work specifically to transplant surgery.)

That doesn't mean that we plastic surgeons *like* having our field invaded. When I was in training, a famous plastic surgeon I worked with wouldn't let ENT residents *near* his operating room when he did a facelift. He didn't approve of the ENT specialty doing such cosmetic operations. Another equally gifted plastic surgeon did not agree and would let any surgeon watch him at work. Regardless of what plastic surgeons think, ENT and eye surgeons are doing cosmetic operations, and you need to know what their specialties are and what they are qualified to do.

Plastic and Reconstructive Surgery. This is my field. Plastic surgeons do all cosmetic operations as well as all reconstructive operations, ranging from removing skin cancers to rebuilding a face or another body part.

Ear-Nose-Throat (ENT) Surgery (Otorhinolaryngologic Surgery). Some ENT surgeons do facial cosmetic operations (facelifts, cosmetic nose and eye surgery) as well as other facial surgery ranging from placing ear tubes to removing major mouth (oral) cancers.

Eye Surgery (Ophthalmologic Surgery). Some eye surgeons do cosmetic eye operations as well as other eye operations, ranging from removing eyelid cysts to repairing retinal detachments.

What Does "Board Certified" Mean?

Each of these three specialties is governed by its own specialty board approved by the American Medical Association (AMA). Each specialty board has strict rules on training requirements and gives examinations that test a surgeon's competence. These exams, which are called board examinations, are usually given after the surgeon has been in practice for a year or so. That way he can demonstrate his competence, or lack of it, by submitting his own results for review. A surgeon has to pass his board exam before he is board certified in his specialty.

Although board certification does not guarantee a surgeon to be competent, it is the highest hurdle a surgeon can vault. Certification reliably attests to a surgeon's achievements. But there are some competent surgeons who are not board eligible or board certified. For instance, a surgeon from another country might be fully trained in his specialty in his home country, but not eligible for board certification by an American specialty board. Or a surgeon might truly be very good, but become so busy so fast in private practice that it never seemed worth his while to take the board exams. Such surgeons used to be common but are increasingly rare because board certification is recognized as such an important credential.

You may find the surgical names and categories confusing, so use this glossary to help you keep all the terms straight.

COSMETIC SURGERY GLOSSARY

Plastic: From a Latin/Greek word meaning "to mold."

Plastic surgery: Surgery that molds the human body.

Reconstructive: For the purpose of rebuilding something damaged.

Cosmetic: Having to do with beauty.

Esthetic: Having to do with beauty.

Cosmetic/Esthetic Surgeon: A surgeon doing "beauty" surgery.

"Boards": Examinations that certify competence in a medical specialty. The recognized "boards" are those approved by the American Medical Association (AMA), which sets standards for medical specialty training.

Board eligible surgeon: A surgeon who has finished a specialty training program and is qualified to take the board exams if he so wishes. A surgeon is usually allowed to fail the exams twice before losing board eligibility.

Board certified surgeon: A surgeon who has finished a specialty training program and has *passed* the board examinations.

Board Certified Plastic and Reconstructive Surgeon: A surgeon trained in all aspects of plastic (including cosmetic) and reconstructive surgery who has *passed* the board exams. (Plastic surgery that isn't cosmetic is automatically considered reconstructive.)

Plastic Surgeon: What most board certified plastic and reconstructive surgeons call themselves.

Board Certified Ophthalmic Surgeon: An ophthalmic (eye) surgeon who is trained in all aspects of eye surgery (often including cosmetic eye surgery) who has *passed* the board exams. This is a different board and different exam from the Plastic and Reconstructive Surgery Board.

Cosmetic Eye Surgeon/Cosmetic Ophthalmic Surgeon: What most board certified eye surgeons call themselves if they do cosmetic eye surgery.

Board Certified Otorhinolaryngologist: An otorhinolaryngologic (ear-nose-throat or ENT is easier to say) surgeon who is trained in all aspects of ear, nose, and throat surgery. This often includes cosmetic surgery of the face. He has *passed* the board exams for this specialty, but again, these exams are not the same as the eye or plastic surgeons' exams.

Facial Plastic Surgeon: What most board certified ENT surgeons call themselves if they do cosmetic surgery on the face.

Board Certified in Cosmetic and/or Esthetic and/or Facial Plastic Surgery: This tells you *nothing.* There are no accrediting or examining boards recognized by the AMA with these names.

WARNING: *Any* doctor can call himself a plastic, facial plastic, or cosmetic eye surgeon. To evaluate his expertise, you need to know whether he is *board certified* or *board eligible* and, if not, what training he has had.

For example, I took my board exams with a brilliant Canadian surgeon who had developed new plastic surgery operations. He had passed the Canadian Board exams in plastic surgery but not the U.S. boards, which include multiple-choice questions and require a different kind of preparation. This surgeon was taking the U.S. boards but, at the same time, he was giving lectures to prepare other plastic surgeons for exam questions in *his own new operations.*

The problem comes up most often with new young surgeons who have just started out in practice. Before I was board certified, some patients wanted me to explain my lack of certification. They were entitled to ask. So are you.

Remember this: A surgeon may be qualified to "touch" you even without board certification—*if* he has the training and ability. It's true that board certification makes it *much easier* for you to assess a doctor's training. Think of it this way: If a surgeon isn't board certified, you *should* know why, and what his "just as good" credentials are, *before* you let him touch you.

What Are "Hospital Privileges"?

Two additional terms that are useful to know deserve some explanation: **hospital privileges** and **curriculum vitae.** Having "hospital privileges" or "admitting privileges" at a hospital means that a doctor is allowed to admit and treat patients in that hospital. Reputable hospitals tend to have fairly strict rules for their staffs. For instance, I could do *any* operation in my own clinic (even brain surgery!), but at a major hospital I would only be allowed to do operations in my field of specialty. I might also be required to have passed my boards to *keep* my hospital staff privileges. Most good surgeons have privileges at a major hospital, and having them is some indication of a surgeon's credentials, even if your surgery is done in his office or an outpatient surgery center. What if you don't like the hospital your surgeon uses? If he has privileges at several hospitals, you'll have a choice. If not, unless you consider the hospital dangerous (as opposed to unfriendly) dislike of a hospital is rarely grounds for choosing another surgeon.

What Is a Curriculum Vitae?

A curriculum vitae, commonly called a C.V., lists what your surgeon has done professionally. It may be one or ten pages long, depending on how many details he includes. A C.V. lets you study your surgeon's qualifications, as opposed to trying to remember them. At first glance, any C.V. will look impressive, but don't be intimidated. It should list college and medical school. Are there gaps? You might want to know why a surgeon took two years off after finishing his training. (Maybe he had a nervous breakdown.) Where did he do his training? How long has he been in practice?

Danger signals on a curriculum vitae include too much insignificant information: is he trying to impress you with trivia? For instance, a long list of conferences attended is padding on a C.V. Some C.V.s will tell you about a surgeon's family and hobbies. That is fine, if noted. But if the hobbies go on for more than a few lines, it begins to look like padding.

One of the most impressive C.V.s I have ever reviewed was one-page long: a lawyer who became a doctor and a specialist. It listed only the highlights of her career.

What About Professional Organizations?

Suppose the surgeon you are considering belongs to the *Association/Academy/Society of . . . Whatever*? There are dozens of organizations. Some are for the elite of a specialty. Some have virtually no standards. Some are for surgeons with certain interests. It is difficult to know what to make of the organizations to which your prospective surgeon belongs, unless you happen to do cosmetic surgery yourself. But you can and should feel free to ask him what a society means. For instance, A.S.P.R.S. is the American Society of Plastic and Reconstructive Surgeons. Membership is open only to surgeons who are Board Certified in Plastic and Reconstructive Surgery, plus a few distinguished plastic surgeons from other countries. On the other hand, the American *Academy* of Plastic and Reconstructive Surgeons doesn't exist. You have to be familiar with these organizations to know whether they're worth anything. If a surgeon wants you to accept membership in an organization as a substitute for board certification, I would be wary. All the reputable organizations I'm familiar with require board certification for membership.

Recognizing Professional Feuds

Competitors anywhere tend to speak against each other. I have heard excellent surgeons who usually act professionally inveighing vehemently against competing surgical fields. They may be right—or wrong. You can often tell when a surgeon whom you consult for cosmetic surgery is talking down colleagues in another specialty. You can also tell when a doctor is trying to convince you that he is qualified when he may not be.

Are Plastic and Reconstructive Surgeons Better Than Other Cosmetic Surgeons?

Please! As a plastic surgeon myself, I think we're the *best*. I tend to see the problems in the other specialties. I don't want to be accused of taking cheap shots at my competition, so let me explain what is going on. Plastic surgeons created the specialty of cosmetic surgery. However, physicians who are not plastic surgeons *have* developed some cosmetic techniques. For instance, liposuction (suctioning of fat) was developed by plastic surgeons and a dermatologist in Europe. But in the United States, plastic surgery is the only surgical residency that offers complete training in liposuction and all other cosmetic procedures as well as the psychological aspects and complications of cosmetic surgery. I could give you examples in which cosmetic surgery done by specialists in other fields fell short of what a plastic surgeon would consider standard: a scar revision in which the suture used made the scar worse, not better . . . a patient who should not have had a facelift because of psychological problems . . . a patient whose surgeon did her nose operation and admitted he didn't really know how to do it—afterwards.

Even so, plastic surgeons aren't perfect. There have even been lawsuits against plastic surgeons by ENT specialists who claim they are slandered by what these plastic surgeons are saying about them. The ENT specialty wants its board certification to include cosmetic surgery along with other procedures not traditionally in their field. However, their right to do so is currently being suspended by a court order until the AMA, which supervises the Specialty Boards, evaluates the conflicting views of ENT surgeons, allergy specialists, general surgeons, and plastic surgeons.

I think that, taken as a group, we plastic surgeons are more attuned to problems in cosmetic surgery and take it and our patients more seriously than those from other specialties. I myself would only feel comfortable putting myself in the hands of a plastic surgeon, if and when I turn to cosmetic surgery. Training is not the only issue; experience also counts. Plastic surgeons tend to do a much higher proportion of cosmetic surgery because we do all cosmetic surgery and don't limit it to one area.

You don't have to feel the same. If you read this to an ENT surgeon, he may be enraged with me and all plastic surgeons, saying, "They're just arrogant. We know as much as they do." If you show this to one of my plastic surgery colleagues, he may be equally upset: "Why does Elizabeth even have to *mention* the other guys? We're better." The fact is that you may or may not choose to go to a plastic surgeon for various reasons. You are entitled to know the facts, as objectively as I can state them, given my personal bias.

How Do I Deal with Professional Feuds?

Remember that there is professional competition. Doctors are people first, whether they'll admit it or not. If a surgeon you see for cosmetic surgery talks against another surgeon, ask him to explain how his qualifications differ from the other surgeon's. If the complaint is that the other surgeon is in a competing specialty and therefore not as good, take these objections as opinion, not fact. The same applies to me—I've tried to make it clear what the facts are, and what my opinions are. In time, plastic, ENT, and eye surgeons will agree on the proper credentials for cosmetic surgeons, and then we will have Board Certification in Cosmetic Surgery.

Where to Get Names of Reputable Plastic Surgeons

You can make your search as simple or as complicated as you wish. Like all good surgeons, I have patients who come to me because they know my reputation and my credentials, know patients on whom I have operated, and know that I will treat them well. I also have patients who have done hours or days of research looking for the right plastic surgeon, and they interview me as one of a list of possibles. But if I needed a surgeon and didn't know where to start, I'd try the following sources:

The *Directory of Medical Specialists*. Your local library ought to have the *Directory of Medical Specialists*, which lists every board certified doctor in the United States. If you are checking on a particular doctor, look for his name in the Index (Volume 3). If you are looking for cosmetic surgeons in your area, you want Volume 2. This lists all board certified plastic surgeons, eye surgeons, and ENT surgeons state by state. Find your state, then look up the town nearest you. If you live in a big city, New York for instance, the surgeons will be listed under New York City if their main office is in Manhattan. Brooklyn, the Bronx, Queens, Flushing, and Fresh Meadows are all listed separately.

The print is small. The information will be:

- Date of board certification
- Date and place of birth
- Where, when, and in what field the physician was trained
- Where he or she practices
- Whether he or she is associated with a medical school
- To what medical societies he or she belongs.

If you find only the name and address for a particular physician, it means the information was not sent in in time for publication. This may be an oversight, or it may mean that he or she is only recently board certified or is retired.

You can buy the directory from Marquis Who's Who, Inc., 200 East Ohio Street, Chicago, IL 60611, but I would keep my money for something fun. This directory costs almost $200. It is in almost all libraries, and new editions are published every two years, so if you buy one, it will soon be out of date. The beauty of the directory is that you can pick and choose. You can look for surgeons near you, or those who went to your university, are your age, trained at a hospital you are familiar with—whatever. If you don't have a surgeon in mind already, choose three who seem right for you. For instance, I chose my gynecologist by searching in the directory. I wanted someone from Yale, if possible. I went to Yale Medical School and they had a great gynecology department. When I walked in for my appointment, the gynecologist remembered me. He had been one of my medical school professors!

Your County Medical Society. If the directory search seems too much bother, here's a shortcut. Call your County Medical Society. Explain that you are considering cosmetic surgery and ask them for the names, addresses, and qualifications of three board certified surgeons. They will probably give you only the names of plastic and reconstructive surgeons, so if you want to consult with an ENT or eye cosmetic surgeon, you should say so. Most medical societies are friendly and helpful. Doctors are not required to belong to their County Medical Society, but most of us in private practice do belong.

Other Doctors. Ask your doctor, if you have one, to recommend a cosmetic surgeon. Make sure the one recommended is someone your doctor really knows. Has your doctor had other patients who got good results with a cosmetic surgeon? If your doctor has only "heard about" but doesn't know the surgeon he recommends, be wary. Sometimes a doctor stays a step ahead of a bad reputation for a while. For example, I knew of a doctor who had a good reputation for some years. Doctors recommended him because other doctors had mentioned his name at meetings. His practice flourished . . . until he was discovered to have forged his medical school diploma, and had a series of lawsuits from dissatisfied patients!

Nurses. You'll find that nurses can also be helpful. A nurse you know may have worked in an operating room or may have friends that do. Nurses are friendly and keep in touch with one another. They hear all the "inside information" about who is competent, and they tend to be more candid than a doctor would be about a colleague. Nurses are no more infallible than doctors, but they do know the surgeons who are conscientious, meticulous in their surgery, and thoughtful. A number of surgeons are on their good behavior with colleagues and reveal their true personalities in the privacy of an office or operating room.

Friends. Friends or friends of friends who have had cosmetic surgery also can help, if your questions aren't too intrusive. You should ask how the surgeon treated them. What was his office like? What was the surgeon's training? Did your friend find out, or did he or she take it on faith? Were there complications? If so, did the surgeon blame your friend for causing the complication or did the surgeon show concern and act quickly to treat it?

Helen had a facelift. Two days after the surgery, she came back to have the bandage removed. Her surgeon was not there. His office nurse removed the bandage. There was an infection behind one ear.

"It's going to be okay," said the nurse.

"Where's my surgeon?" asked Helen, who had expected to see him that day.

"He's not available."

"Can't you find him and ask him what to do?" asked Helen, who was worried.

"I know what to do. He's trained us."

"Can't you reach him?"

"No. He took five days off to go skiing. He has to have personal time, you know. He can't spend every minute of his life looking after patients."

This surgeon might have been fine in the operating room. I don't know. But I do know, from the way he treated his patients, that (1) he had little concern for his patients, or he would have told Helen that he would be out of town, and (2) he and his staff regarded his patients as less important than himself.

You might go to a surgeon like that. I wouldn't care to do so. What if he were operating on me and he wanted to go skiing? If he, not I, came first, he'd be tempted to hustle through my surgery, maybe doing a sloppy job. No thank you.

Beauticians. Hair and makeup professionals may sometimes be helpful, if their clients confide in them about their surgery. Some beauticians are very astute, but you should also know that a number of beauticians have commercial relationships with cosmetic surgeons, getting free cosmetic surgery or even commissions for patients referred.

Is Advertising or Publicity Helpful?

Only for the *facts* it gives you. Advertising is open to good, great, terrible, and every other kind of cosmetic surgeon. An advertisement about me only tells you what I want you to know, e.g., where I practice, what kind of surgery I perform and as much about my qualifications as I care to tell you. (It would also tell you that I had enough money to pay for the ad.)

How about write-ups and TV interviews? I wouldn't rely on these. You should be a little cynical about such publicity. Many cosmetic surgeons hire publicity agents to promote their surgical practices. Or the publicity may result from a book the cosmetic surgeon has written (including this one) or because the surgeon comes from a prominent family or has relatives in the media. Good, great, and terrible cosmetic surgeons get publicity, and some patients have come to me because I seemed to be sympathetic, caring, and honest in a TV interview. It so happens that I am—but it worries me because I know of doctors who also appear kind, caring, and honest on TV who are in fact hard, cruel, and crooked. Besides, many of the best surgeons I know appear to be wooden, boring, and even stupid on TV. I would treat publicity like advertisements.

Are Popular Guides Helpful?

I don't recommend them. Guides to all kinds of physicians appear periodically in magazines and newspapers. For example, a magazine recently published a nationwide guide to the "best" doctors. I knew all the plastic surgeons they listed. Some were *great* surgeons, some were definitely not. Some were retired, some should have retired years ago. Some did brilliant laboratory research but were unreliable with a scalpel. One was an alcoholic. One was mentally disturbed. A number were good reconstructive surgeons but not skillful in cosmetic surgery. Others were renowned for their cosmetic work only. How did such a hodgepodge get into this directory? Because they were professors at "name" medical schools. Or because they had good publicity agents. A PR firm *promotes* a cosmetic surgeon, it doesn't *qualify* him. As for professors, many are so busy traveling, talking, and writing textbooks that they don't do much of their own surgery. Such directories are not much help to you in finding the right cosmetic surgeon.

YOUR "CHECKING-ON-YOUR-COSMETIC-SURGEON" CHECKLIST

To determine if you've done a good job of finding a surgeon, ask yourself these questions. The more "yes" answers you have, the better.

- Did I look in the *Directory of Medical Specialists*?
- If not, did I check his credentials through my County Medical Society?
- Is he board certified or board eligible?
- If he is *not* board certified/eligible, have I seen his curriculum vitae? Does it satisfy me about his training and competence?
- Did I ask his office for a C.V. and get one? (Or did I get excuses as to why I can't or shouldn't have that information?)
- If I have done none of the above, do I at least know where he went to medical school, where and in what field he did his surgical training, and how long he's been in practice?
- Did I learn of his reputation through a doctor, a nurse, or a friend?
- If I chose this surgeon *only* because of good publicity or ads, is my choice based on the *facts* I know about the surgeon, or only the *impressions* that the publicity/ads gave me?

- Have I selected two other cosmetic surgeons, in case, after the initial consultation, I don't care for my first choice, or in case it turns out that he isn't as qualified as I thought he was?

Still anxious? Don't be. Once you have found a well-qualified surgeon who is polite and patient, and who explains what he wants to do—relax!

WHEN TO SCHEDULE YOUR SURGERY

You are probably wondering when the best time is to schedule cosmetic surgery. Should you first consult a surgeon a week before you want your surgery? A month? A year? Scheduling depends partly on the time of year: Fewer people have cosmetic surgery in the fall (October, November) than at other times of the year. Also, scheduling depends on the number of operating rooms available to your surgeon. If all the operating rooms are booked for other surgery, there may be no place to do your operation, even if he and you are free on a certain date.

Your surgery can probably be booked two months after your consultation, but I have seen patients who had consultations three years before they were ready for surgery and others who wanted it the next week—and a cancellation made it possible to schedule it! If you are on a tight time schedule, you might mention it when you call for a consultation. What's more, it may be a month or two or three between the time you call for a consult and the time you can get into the office. In the meantime, you can read, and reread this book.

When is the best time to have surgery? It depends on you. People have surgery in the beginning of the year to start the year right, for them; in the spring to get ready for summer clothes; in the summer during vacation time. The fall is least popular because school and college schedules make it inconvenient for students and parents, vacation time is used up, and people are saving money for Christmas spending.

WHERE TO HAVE YOUR SURGERY

Medically speaking, it doesn't matter where you have your cosmetic surgery done, so long as the operating room in which you have it is properly staffed and equipped for your particular operation. Your basic choices are:

- Cosmetic surgery clinic
- Cosmetic surgery office operating room
- Surgery center
- Hospital

Your final choice will depend on what your surgeon recommends, and on what kind of anesthesia you need (fully awake, awake but sedated to a twilight sleep, or fully asleep).

When Do I Stay Overnight After Surgery?

You can go home the same day after most cosmetic operations, *even if you have had general anesthesia.* Some operations require a hospital stay for nursing care and pain injections. Breast reduction surgery, thigh lifts, and tummy tucks are the common *cosmetic* operations that require overnight hospital care.

Is Office Surgery Really Safe?

Hospitals and surgery centers have to meet local and national standards for safety. Surgeon's office operating rooms and clinics are not well regulated. You need to rely on your surgeon's good judgment to decide where you should have your surgery.

As an example, my present office operating room is used for cosmetic operations that can be done with either straight local or local/sedation using minimal sedation—to lessen anxiety, not to truly sedate. I do my major cosmetic surgery in one of various hospitals or a surgery center.

A properly run doctor's operating suite is convenient for you and your surgeon. But such an operating room is expensive and time-consuming to run safely. (It raises the overhead cost for the office from 30 to 60 percent!) In most cases, the cost of surgery in a doctor's operating suite will not be less than the cost for the same surgery done at a hospital, clinic, or surgery center that specializes in outpatient surgery—assuming that the office operating room is as well staffed and equipped. If you have any doubt, ask to see the surgeon's operating room.

- Is it tiny?
- Is it dirty?
- Is it disorganized?
- Is there a stretcher available?
- Is there a recovery room?
- Is a heart monitor used?
- Who are the nurses, and how many nurses work with the surgeon? One nurse is necessary for moderate surgery (upper lids, chin implants) and two for major cosmetic surgery.
- If you are having heavy sedation and/or major cosmetic surgery, is there an anesthetist available?
- How close is the nearest hospital?
- Who runs the operating room? (A nurse should be in charge of the day-to-day supervision. A busy cosmetic surgeon cannot manage it by himself.)

Are There Any Standards for Office Operating Rooms?

The A.S.P.R.S. (the plastic surgery professional society) has sponsored the AAAAPSF. This mouthful stands for American Association for Accreditation of Ambulatory Plastic Surgery Facilities. This accreditation is only available to board *certified* plastic surgeons. To have an office operating room accredited for local/sedation, the surgeon's operating facility must meet rigid standards for staffing and equipment.

Rules of Thumb for Office Operating Rooms

- *Trust your first impression.* If the operating room doesn't look right, say that you prefer a hospital or surgery center.
- If you have a good surgeon, *trust him.* Good surgeons take good care of their patients. A conscientious surgeon will do your surgery where it is *safe for you.* You can't be an office accreditation committee.

CHAPTER   3

"Who Needs This Operation: Me? or My Surgeon?"

This is the chapter that is most likely to distress your cosmetic surgeon, but it has information that you must know. Cosmetic surgery is very commercial, just as commercial as interior decorating. No one ever *needed* to wallpaper a home, but manufacturers of wallpaper need you to buy it so that they can make a living. The same is true for cosmetic surgery. You may want—even feel you need—cosmetic surgery, but unlike food, it's not vital: You won't die without it. But your cosmetic surgeon needs to perform operations in order to make a living. If you don't use his services, someone else will, but financially he's better off if both you *and* someone else let him operate.

The *commercial* goal of cosmetic surgery is to make you want the most extensive surgery at the highest cost that you can afford. This goal directly contradicts the *medical* goal of cosmetic surgery. All surgery is hazardous, and to minimize your risk, the doctor should be helping you decide what *not* to have. If you can get the same, or nearly the same, psychological improvement from a facelift alone, you should not be persuaded to add nose surgery, a chemical peel, and an upper-lid "tuck" to your surgical agenda.

In my experience, as many as 15 to 20 percent of Board Certified Plastic and Reconstructive Surgeons who perform cosmetic surgery may tend to put their commercial goals ahead of your goals. And among cosmetic surgeons who are *not* Board Certified in Plastic and Reconstructive Surgery, I'd say the percentage is considerably higher—well above 25 percent.

When you consult a cosmetic surgeon, you are assuming that he will forget his profit and his net income. You think he will advise you on what you need, what is *best* for you, without regard to how much money he can make from you. Is this unrealistic? No . . . and yes.

I am a member of the prestigious American Society of Plastic and Reconstructive Surgeons, the A.S.P.R.S. You can become a member only by being board certified in plastic and reconstructive surgery *and* being voted in. (This can prove unexpectedly difficult.) After I applied to become an A.S.P.R.S. member, one requirement was that I attend a marketing seminar. The topic was a nationwide survey showing that the rising numbers of cosmetic surgeons in other specialities were in direct competition with board certified plastic and reconstructive surgeons doing cosmetic surgery. Therefore, we were told, we would have to create a desire for cosmetic surgery in those middle-class Americans who weren't yet "into" cosmetic surgery—or there would not be enough money in it for us all. In other words, this "professional seminar" was about *money*: marketing, advertising, sales techniques. Patients' needs weren't even mentioned. Was it a turnoff? To most of us, yes. Like the majority of cosmetic surgeons, I spend much of my time helping people decide to either have or *not* to have cosmetic surgery. But . . . buyers beware. Those 15 to 25 percent of cosmetic surgeons leaning toward making themselves richer (and you poorer) use many sales techniques to convince you to have surgery. To tell when you're merely a dollar sign on your cosmetic surgeon's bank deposit slip—instead of a patient—you need to know when you're being targeted by a sales technique that can hurt your psyche as well as your pocketbook.

AM I BEING "SOLD"?

The Off-the-Street Approach

A tall, dark, and handsome cosmetic surgeon wanted more money. In the evenings he'd stop promising suspects in supermarket aisles by saying: "Hi.

I'm Dr. Z. I just happened to be here doing my shopping—and believe me, I don't usually do this—but you could be so lovely, if you had your nose [or whatever] corrected. I couldn't stop myself." He'd smile charmingly. "The surgery is so easy. It's not expensive. And what a difference it would make to your life!" Graciously he'd press his business card into the hand of the unsuspecting shopper. Business boomed.

When I was looking for a new office, my real estate agent asked, "Do I need my eyes done?" I studied her face. "I'd say no for your upper lids. Your lower lids could be done, but it would be early. If it bothers you, I'd say yes. If it doesn't, I'd wait." She looked puzzled. "I was at a cocktail party last night. A Dr. ——— came up to me and told me I urgently needed my eyes done. He gave me his card. Why would he tell me that if they didn't really need doing?"

Why indeed? It's worth a thousand dollars or more to him, that's why. However, exceptions *do* exist.

A cosmetic surgeon knew that a teenage boy in his daughter's class was badly teased about his ugly nose. The surgeon cautiously approached the boy's parents and explained what cosmetic nose surgery might do to help their son. They had thought that their son was too young to have the surgery and that it was so expensive that they could not afford it, anyway. This was not the case. Their son ended up having the operation and was happy. This was an "off-the-street" approach, but it was not a sales technique. It was the act of a physician who wanted to help someone who was suffering.

How to Handle the Off-the-Street Approach. If a cosmetic surgeon approaches you to *sell* you cosmetic surgery, he is lured by your money. *Do not go to that cosmetic surgeon*, even if you decide to have the surgery he recommends. If money comes first to him, you'll come second.

The Psychic Destruction Approach

Madeline, a lanky secretary new on the job, was referred to a cosmetic surgeon to have a facial mole removed. She was sitting on the exam table in the surgeon's office when he walked into the room and stopped short.

"Oh yes, oh yes," he said, his voice oozing with concern. "It's a pity, but certainly I can help you." Madeline was puzzled. "Your nose is deformed. Of course you feel ugly," the surgeon went on. "No wonder you're not married." Madeline was smart enough not to sign up for surgery on the spot. She got a second opinion. It happened to be from me. "I have never been so depressed in my life," Madeline told me. "He destroyed my self-image in ten seconds. I walked down the street from his office in tears. At this point I hate myself. I'd like you just to cut my nose off."

What was shocking about this situation was that Madeline had a delicate, well-shaped nose. Surgery would not have improved either her nose or her looks in general. I removed the facial mole that had started this journey for her. I photographed her nose and pointed out why it was good and why she shouldn't have cosmetic nose surgery. I didn't add that, in my opinion, this "respectable" cosmetic surgeon had not been truthful and had tried to humiliate her into having cosmetic surgery that would not help her. I can imagine few things worse for a doctor to do to a patient than to inflict suffering on her for his own financial gain.

Bob consulted a cosmetic surgeon about gynecomastia—enlargement of the tissue around his nipple, giving him the appearance of female breasts. "This doctor took one look at me and laughed and said, 'What are you? A C cup?' Half of me wanted to punch him, but the other half made me feel so sick with myself that I found myself almost begging him to operate on me." Bob's wife was so outraged for her husband that she insisted that he find a different surgeon.

How to Handle the Psychic Destruction Approach. If a cosmetic surgeon criticizes a feature that you didn't ask him about and urges you to pay him to "fix" it—and above all if he leaves you feeling demeaned or humiliated—you are his *victim*, not his *patient*. Find a new surgeon.

The "Why Not!" Approach

Marsha consulted a cosmetic surgeon about a dermabrasion. "What about your ears?" he demanded. Marsha shrugged. "I know they stick out, but I don't want them changed. I'm used to them."

"Why not have them changed?" argued the surgeon, *as though she were crazy.*

Marsha complained to me later: "He made me feel so dumb. Why not? I don't know why not. They just don't bother me. But it upset me. He made me feel so weird for not wanting them done, that I almost told him to go ahead and do them!"

Mark went to a cosmetic surgeon about a scar on his face. "First she examined the scar," he told me, "and then she started on my eyes. I said, 'Wait a minute. My eyes have bags, but what the hell. I don't want them fixed.' She practically fell over and said, 'Why not?' like it was an insult to her. She made me feel so ridiculous, I couldn't think 'why not.' I scheduled the surgery. Then I got out of there and the clouds cleared and I thought: 'What the hell am I doing? They don't bother me and it costs two thousand bucks and I need a new car. That's why not.' "

How to Handle the "Why Not!" Approach. "Why not?" is an aggressive, somewhat hostile sales approach. The cosmetic surgeon here is asking you why *you* are not spending more money on *him* (or her). Of course, the truthful answer is, "Why *should* I pay you money for something I don't want done?" Aggression and anger are not helpful traits in your surgeon. Avoid them. If you were to be the patient of such a surgeon, and you had, for instance, a complication or if you complained of your result, you might find yourself treated aggressively and angrily. No one needs that!

The Inspirational Evangelical Approach

This is the most difficult technique for a cosmetic surgeon to practice on you. The surgeon has to be a natural psychologist. The technique is seductive, so be careful. Caught unawares, you can end up agreeing to almost anything. The "logic" of the technique is this: You came to see me, a doctor and a cosmetic surgeon, for advice. My advice is to have your face and body redone surgically. If you take my advice, you will be successful and happy. You will find inner peace.

Mary went to Dr. X. She had had a number of disappointments in life, as we all have had. Now she was starting over. Dr. X walked in, solemn but reassuring, a friendly high priest.

"I guess what really bothers me," said Mary, "is my cheekbones and my chin. They're so flat. What do you think?"

"Stand up and walk around," said Dr. X. Mary stood up and walked around for him.

"Sit down," said Dr. X. He studied her face intently. He took photographs. "Life is hard, isn't it?" He looked into her eyes, soulfully.

Mary sighed. "It has been for me."

"But you're determined to make the best you, aren't you? Wonderful." He continued to gaze at Mary solemnly. "My advice has nothing to do with money. I never think about money. You do that. I think only about you, what you need. For your own sake, you need breasts a little fuller to express the woman in you. You need thighs a little slimmer, to make you graceful. Your face?" He stood back, a Renoir looking over a canvas. "Yes, the cheek and chin implants will show the strength inside you. Your eyes? Don't hide them from the world. Have them done, upper and lower. A facelift is essential to show the rejuvenation in your soul. That way, I could tell you, 'Mary, you are healed. You are whole. You are the you that was meant to be.' Please, for your own sake, do this for yourself. You need it. Please."

"How much money are you talking about, Doctor?" asked Mary.

Dr. X held up a deprecating hand. "I'm a physician," he said solemnly. "My staff takes care of all the details. I don't believe in money. I can't be your doctor, counseling you, and let money stand in our way, can I?"

So, since Dr. X didn't think about money, the nurse explained the cost to Mary:

What Mary Wanted		What Dr. X Wanted	
Chin implant	$1250	Chin implant	$1250
Cheek implants	$1250	Cheek implants	$1250
		Facelift	$5000
		Upper lids	$1500
		Lower lids	$1500
		Breast implants	$3000
		Fat suction, thighs	$2000
Mary's total	**$2500**	**Dr. X's total for Mary**	**$15,500**

Dr. X claimed that he didn't think about money, but his office staff called Mary repeatedly, begging her "for your own good," "for your own sake," "for your future happiness," and "for your success on the job" to please have the surgery, as a favor to herself.

Where did I come in? Mary wasn't easily sold anything. She came to see me for my opinion. I thought her idea of cheek and chin implants was reasonable. She was young and attractive, but the operations she had thought of entailed a short recovery for her, at a price she could afford, for something that she wanted psychologically, and that would improve her appearance. It seemed worthwhile. The rest was $6000 of surgery she didn't want and certainly didn't need. Her eyes and her face were youthful and charming. Her small breasts fitted her small frame and anyway, they didn't bother her. Her thighs might have been a little thinner if she lost a few pounds, but $2000 of fat suctioning was ridiculous.

What about Dr. X's statements that he was a doctor and never thought about money? First of all, a doctor has to consider a patient's overall welfare, and instant poverty for a young working girl having cosmetic surgery isn't exactly doing her a favor. Even if Mary had been rich, Dr. X's statements were preposterous. Of course he thought about money—any doctor in private practice *has* to be aware of finances. (Besides, he drove around in a $60,000 car.) A lot of suggestible people fell for his approach. Many of them, after their surgery, felt rather cheated that all the life-changes promised to them hadn't come to pass. Were they gullible? Yes. But we're all inclined to believe what a doctor tells us, especially if it seems that it might give us a boost in life that is a tiny bit magical.

Emma, a girl of 19, had been in high school when a classmate's father, a cosmetic surgeon, told Emma that she would have a wonderful career ahead of her as a high-fashion model if she could only persuade her parents to let him "perfect" her features. Achieving perfection included cheek and chin implants, nose surgery, and upper and lower eyelid surgery. But what had most inspired Emma had been the virtual guarantee that the surgery would open up an exciting, glamorous life in Manhattan as a model. Her parents had money. So she had the surgery. When she finally discovered she couldn't get a job as a model, Emma wanted to know how the surgery had failed her. It hadn't—but the surgeon had.

How to Handle the Inspirational Evangelical Approach.
Inspirational cosmetic surgeons tend to deceive themselves, as well as their patients, about what cosmetic surgery can achieve. These cosmetic surgeons tend to be dreamers, not doers. You may feel inspired to have operations they recommend, but you may get a below-average result, even for the surgery you want. Besides, let's be honest. Anyone who claims he doesn't *think* about money is either poor or telling you a lie so big it should leave you breathless. Deception is *not* a good trait in a surgeon.

The "Do-It-Before-It's-Too-Late" Approach

Maude consulted Dr. Y about a breast enlargement.

"How old are you?" he asked her during the consultation.

"Thirty-five." He inspected her face closely. "You want to have your facelift soon," he told her. "You don't want to leave it too late. Don't want you to wake up one morning and find your face has fallen off. Can't do much for you then."

Maude signed up for a facelift, as well as breast surgery, immediately. However, she moved away before her surgery could be done. She was in a panic when she came to see me.

"Dr. Morgan, I don't want to wait until there's nothing you can do for me."

"Do you know when that would be?"

"I don't know—a year or two?"

"A bit later than that," I told her. "Though, in my experience, once you're over seventy or seventy-five, it's very hard to get a really good facelift result, at least with one operation. It usually takes a second one at that age."

"Seventy? I won't care how I look at seventy."

"A lot of people care how they look at seventy. But you're asking me how long you should wait. Roughly speaking, a first facelift is usually done somewhere between the ages of forty-five and fifty-five. It can be done sooner for some people, but you aren't one of them."

"Won't a facelift keep me from aging?"

"No. The only thing for that is the Fountain of Youth, and we haven't found that yet. A facelift tightens what has loosened. It won't stop aging. It won't stop the hands of time."

Why would a cosmetic surgeon tell you, at age 35, to have a facelift you didn't need or want and hadn't even thought of? Possibly to stampede you into having costly surgery. I have even seen unscrupulous cosmetic surgeons give patients false information in order to persuade them to have surgery.

Jennifer took herself to an ENT surgeon for treatment of an ear infection. This surgeon also happened to do facial plastic surgery. He didn't even bother to examine her ears but zoomed in on her nose. "You'd better get this fixed," he advised her, after looking inside her nose at the septum. "I'm surprised you can still breathe. I don't know how much longer you can leave it. Pretty bad. When I do this, I'll refine your nose a bit too. Let's get rid of the little bump."

What Jennifer Wanted	What Dr. X Wanted
Treat ear infection: $35 to $85	Cosmetic plus Septal Nose Surgery: $3,000, half paid by Jennifer, half by insurance

I hate to keep coming back to money, but when you are having cosmetic surgery, you must remember that cosmetic surgery is a strange blend of medicine and commerce. For your own good, you have to note how your cosmetic surgeon deals with it.

Jennifer came to me for a second opinion on her nose surgery. I hesitated to contradict another doctor's opinion on the septum. The septum is often curved and irregular and a misdiagnosis of obstruction can easily be made in good faith. Alas, not this time. Jennifer had a broad nose with wide-open nasal passages. She had no allergies and no breathing problem. And the cosmetic surgeon who had told her that she *did* need the surgery was competent and must have known that he was lying to her about what he saw when he examined her nose. I told her that I did not see any obstruction. Besides, even if the septum were curved, there would be no reason for her to have surgery unless she had symptoms or wanted to change her appearance.

"Are you saying that he lied to me?" she asked. I replied, "I am saying that I don't see what this doctor told you that he saw." She looked dissatisfied. "My ear still hurts. Now what do I do?" I gave her the name of an ENT surgeon in whom I had confidence. He also did cosmetic surgery, but I didn't think he'd try to hustle her. She called back to thank me. Her ear was fine, and the new ENT surgeon had agreed that her septum was normal. "Why would the other guy lie to me?" she insisted. I thought the reason stood out a mile, but I didn't like to say so. "You'll have to ask him," I said. She laughed. "I think we know the answer, don't we? It's just that you doctors will never say so. It's money."

How to Handle the "Before It's Too Late!" Approach. If something works fine for you, think twice before you believe the cosmetic surgeon who wants to fix it. And if it looks fine to you, think more than twice if the cosmetic surgeon wants to improve it.

Sometimes, of course, there are valid reasons for having surgery sooner, not later. For instance, a big-chested young woman may not be able to take part in sports during college or high school. Breast reduction surgery can change that. Having breast reduction surgery after college would be too late for her to enjoy school or college sports, even though there may be no urgent medical reason to have the surgery in her teens. Also, some people come from families that age unusually early and in a particular way, such as having the neck muscles loosen into saggy folds. A face/neck lift at the age of 55 would come too late for such people to enjoy the results of cosmetic surgery in their forties. Thus, timing is important, but it should be determined with *your* best interests in mind.

The Sexual Seduction Approach

Sexual seduction is used, in my experience, only by male cosmetic surgeons on female patients. I haven't heard of its being used by a woman surgeon on a male patient—but it could happen. No one knows how common this technique is. No one talks about it. Just bear in mind that a recent survey showed that 10 percent of psychiatrists have sex with their patients. Merely being a doctor does not guarantee a well-adjusted attitude toward the opposite sex.

It is *grossly* unethical for any doctor to make sexual advances to a patient. No one would object if you went to a plastic surgeon you knew, or even one you had dated. That is your choice, and the surgeon's choice if he decides to look after you. And no one would object if a cosmetic surgeon asked you out for a date (assuming he was single) *after* you were released from his care. But sexual advances are a gross abuse of a doctor's authority when he inflicts them on a patient. Patients are vulnerable, and the doctor is in a position of trust. This is especially true of cosmetic surgeons because you go to a cosmetic surgeon at a psychologically important and vulnerable time in your life. Common sense may make you wary of other sales techniques, but this one can catch you off guard, especially:

- If you are a teenager, and possibly do not have the sophistication or the experience to deal with a sexual affront.
- If you aren't currently involved with someone sexually, but would like to be. Why? Here you are especially vulnerable to a sexual advance that reassures you that you are desirable.
- If you are recently divorced or otherwise rejected by a man. Why? Again, you are especially vulnerable to sexual advances that reassure you that you are desirable.

Remember, if your cosmetic surgeon is recently divorced or otherwise rejected, he may be using *you* to reassure *himself* that he is desirable. Well, don't cry for him. No matter what his motive, it is still unprofessional.

Angela was a lovely young woman who consulted a cosmetic surgeon about a breast enlargement. She was at a particularly vulnerable time in her life, having just ended a romance. The cosmetic surgeon talked to her and examined her. He was an older man but very charming. Angela couldn't decide for or against the surgery. She called back to make a second appointment to go over the possible complications once again. Angela described that visit to me like this:

"He said he needed to examine me again. This time his nurse wasn't in the room, but frankly he seemed so old to me that I didn't think twice about it. I said I wasn't sure if I should have the surgery, if the risks were worth it, considering that I didn't want my breasts to be all that much bigger. That's reasonable, isn't it? He had me lie down, and this time the exam was totally different. You can tell. It wasn't like a doctor—it was like a caress. Then he pinched my nipple hard, winked at me, and said, "We'll make you quite a little handful in bed."

She stopped talking. Thinking about it again was so humiliating that she was about to cry. "All I could think was that he wasn't a doctor—he was just a dirty old man. I should have slapped his face. I got up and put on my clothes and walked out. What did he think I'd do—sign up for surgery because he thought I was sexy?"

Quite possibly. When you are vulnerable, that kind of sexual advance could make you do things you would not otherwise decide to do. Fortunately for Angela, she saw the doctor's technique for what it was—pure unprofessionalism.

There is a saying that all patients fall in love with their doctors. Well, if *you* choose a cosmetic surgeon because you think he is sexy, that's your judgment, good or bad. But if your cosmetic surgeon approaches you as a sex object, he is using his privilege as a physician to assault your body and perhaps get at your pocketbook.

Blowing the Whistle on the Sexual Seducer

If you believe that your doctor has acted unethically, of course you should go to another surgeon. But for the sake of other people, you also should consider writing a letter of complaint to your State Medical Licensing Board and the County Medical Society. (The County Medical Society will be listed in the phone book. Ask them to give you the address of the licensing board as well.) Your letter should be brief, objective and factual. For example:

> This is a letter of complaint against Dr. _____. On [date] at [time] I saw him at [address] as a patient. During the medical visit, Dr. _____ said/did the following: [briefly describe the event]. I feel that this behavior was wrong. Please let me know *in writing* if such behavior is consistent with ethical medical care.

Why write instead of calling? Because a phone call may not be taken seriously. Why ask for a reply in writing? Over the phone, things can be said vaguely or ambiguously. A written reply means your complaint has received some thought. If your surgeon was in the wrong, the Society or Board is more likely to censure him and to protect other patients. If you are mistaken, they will take more trouble to explain the reason, which in turn reassures you.

APPROACHES YOU CAN TRUST

Now that you know what should warn you away from a cosmetic surgeon, here are some examples of approaches that should reassure you that your surgeon has *you* in mind.

The Old-Fashioned Approach

I trained with one famous and wonderful plastic surgeon who conducted his cosmetic consultations like this:

> *"Doctor, I think I want a facelift."*
> *"Fine."*
> *"Should I have my eyes done too?"*
> *"If you want."*
> *"Well, Dr. Z said that I should have my eyes and my face done."*
> *"Then go to Dr. Z."*
> *"Am I ready for a facelift?"*
> *"I'll do it if you want it. I can't promise you a thing."*
> *"What will it do for me?"*
> *"I'll pull you as tight as I can."*

And so he did. He was a fantastic surgeon and a wonderful man. His patients believed in him, not because he explained a thing, but because they *knew* he wasn't trying to take advantage of them. Of course, if you wanted a cosmetic surgery *opinion*, he wasn't exactly a big help.

The Honest and Modern Approach

A friend of mine, another board certified plastic surgeon who does cosmetic surgery, handles a cosmetic consultation in a way I think is terrific. His approach is not exactly like mine, but it has the feel you should get from your consultation. He says:

> Elizabeth, I think the cosmetic consultations are tough. People come in with ideas of what you can do for them that aren't realistic. Or, they

come in because you operated on their best friend and she looks so good, they want the same result. I examine them and I sit them down and I really give them a kind of no-holds-barred idea of what could go wrong. I want teenagers to know that if I do their nose and their septum, they could get a sunken nose and look pretty terrible and need more surgery to change it. I don't think it's fair for someone to trust me to do a good job and have no idea that they could get a horrible result. What could I say? "Oh, yeah. It happens"? They need to know *before* that it could happen, even in the best hands. And if they want something I don't think I'd personally like, I feel uncomfortable. If a lovely woman wants her nose done and I know I won't like the result unless I fill out a weak chin, I try to lead her around to telling me how she sees herself. I'll study a picture of her profile with her. Maybe I'd point out that her chin is weak and that her nose surgery won't change that. I won't tell her to have anything done to her chin because I think that's pushy. But if she asks me *my* opinion, I'll tell her that if it were my face, I'd make the nose smaller and the chin stronger, but that a lot of my patients don't want that. If a woman comes in for a breast enlargement and wants to know how large they should be, I have to tell her I'm not the right man to consult. She has to decide that for herself. I love my wife and she has small breasts and I don't want her any different. But if I make a patient look like my wife, and she doesn't happen to admire that kind of look, well, we're in trouble, aren't we? I can tell a patient what *I'd* do, or what I'd want my *wife* to do, but I can't tell a patient what she—or he—should do. I'm just a guy who loves cosmetic surgery. I love what it does for people. I love the fact that I can do this and make a really good living for my family. I feel too lucky. How many people can say as much?

One day this surgeon was out of town and a patient of his had to see me instead of him when her son mistakenly hit the stitches that had just been put in. The patient, Barbara, only needed me to change her bandage, but it was clear that she considered me a poor substitute for her own surgeon. *You* want to feel that way about *your* cosmetic surgeon, too.

YOUR "AFTER-THE-CONSULTATION" RATING SHEET

Now that you know all the sales techniques to look out for, here is a rating sheet to use after the consultation to see if, and how, you are being "sold":

"Pluses" Add the number of points given for each "yes" that applies.

1. Did your cosmetic surgeon treat you politely and with respect? (+10) ( )
2. Did he discuss the risks with you, giving you some idea of what might go wrong, how common that would be, and what would be done to treat a complication? (+10) ( )
3. Did he or his staff make the cost clear to you so that you know how much the whole cost will be? (+1) ( )
4. Did he suggest that, if you haven't made up your mind, you could wait and think before committing yourself to surgery? (+1) ( )
5. Did he listen to your reasons for having the surgery? (+1) ( )
6. Did you leave the office feeling calm and reassured? (+1) ( )
7. Did you feel in control and not "programmed" by the cosmetic surgeon? (+ 10) ( )
8. Did you feel better when you left than when you came? (+1) ( )
9. Did you feel your decision was reasonable? (+1) ( )

Total "pluses" ( )

"Minuses" Subtract the number of points given for each "yes" that applies.

1. Did he make you feel uglier going out than when you came in? (−1) ( )
2. Did he tell you that you *needed* cosmetic surgery before it was too late, or that you *had* to have it done? (−1) ( )
3. Did he tell you that you *needed* more surgery than you thought you wanted? (−1) ( )
4. Did he make sexual comments or touch your body in a way that made you feel humiliated? (−20) ( )
5. Did he tell you to "fix" something that wasn't wrong or urge you to have cosmetic surgery that you hadn't thought of having? (−1) ( )
6. Did you go to him because he met you socially and suggested the surgery? (−5) ( )
7. Did he urge you to have cosmetic surgery for a specific goal, such as a better life, a better job, a happier you? (−5) ( )
8. Did you feel hustled, sold, or suspicious of him in any way? (−10) ( )

9. Did you feel your cosmetic surgeon would be angry, disappointed, or would otherwise reject you if you did not have all the surgery he suggested? (-1) (   )
10. Did you go to him for a noncosmetic consultation and find that *he* turned it into a cosmetic consultation? (-1) (   )
11. Did anyone else in the cosmetic surgeon's office do anything as described in Questions 5 to 10? (If "yes," score the same way for each item and fill in the total.) (   )
12. Did he tell you that he never considered money or make any other breathtakingly preposterous statement? (-20) (   )

Total "Minuses" (   )

What your score means:

Subtract the "minuses" from the "pluses" to arrive at a final score. For example, if the "pluses" totaled $+25$ and the "minuses" totaled -10, that surgeon's score would be $+15$.

1. Plus 30 or more: You probably don't need a second opinion.
2. Plus 20 to plus 29: It wouldn't hurt to get a second opinion.
3. Plus 10 to plus 19: You *definitely* need a second opinion.
4. Plus 10 or less: You need another surgeon.

You should now feel confident that you can recognize and appreciate what to look for in a cosmetic surgeon. Just remember these rules:

- *Don't* trust a surgeon who pushes his services without being asked or insists money is of no importance to him.
- *Don't* trust a surgeon who promises you perfection or a "whole new you."
- *Don't* trust a surgeon who insists you have more surgery than you think you really need or makes sexual advances toward you.
- *Do* trust a surgeon who is honest about the possible risks involved in any cosmetic surgery procedure.
- *Do* trust a surgeon who listens to your feelings and helps you examine your motives.
- *Do* trust a surgeon who treats you with the dignity and respect you deserve.

CHAPTER 4

The Truth About "Before and After" Photos

In 1981, the *Journal of Plastic and Reconstructive Surgery* published a fascinating article. It contained "before-and-after" photographs of cosmetic surgery patients who had had a "facelift," "nose surgery," and "eye surgery." All the patients had lovely results. The catch was that no surgery had been done! Only the photographic lighting, camera angle, and film had been changed between the "before" and "after" pictures.

I don't like to look ridiculous, but to show you how extreme the difference can be with photographs, see my "before" picture taken with a Polaroid SX-70 camera (Figure 4-1) and a closeup of my face taken under more favorable circumstances (Figure 4-2).

I haven't had any surgery done, just a change in clothes and camera technique. I'm gullible: If I weren't a cosmetic surgeon and those were presented to *me* as my "before" and "after" photographs, I'd love the difference and I'd accept it *unhesitatingly* as the direct result of surgery. Understanding your cosmetic surgery photographs (and those of other patients you might be shown) is what this chapter is all about.

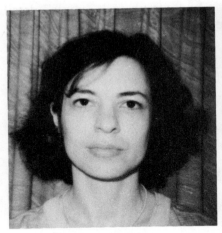

Figure 4-1. The "before."

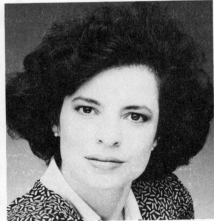

Figure 4-2. The "after."

The Surgeon As Photographer

Although a few doctors (including several plastic surgeons) are competent photographers, there are not, to my knowledge, any great portrait photographers among them.

At Harvard, one of my plastic surgery professors trained me in the importance of closeup medical photographs. Trial and error and a lot of helpful camera salesmen taught me what I know. One of my most consistent experiences is this: As soon as I've developed a reliable system for photographing my patients . . . my camera breaks down. So I keep four cameras in my office: a Canon with closeup lens, a Canon with a standard lens, a Polaroid SX-70, and a Polaroid portrait camera. Whichever camera I use, I try to use that same camera for the "after" photos, under the same conditions if possible.

The Polaroid Faint

For me, and for many plastic surgeons, the most reliable camera is the SX-70, or similar camera, which produces instant pictures for the consultation. It's affordable. A surgeon doesn't need to be a genius to use it. The instant pictures allow your doctor to explain the surgery and the results you can expect. Great. But like anything else, the SX-70 has drawbacks. The lens causes distortion in a closeup picture.

The flash gives a harsh look to the photograph and "erases" detail with its sudden bright light. Scars and color don't show up well. Regardless of the camera used, scars are often hard to show photographically.

A closeup photograph of your face taken with the SX-70 can make you look surprisingly plain. I like to show my patients these photographs when they are sitting down! Otherwise the immediate reaction might be to faint or to sign up on the spot for every known cosmetic operation. Please don't judge your looks by *any* medical photograph, especially not by a medical instant photograph.

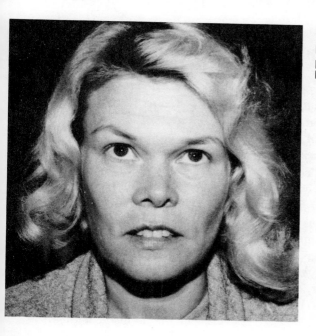

Figure 4-3.

Here is a typical "after" photograph. The patient hardly looks her best.

Figure 4-3 is a typical "after" photo of a woman who underwent scar revision surgery. It was taken with a 35mm camera. As a clinical medical photograph, it is adequate. But it shows her at anything but her best. Please don't decide, on the basis of an "after" photograph like this, that your surgeon didn't do a good job. Use such a photograph to assess and compare *outlines* and *major features* such as sagging of a neck or a bump in a nose. Don't use it to judge overall looks.

One solution to a surgeon's photography problems—having a professional photographer take the "before and after" photos—turned out to be a nuisance for my patients and unnecessarily expensive. Every surgeon works out what works best for him.

Here's how *I* took the "before and after" photos shown in this book:

- Almost all the "befores" are taken at the first consultation.
- Almost all the "afters" are taken six weeks after surgery.
- The lighting is a flash or strobe against a dark background.
- The film and camera are the same in before/after sets unless I indicate otherwise.

Photographic Pitfalls "Before" and "After"

It is 7:00 A.M. the morning of your surgery. You are about to be wheeled into the operating room. You are dressed in a blue paper surgical cap and a dark green surgical gown. If you are a woman, you are allowed no makeup. If you are a man, you may not have shaved. You have had nothing to eat or drink since midnight. You are barely awake. You are nervous about the surgery. You are probably already sedated, so your eyes droop and you can't sit straight. Needless to say, you are not smiling. You are illuminated by overhead fluorescent lighting. Your surgeon, or the nurse to whom he has assigned the photography, is in a rush. He whips out the camera (most likely an instant flash one) and takes your "before" picture now, instead of during your office consultation. No matter how beautiful or handsome you may be, you can be sure you will look your worst.

Two to six weeks later, the surgeon will take your "after" photo. You are dressed in street clothes. You are rested. You are no longer nervous. In fact, you feel relieved: The surgery is over! *You are no doubt smiling.*

When you compare such "before" and "after" pictures, your "after" will look so much better, that (1) you won't be able to look at your frightful "before" pictures without wincing, and (2) you will attribute your great improvement to your surgery.

Figures 4-4 through 4-31, with my comments, will give you an idea of how a picture can mislead you—for better or worse.

Most surgeons don't have a rigid schedule for when to take "after" photographs. I take mine about six weeks after surgery, to allow the swelling and bruising to fade. Ideally, for scientific purposes, every

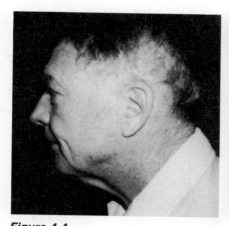

Figure 4-4.

This patient had a face-neck lift. Note the slack jaw and the loose neck skin in this "before" photo.

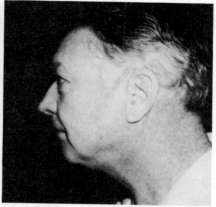

Figure 4-5.

"After" the face-neck lift. The improvement shows up dramatically in this profile photo. It might not show up nearly so well in a face-on photo, though it is obvious in real life.

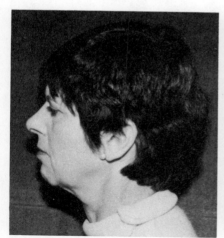

Figure 4-6. "Before."

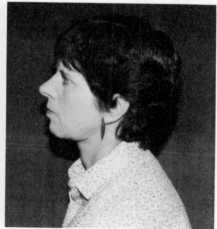

Figure 4-7. "After."

This patient had a face-neck lift. These profile shots show a dramatic improvement, but the patient is farther from the camera "after" than "before," so scars and irregularities are less noticeable. This patient is extremely attractive and was especially enhanced by her surgery. She is not photogenic, and so photos do not reflect the true result.

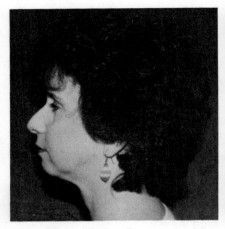
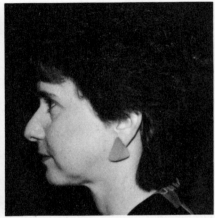

Figure 4-8. "Before."   **Figure 4-9.** "After."

This patient had a chin implant and submental lipectomy (removal of fat under the chin). In this case, surgery perfected the profile of a very attractive woman. But note that in the "after" photo she has her eyes open and is wearing earrings and a more fashionable hairstyle. The "after" photo reflects her true attractiveness; the "before" picture diminishes it.

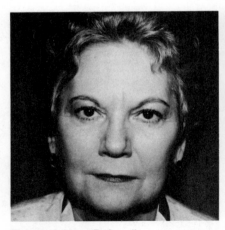
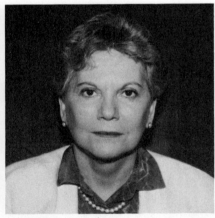

Figure 4-10. "Before."   **Figure 4-11.** "After."

This patient has an unusually expressive face with great charm, which does not show on either photo. She had a face-neck lift, an upper lid lift, and collagen injections. The deep frown lines that gave her a stern look do not show in the "before" photo. Neither does her chief problem—a sagging lower face and neck, and the improvement cannot be seen in this face-on "after" photo. Correcting the frown lines with collagen made a startling real-life improvement— not visible on the photo.

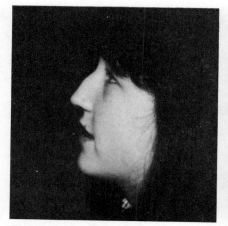

Figure 4-12. "Before."

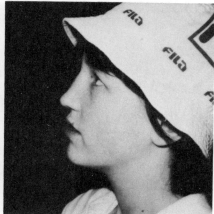

Figure 4-13. "After."

This lovely teenager had nose surgery with a good surgical result. However, the most noticeable change in the "after" photo is her hat and her swept-back hair. These give the "after" photo a lively charm lacking in the "before," making it appear that surgery changed her personality as well as her nose. In fact, her vivacity did increase as her confidence improved after surgery, but it distracts from an objective assessment of her face.

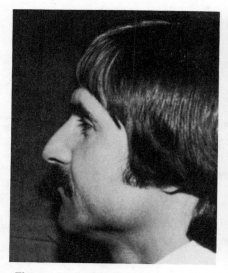

Figure 4-14. "Before."

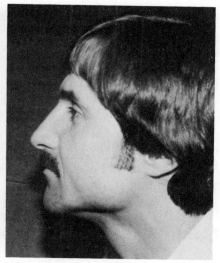

Figure 4-15. "After."

This handsome man had a "nose job." The photos make the before/after difference look subtle, because his face is turned slightly away in the "before" picture. This diminished the hump in his nose profile. The improvement is far less than in real life.

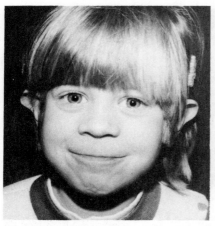 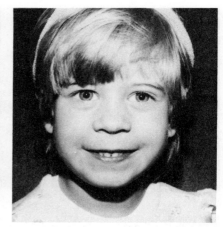

Figure 4-16. "Before."   **Figure 4-17.** "After."

This adorable girl had ears that stuck through her hair. In the "after" photo, the band holds her hair back, but not her ears. "Before," the close-up distorts her face, and she has an anxious smile. The "after" leaves the deceptive impression that surgery not only corrected her ears but made her prettier and more poised.

patient should have photographs at two weeks, six weeks, six months, and one year after surgery. (This isn't usually practical, being expensive and time-consuming.)

The *two-week* photograph tends to be the least reliable. However, I may take a photo at two weeks because a patient may not return for a six-week check or I may forget to take a photograph at that time. The disadvantages of the two-week photo are that your bruising is gone but the swelling is not. As a result, the swelling may conceal a real result, especially after a facelift or "nose job." (The swelling will fill out face creases and straighten the top of the nose; only time can reveal the true result.)

Is Such Photographic Deception Intentional?

Most often it is not. I myself have set off for an operation with no "before" photographs for various reasons. Perhaps the pictures didn't develop, or the patient refused to have photographs taken at the consultation. Occasionally, none of my cameras were working on the day

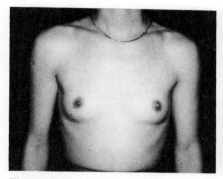

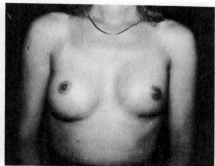

Figure 4-18. "Before."   **Figure 4-19.** "After."

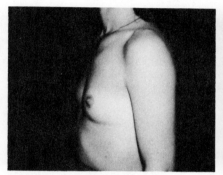

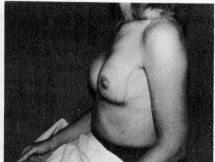

Figure 4-20. "Before."   **Figure 4-21.** "After."

These photos show a way-above-average result for a breast reconstruction after mastectomy of the left breast (our *right*). The reconstruction method can only be used in a few patients. The scar seen in the profile "after" view and the preservation of the patient's own nipple make this an unusually liveable result. The "after" photos are more close-up, so the "after" breasts appear disproportionately larger. However, the "after" photos do not show that the reconstructed breast lies too high. This did not bother the patient, but she *was* bothered by the implant pocket being too large, so that the implant shifted under her arm when she lay down. This is *not* shown by the photo, yet it required a corrective operation.

of the consultation. Sometimes the patient decides on a different operation, and the photographs don't show the right part of the body. In such cases, I have little choice but to take photographs just before surgery, no matter how poor these photographs will be.

When your body—as opposed to your face—is being operated on, even last-minute photographs may prove to be adequate. When

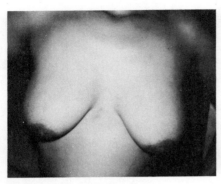
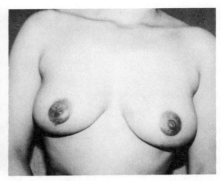

Figure 4-22. "Before." ***Figure 4-23.*** "After."

This patient has had a breast lift. The "after" photo was taken at six weeks. Notice that in the "before" photo the patient has her arms out at the side, and the breast fullness in her underarm area is not apparent. (This was caused by misplaced breast tissue, and the patient did not want it removed.) In the "after" photo, her arms are down, pressing the fullness forward and making it obvious. It looks as though the surgery had enlarged the patient's breasts, yet nothing was done in this area. Thus, a change in position can make something "appear" in the "after" photo when it was present the whole time.

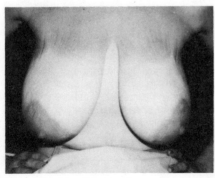
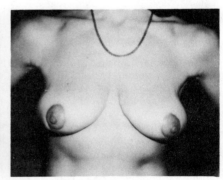

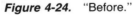

Figure 4-24. "Before." ***Figure 4-25.*** "After."

This patient had a breast reduction. Her breasts were large and unequal in size; surgery made them smaller and more symmetrical. The "after" photo was taken three months after the operation, yet the scars are barely noticeable. In real life the scars were obvious and took several more months to fade. The close-up "after" photo makes the breasts look slightly larger than they are. The camera used for the "before" picture shows less detail than the one used for the "after" picture; had it been used "after," the scars would have looked even more deceptively faint.

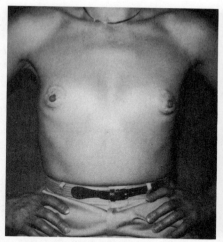

Figure 4-26. "Before."

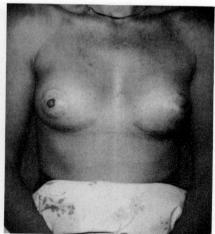

Figure 4-27. "After."

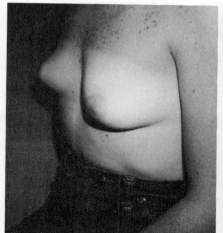

Figure 4-28. "Before."

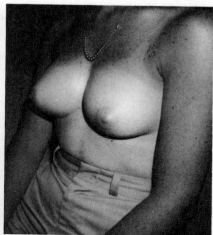

Figure 4-29. "After."

These two patients had a breast augmentation. Here, the "befores" and "afters" were taken with the same camera, at the same distance, with the patient in the same position and wearing the same clothes. In these respects, the photographs are comparable. However, the "after" photographs were taken two weeks after surgery, when the breasts were still swollen. The breasts therefore seem fuller, rounder, and less natural than they will when healing is complete. Thus, not only photographic technique but also timing is important in evaluating a surgical photograph.

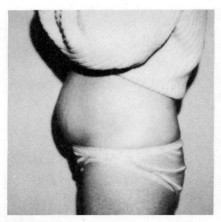 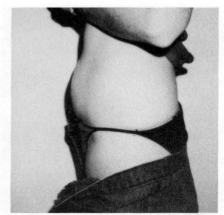

Figure 4-30. "Before."   **Figure 4-31.** "After."

This patient had a "mini tummy tuck." Her abdominal muscles were stretched loose, but otherwise she had a perfect figure. Hence, only a "mini" tuck to repair the muscles was needed. (This is still a lot of surgery.) The "after" was taken a few weeks after the operation. The abdomen is still swollen. Also, photographic shadows make it hard to see the true "before" profile. The sweater makes it impossible to see whether the patient is slouched forward (she is not). Thus, it is impossible to see how much of the "after" improvement is real, from surgery, and how much is from standing straighter. Close-up midriff photos are not flattering—this is a petite, youthful dancer. Those of us in less perfect shape can't bear such photos of ourselves. They aren't pretty before *or* after.

it is your face, such last-minute photographs are taken only because they will be better than no photograph at all.

If your surgeon takes last-minute "before" photos, you should conclude:

1. He has done it for the reasons I mentioned above, *or*
2. He is abysmally ignorant of the simplest rules of photography and takes "last-minute befores" merely because it is *convenient* for him, *or*
3. He is *deliberately* taking "last-minute befores" (and probably elegant "afters") just to dazzle you with the miracles of his surgery —usually because he is either lacking in skill or confidence and cannot be honest with you or himself.

Is this deliberate deception a common occurrence? I don't think so. Is there *any* excuse for it? Occasionally.

A patient Sheila once walked into my office for a second opinion. She had had a facelift, hated the result, and wanted to sue the surgeon. My examination indicated that she had a good surgical result. Sheila had been operated on by an excellent plastic surgeon. Her "before" photograph was a "last-minute before": she was on a stretcher, slipping sideways from sedation, every flaw in her face revealed. Her "after" was an in-office photograph with her nicely dressed, and well made up. Why?

The surgeon's medical notes indicated that Sheila had told him of several lawsuits she had filed against other professionals. He thought he could help her with surgery, but he was concerned that she might include him on her list of "people to sue." (He had been right.) But why the photographs? He was protecting himself legally. Any juror who compared her "before" and "after" photos would conclude that the surgeon had done a great job.

Even the very best doctors are afraid of lawsuits. Deceptive photographs may be part of your surgeon's legal defensiveness. They may have *nothing* to do with his skill or honesty as a surgeon.

Your surgeon may also take "deceptive" photographs for your psychological support. The line between this and deliberate deception is a fine one, but it exists. The surgeon who is doing this to help you will point out the difference in photographs honestly. The surgeon who is fooling you or himself will imply or even state that the photographs are comparable. A deceptive "after" photograph can be helpful because many people get terribly discouraged during the long healing period. There is a tendency to look in the mirror and say: "Yuck! I'm bruised. I'm swollen. I can't tell any difference." Nothing makes such a discouraged patient feel better than to look at a terrible "before" and a flattering "after" picture.

Terry had cosmetic eye surgery. Afterwards his bruising and swelling were greater than normal. His "before" pictures had not returned from the developer before surgery, so I took a set of "last-minute befores." After his surgery, when the bruising was at its worst, Terry demanded to see his "before" photographs. I explained to him that the only ones I had were the "last-minute befores." I suggested that we wait until the better "before" photographs came back from the developer. Terry's response? "Show me at my worst, Doctor. I don't care how accurate it is. I just want to feel better!"

I showed him the "last-minute befores," which made him look dazed and drunk. He was thrilled with the surgery, because, bruises and all, he looked better now than in the "before" photo.

Getting the Best From Your Photos

Here are your guidelines for getting the *best* from your photographs.

- Don't object to your surgeon taking "before" photographs of you.
- Ask your surgeon to take your "before" photographs in his office, not right before surgery.
- Jot down on your calendar what clothes you wore for that photograph.
- For all photographs, look straight into the camera, neither smiling nor glum, but serious.
- Use the *same expression* and wear the *same clothes* if possible for your "after" photograph.
- Ask your surgeon to review your photographs and *show you* in what ways the "before" and "after" photographs differ in surgical results and in camera technique.
- *Don't be dazzled!* If you are an astute observer of photographic detail, study the photographs a cosmetic surgeon shows you so that *you know what the photograph is saying.*
- If you aren't an astute observer, or if you are easily influenced by general impressions, take "befores" and "afters" with a healthy dose of skepticism.

The Surgeon's Workbook: Other Patients' Photos

Many of my patients, on their consultation visit, ask me to show them "Before"/"After" photos of some of my other patients. Most plastic surgeons—including myself—will not do this. We will teach you about your surgery using diagrams, drawings, or textbook photographs, but not by showing you one or two photographs of our other patients. What are we hiding? Nothing. We are trying to protect you from an error in judgment and from being misled, intentionally or not, by great results in another patient who had an unusually good result, a different problem, or even a different operation from you.

Zoe was referred to a cosmetic surgeon for a reconstructive breast operation. She was doubtful about the operation and wanted it only if it gave her a good chance of really normal-looking breasts. The surgeon showed Zoe his "Workbook" of "before" and "after" photographs of other patients having breast surgery. But Zoe wasn't told (1) that the photographs were of another surgeon's patients, not his, and (2) that the photographs were of patients who had had cosmetic breast enlargement, not breast reconstruction. What convinced Zoe to have the surgery? The photographs, of course.

Zoe had the surgery and was bitterly disappointed. Neither her surgeon's skill nor the operation he performed was what she had been shown. She had a mediocre surgical result for an operation she would never have had, if she hadn't seen the "Workbook."

Such deception is rare, but it illustrates how easily you can be misled if your decision is based on other patients' photographs.

Even an Honest Surgeon Will Show You His "Best"

Please don't expect your surgeon to be superhuman. If you consult any cosmetic surgeon and persuade him to show you samples of his work, you are *asking that surgeon to advertise himself to you*. Do you really think he is going to pull out a photo of a poor result in a plain, grouchy patient, scowling at you? Or is he going to produce a great result, in a confident, satisfied, good-looking patient? The essence of advertising is to make you want what you see. If you ask your surgeon to show you photographs of other people, you are asking to be sold.

What's so bad about being sold? Nothing, except that it is not objective. You are seeing your surgeon's best results. The photographs are of people who agree to have their photographs shown to strangers, which means they are likely to be naturally photogenic. The faces and bodies you see may not resemble you at all; therefore, they are no indication of what *you* will look like after surgery. Finally, you are virtually asking your surgeon to invade *your* privacy. If you see another patient's photographs, you may find it hard to say no when you are asked if yours can be shown to others, because that seems only fair.

How to Protect Your Privacy

If your surgeon takes a photograph of you, do you know how he intends to use it? My patients sign a general permission form, letting me use their pictures "for medical and scientific purposes, including publication." Displaying your photo in an operating room may be publication in the legal sense. It is also publication if I show the photo to another surgeon for an opinion. Few patients object to such medical use of photos.

Your cosmetic surgeon cannot legally publish your photographs in any book or journal without your *specific* permission for use in that book or journal. (General forms are not enough.) Thus, you won't turn up in print unexpectedly. However, if you give permission for your photo to be shown to other patients, think carefully. You can end up embarrassed.

Allen had cosmetic face surgery done by another plastic surgeon. He had insisted on seeing other patients' "before" and "after" pictures, and his surgeon had agreed. He had his operation. He didn't mind his photographs being shown to other patients—so he thought. His photographs were shown to Jake, who came in for the same operation. Problem? The two men happened to know each other. Allen had lied to Jake about his surgery. Jake thought it was very funny and told all their mutual friends about what a liar Allen had been.

So Why Am I Showing You Photographs in This Book?

Reading about an operation can be confusing. The illustrations and photographs in this book help to make surgery real for you. When you see a bump on a nose, and see it gone, you can *understand* what the surgery does. I have tried to make the photographs in this book represent the kind of result *any skilled Board Certified Plastic Surgeon could be expected to achieve in that patient.*

Am I Advertising Myself to You?

No, so long as you go to another surgeon. If you were to come to me for surgery, which is statistically highly unlikely, I would show you *pictures from surgical textbooks*, because I want you to know what a skilled cosmetic surgeon can accomplish. I don't want you to conclude: "Dr. Morgan got this result for this patient. Therefore, I will have the same result." What you should conclude instead is: "I understand what the surgery can do. Given *my problem* and *my understanding of the surgery*, I know what to expect *for myself.*"

Textbooks Can Be Helpful

There are many plastic surgery textbooks written by many plastic surgeons. Your plastic surgeon can pull out textbooks to show you lots of different photographs taken for scientific documentation in a textbook. Once you have seen dozens of photographs, you have learned how complicated and how different faces and bodies can be.

One of the textbooks I use with my patients is *Aesthetic Plastic Surgery*, by Thomas Rees, M.D. (W. B. Saunders). It has lots of pictures and is honest. Bad scars and disappointing results are included in the many photographs. One illustration (on page 649 of the 1980 edition) shows a patient who had a facelift but showed virtually *no* difference between before and after. The text discusses the reasons. Because a textbook does not represent the work of your surgeon, the two of you can discuss and criticize results without hesitation.

If you are especially worried about complications, dip into the second edition of *The Unfavorable Result in Plastic Surgery*, by Robert Goldwyn, M.D. (Little, Brown). Dr. Goldwyn teaches at Harvard Medical School. This book has some gruesome pictures of what can go wrong with surgery. There is a risk, though, in asking your surgeon to review with you the parts in this book that concern your surgery. Dealing with complications is routine for surgeons, but unless you're the kind of person who feels comfortable only by knowing all possible problems, you could end up just depressed.

"Painting" Your Dream Image by Computer

You might have heard about computers that can reproduce your face on a TV-like CRT screen while you and your surgeon "operate" on your picture. I love computer imaging—because it's fun. It may give you a more realistic idea of what surgery can do—or it may mislead you. Suppose your nose has a bump you don't like. On a CRT screen you can create the perfect nose—exactly what you want, down to the last millimeter. It's marvelous—but it's technically impossible for your surgeon to do. For one thing, computer images don't bleed, swell, or scar. For another, a bit of the "computer you" can be taken off, put back, taken off again. We can't do that on the real you.

You *Can* Expect the Computer Imager:
- To show your surgeon what *you* have in mind.
- To show you the *kinds of things* surgery can do.

You *Can't* Expect the Computer Imager:
- To show you exactly how you will look after surgery. It can't.
- To show how your scars will look. It can only show where they will be.

Computer imaging takes time to learn. The longer your surgeon has used it, the better he will be able to use it with you. In other words, your computer image result is only as accurate as your doctor's expertise on the machine.

You Are Not a Computer Image

You are three dimensional. You have color in your face. Your face moves in a thousand intricate ways. All these are "you." The computer image is a two-dimensional picture of you made of a million tiny dots. Judge yourself by the way you look—not by the way your computer image looks.

My own appearance is a good example of computer "looks" versus real life. In profile, I have bimaxillary protrusion. In other words, my lips jut out. My computer image shows that I "need" to have my upper and lower teeth set back and/or to have my lips reduced. But the *real me* doesn't need this. The balance of my face, the way it moves, and the depth of my face show that fixing my bimaxillary protrusion wouldn't help my looks. In fact, it might make me look rather ordinary, boring, and weak—not my surgical goal.

I think that *in time*, computers will be used more and more in cosmetic as in other fields of surgery. So far, they are far from necessary.

Sketching Can Help

Few plastic surgeons, including myself, are gifted artists. However, we can help you understand your surgery by drawing a sketch or by drawing on your photograph. For instance, often I find it helpful to draw the anatomy for my patients, so they understand what surgery does. I may find it helpful to draw on the preoperation photograph, to show what I would hope to create.

I use my photograph drawing to show where scars will be and where outlines will change *on that patient*. That helps my patients to imagine what will change on their faces.

Wouldn't You Like to Look As Good As a Model?

You may not be photogenic. You may hate seeing your photographs —before or after surgery. But don't let that hurt your self-image. Real looks and photographs are not the same.

Barbie wanted me to operate on her nose. She had a rather thin, delicate nose with a very big hump. She brought in a photograph of a high-fashion model. The model had her head turned partly away from the camera. I could clearly see the boxy look of her nostrils, which was the result of nose surgery. Also, I could clearly see that the camera had been angled to conceal the fact that the model's nose was much too small for her face. When I pointed this out to Barbie, she was horrified. "I don't want to look like that. How can that girl earn a living as a model?"

Answer? First, the model's skill was in selling her image, not merely her nose. Second, the camera could conceal the defects of her overoperated nose. In real life, her nose did not fit her face. But she put up with that, because she earned thousands of dollars as a model. Too small a nose is better than too big a nose—for a model. *It is more important to a model that her nose photograph properly.* Most of us, though, want our best to be the reality, not the illusion!

The trouble with reality after surgery is that it changes from day to day and week to week while you heal. A photograph may be helpful, especially if it encourages you during the healing period. Photographs don't reflect how most people really look, though. You will almost certainly find that even when you don't look good in the "after" photo, you see the improvement in the real you. It just takes a little time.

CHAPTER 5

The Right Way to Prepare for Your Surgery and Recovery

While you can and should rely on your surgeon for *surgical information*, there's so much your surgeon won't know or won't have time to tell you. Ask your surgeon about nutrition and exercise that will help you get ready for surgery, and you're likely to see a glazed look come into his eye as he struggles to remember the "Seven Basic Food Groups." There is so much that you can do—on your own—to get ready physically and psychologically for your operation. The following guidelines are based on my patients' experiences. They are designed to get you ready to go through your surgery as easily and as comfortably as possible.

PREPARING PHYSICALLY FOR YOUR SURGERY

The seven areas of physical preparation are related to: (1) fitness, (2) dieting, (3) nutrition, (4) drugs, (5) medical checkups, (6) smoking, and (7) blood flow.

Fitness

Surgery depletes you physically. Exercise is an important way to prepare yourself for surgery. If you get regular exercise, *keep it up*. "Regular" means three or more sessions of exercise a week. Walking to the bus stop does not count. A brisk half-hour hike in walking shoes does count.

If you don't get regular exercise, start now—gently. If your surgery is less than three weeks away, spend 10 minutes a day bending, stretching, and deep breathing every other day. Walk briskly on alternate days.

If you have three weeks or more before surgery, start out at 10 minutes a day every day, the first week, of stretching and exercise; the next week, 20 minutes, alternate days, of vigorous exercise. The third week and after you can do a half hour of vigorous exercise three times a week.

Be kind to yourself. You are not trying out for the Olympics or trying to turn pro. Don't exercise to soreness, especially if surgery is near. "No pain, no gain" is not your motto. Sore muscles are hurt muscles. They have to heal. Save your healing for surgical healing. Don't waste your energy and body protein on repairing damaged muscles from misguided, masochistic workouts. Your fitness goals are:

- Increased *lung power*, for stamina on the operating table.
- Increased *skin blood flow*, to heal surgical incisions.
- Increased *joint looseness* for your comfort. Your joints will stiffen after surgery from lying on the operating table for several hours. Then you will be relatively inactive for 3 to 14 days after surgery. A loose joint is a happy joint. Stiff ones hurt.

Dieting

Forget your diet during the two weeks before your cosmetic surgery. When you diet, your body goes into a *catabolic* (breakdown) gear, burning up stores of protein, carbohydrate, and fat, so that your reserves diminish. But your body also goes into catabolic gear after surgery. The stress of surgery makes your body break down fat, carbohydrate (glycogen) stores and even muscle protein. You will hurt yourself if you stress your body twice over: diet *plus* surgery. You will end up exhausted. You are then susceptible to flu and whatever infection is going around. Also, you will have more pain than you ought to have. Be kind to your body. For those last two weeks, throw out the diet and maintain, don't lose, your weight.

Dieting before surgery is pointless anyhow, because the catabolic phase caused by your surgery will be immediately followed by the rebuilding phase of rebound hunger and uncontrollable eating until you gain back all the weight you lost from surgery. If you are dieting up to the day of surgery, your rebound hunger will direct your body to gain back all your diet weight loss, too. Your body can't tell your diet stress from the surgical stress if the two events occur close together.

Must I Be My Ideal Weight Before Surgery? Ideally, yes—but we don't live in an ideal world. Most of us who want to lose or gain weight have a hard time doing it. It can take years. Often, people can't diet until something happens that changes them. I have had patients who couldn't lose weight before surgery, and who, after cosmetic surgery, felt stimulated to improve in other ways and went on successful diets.

With modern surgical techniques, even if you are overweight, you can have a good cosmetic result from surgery. But you may need to plan your surgery around future weight loss.

Evelyn was a lovely, but overweight, mother of four children. She had flat, flabby breasts after her last pregnancy. She wanted a breast enlargement. She wanted to lose weight—about 40 pounds—but she also wanted her breasts to look better now. Evelyn was worried because her correct breast size for her overweight shape was a D cup, at least, but if she lost her weight, she wanted to end up a B cup. What I did was to put in breast implants that were too small for Evelyn in her overweight condition, although still an improvement on what she had. These breast implants made Evelyn a C cup when she was fat—too small. But they made her a full B cup (what she wanted to be) once she lost her weight after surgery.

Sam was overweight, middle-aged, bull-necked and going to stay that way. All his brothers were the same shape. Sam didn't mind except he hated his double chin.

Ten—even five—years ago, it would have been hard to help him. We didn't know how to treat fat in the neck, and we didn't have the instruments that we have today. I would probably have advised Sam to diet first, and then have a facelift. It wouldn't have helped him because Sam couldn't diet and knew it.

Today we can remove neck fat by cutting and suctioning it away. I did a facelift on Sam, in which I first removed the fat and then cut off the skin that was flabby when the fat was gone.

Without his double neck, Sam looked thinner, felt thinner, and could wear shirts without his chin hanging over the top.

Joyce was fat and hated it. She was 18 and was teased for her weight and her very big breasts. She could not diet—it made her depressed. Her mother was sure that Joyce ought to lose weight before breast surgery. She feared Joyce's breasts would be too small if she had surgery before she lost weight. Joyce wanted her overlarge breasts off! She didn't care about "too small." When she became bulimic (bingeing and purging) trying to lose weight for surgery, her mother agreed that surgery came first.

I explained to Joyce that I would make her a *full B cup.* She wanted to be an A—which would leave her with practically no breasts if she lost a lot of weight. Joyce had been a DD before surgery. The change to a B cup was dramatic. She was overjoyed.

Result: Her smaller breasts made her look as though she had lost 20 pounds. Everyone wanted to know what diet she used. With smaller breasts, Joyce could take part in school sports. She didn't diet—but she became much more active and lost weight.

Note: If you have been bingeing and purging, please tell your surgeon. The vomiting depletes your body acid level and can cause heart malfunction during surgery if untreated. He will check your blood electrolyte level, probably shortly after you tell him and again a few days before surgery. If that is normal, you should be fine.

Nutrition

You need all the nutritional help you can get during surgery. Your body will burn up extra protein during and after surgery, so stock up on protein for two weeks beforehand. Animal protein is the nearest to the protein in our own bodies. So preferably increase your *animal protein*: veal, poultry, beef, pork, fish, eggs, cheese.

What about vegetarians? Don't change your eating pattern radically. Just increase your vegetable protein (especially legume) intake. If you rely on eggs or cheese for protein, increase your intake of eggs and cheese. It won't be good for your vegetarian body to suddenly start eating steak if you haven't had any for years. Your increased protein should not be incompatible with your body.

Cholesterol. The fat in red meat is higher in cholesterol than most other protein foods. So if you are increasing your red meat intake, choose lean meat and cook it so that the fat drains off.

Vitamins. If you already take vitamins, *don't increase your daily dose*. You don't need more, and overloading on vitamins can be dangerous. For instance, excess vitamin E can make you bleed.

If you don't usually take vitamins, add *one* multivitamin a day for the two weeks before surgery. This way you'll have plenty to spare for healing, even if you have been run down from an unbalanced diet.

Gelatin. If your nails (or hair) tend to split or break, you should take a pack of gelatin a day for the two weeks before surgery. The protein you lose during surgery depletes what you need for your nails and hair.

Drugs

Illegal Drugs. Surveys show that a *huge* number of Americans take illegal drugs, from marijuana to cocaine. If you take *any* illegal drug, stop for the two weeks before surgery. All such drugs have chemicals that will interfere with your sedation. Cocaine can cause sudden heart failure.

If you try to stop two weeks before surgery but can't because of withdrawal symptoms, be honest and tell your surgeon! You may still be able to have your operation. Or, you may need to postpone surgery *for your own safety* until you are off the drugs and/or under treatment.

Don't be silly and keep quiet if you can't get off the drug. Your life may be at stake. If you do have a drug problem, it is confidential between you and your surgeon. Let him help you. A good surgeon is also a good doctor. If you don't trust a surgeon enough to confide in him about your dangerous drug habit, maybe you shouldn't trust him to operate on you, either.

Legal Prescription Drugs. Tell your surgeon the names and doses of *all* prescription drugs that you take. If they are unusual, or if your surgeon is not familiar with your prescriptions, call the doctor who prescribed them. Ask that doctor to call your surgeon to discuss possible side effects.

Luke was in his early forties and was taking a blood pressure drug that had recently come on the market. I had never heard of it. I called his doctor. Luke's doctor knew of two patients taking this drug who had had fatal reactions to epinephrine! Ordinarily I would give Luke epinephrine at surgery. By consulting with his prescribing doctor, I learned that I couldn't give "epi," but I also learned what drugs I could give, so that Luke could still have his surgery.

If you don't know your drug's name or your dosage, and your prescribing doctor isn't around, call the pharmacy that filled your prescription. Ask them to give the information to your cosmetic surgeon. It doesn't help to bring in your prescription bottle to your surgeon, *unless the drug name and dose are on the bottle*. Some pills can be identified by comparing them to a picture chart, but this only works for fairly common pills, and it wastes time for you and your surgeon.

Do you have prescriptions filled abroad? It may be impossible to find out what is in a foreign drug. If a drug is prescribed for you abroad, get the name of the drug, the dose, and the *name of the manufacturer*.

Legal Nonprescription (Over-the-Counter) Drugs. For three weeks before surgery, take *no over-the-counter drug* except acetaminophen (common brands: Tylenol, Datril). Any other medicine should be approved by your cosmetic surgeon. Why? Many over-the-counter drugs contain aspirin or anti-inflammatory painkillers (analgesics), all of which interfere with the blood's clotting ability and can make you bleed excessively. Take nonprescription pills out of your purse, medicine chest, and pill box. Put them aside until *two weeks after your surgery*. About 2 percent of people can have serious bleeding if they have taken aspirin or such anti-inflammatory painkillers as ibuprofen (Motrin) within the weeks before surgery. Routine blood tests *do not detect this drug-caused bleeding tendency.*

Miranda didn't think that just one aspirin would hurt, if she took it the week before her facelift. She didn't know that she was one of the unlucky 2 percent whose bleeding rate is affected by even small doses of aspirin. Miranda's facelift surgery began with unusually heavy bleeding. Halfway through, Miranda was hemorrhaging (bleeding profusely). She required blood and platelet transfusions to stop the bleeding and was in hospital for days after her surgery.

Even if you don't hemorrhage, aspirin and anti-inflammatory painkillers can cause severe unsightly bruising after your surgery. Isn't it easier to avoid aspirin, rather than to risk being black-and-blue for three weeks or more?

What If I Forget? About 20 percent of my patients forget, even though I warn them and give them a reminder slip. Don't panic. Call your cosmetic surgeon and let him know. Depending on your surgery, on how much you took and on whether you have bled in the past, your surgeon may recommend:

- No action
- Bleeding and clotting tests before surgery
- Consultation with a hematologist (blood specialist)
- Postponing your surgery

By telling your surgeon, you put him on notice to look out for unusual bleeding. Thus, if you start to bleed excessively early in your surgery, he won't expect it to take care of itself. He can stop—or treat you with platelets or plasma to correct the bleeding. This is all very unlikely to happen. Still, it's easier for you if you are one of the 80 percent who don't forget.

Does This Mean That Acetaminophen Is Always Safe? No. All drugs have side effects. Acetaminophen (e.g., Tylenol) sometimes causes liver and kidney damage if taken in excessive amounts. But it is safer around surgery than aspirin because it doesn't increase your risk of hemorrhage.

Even if you ordinarily don't take over-the-counter medicines, buy a bottle of acetaminophen to use after your surgery. You will need a mild painkiller. Many patients after cosmetic surgery need no prescription painkiller and use only acetaminophen for the pain.

If you will be in hospital overnight, you can save a little money by taking your own acetaminophen to the hospital with you. A hospital can charge you 60¢ or more per pill. However, many hospitals have policies, required by their insurance, that patients can only take hospital-issued drugs.

What If I Get a Cold? It sometimes seems like fate: Your surgery approaches and your allergies tend to flare up or you start to sniffle. I usually tell my patients to take *no antihistamines* (cold or allergy pills). They may increase your bleeding risk. From a practical point of view, though, it is important for you to be rested for surgery—which you won't be if you are up all night with a dripping nose. So, I will approve taking an antihistamine for a few days *if* my patient tells me which kind is being used, calls me daily with a report on how much is needed, and understands that a *really bad cold* can mean surgery should be cancelled. Check with your surgeon before you take a cold medicine, so that he can advise you if it is safe.

Constipation. Narcotics and narcotic painkillers slow down your large intestine and make you constipated. After cosmetic surgery you need only a small amount of narcotic. If you tend to be constipated:

- Take a narcotic only when you *must*.
- Drink lots of water after surgery.
- Take a dose of Metamucil or other bulk laxative on the night before and the night after surgery.
- Have a suppository, milk of magnesia, or your laxative available for after surgery.
- Don't strain to have a bowel movement; straining can increase pressure and start bleeding in the surgical area.
- Tell your cosmetic surgeon if you have not had a bowel movement on the second day after surgery. He should help you decide what next to take.

Medical Checkups Before Surgery

Most of us hate going to a doctor (including doctors!). You don't always need a checkup before your cosmetic surgery. Sometimes it is worthwhile. Sometimes it is *necessary*.

Your Breasts. General surgeons are the breast lump specialists. If you are having cosmetic breast surgery and you have had breast lumps in the past, it is usually best to have a general surgeon or your treating doctor check your breasts before surgery. If he finds a new lump, your cosmetic surgeon can do a biopsy (microscopic examination of the tissue) at the same time that he does your cosmetic breast operation. This saves you having two operations.

Your doctor should also be consulted if there was any change on your last mammogram. If you're over 35, a mammogram is often done routinely before your surgery. Suppose you have no lump, but there is an area on the mammogram that doesn't look quite normal. A general surgeon, or your cosmetic surgeon, can biopsy the questionable breast area at the same time as your cosmetic breast surgery. All this is a nuisance. But it makes sense.

Lonny is a charming young model in her late twenties. A general surgeon had checked her before she came to see me for her cosmetic breast surgery. He had found an apparently insignificant lump in one breast. Her general surgeon and I agreed that I should take a tissue sample (biopsy specimen) of this tiny lump when I did Lonny's cosmetic breast surgery. In such a situation, the operation is halted while a pathologist microscopically examines the biopsy specimen. In Lonny's case, the insignificant lump was a breast cancer.

I had done the biopsy first, so I did not go on with the cosmetic breast surgery. Within the week, the general surgeon and I operated on Lonny together. He removed the cancerous breast. I reconstructed her breast and did the cosmetic enlargement of her normal breast.

Ironically, this saved Lonny a lot of money. Insurance paid for all of her surgery. The money was not important. The biopsy of the lump saved Lonny's life.

Your Eyes. Your eye doctor should check your vision before you have cosmetic eye surgery. A change in the pressure in your eyes, eye allergies, or a change in vision should be treated before surgery. Your eyes are valuable and irreplaceable. Something "minor" such as a pollen allergy can flare up and become a painful setback to your recovery, if it has not been diagnosed before surgery. Also, surgery will make your eyes sensitive to everything. You don't want to discover *after surgery* that you need new contacts, and your eyes will be too sensitive for weeks to be fitted for them. Have eye prescriptions filled before surgery. *On the bright side*, cosmetic eye surgery seems to improve your eye allergies, for reasons we don't understand.

Your Skin. Do you have a skin eruption or rash in the area of your cosmetic surgery? Be sure the eruption is treated. Your cosmetic surgeon may be able to diagnose the problem and prescribe treatment. Or, you may need a dermatologist (skin specialist).

A healthy skin is important to your healing. Besides, surgery itself damages your skin. Surgical soaps and bandages can make *any* skin condition worse. An acne or rosacea flare-up could cause an infection that spoils your surgical result or delays your healing. *Take even minor skin problems seriously before surgery.*

Your Vital Organs. Vital organs are ones you need to live: heart, lungs, liver, kidney, essential glands. You should see your treating doctor before surgery *if you have a malfunction of a vital organ* or any ongoing disease condition such as diabetes or hypertension. A full health history is taken routinely before cosmetic surgery. Be sure to tell your surgeon about any chronic conditions.

Lincoln was in his thirties and had mild diabetes. He wanted cosmetic surgery to correct the loose skin and muscle on his stomach which appeared after he lost 50 pounds. Lincoln did not think his diabetes doctor needed to see him before his surgery. I disagreed. Lincoln's surgery was going to be under general anesthesia. Reluctantly, Lincoln saw his regular doctor for a checkup.

Stoical Lincoln's diabetes was much worse than he had suspected. He now needed insulin. His doctor regulated Lincoln's diabetes before the surgery. Lincoln had general anesthesia, a successful operation, and a rapid recovery.

Without the checkup and insulin regulation, Lincoln would have ended up in the hospital with diabetic complications and possibly even a temporary diabetic coma, brought on by the stress of surgery, anesthesia, and his unregulated diabetic condition.

Smoking

If you don't smoke, of course you won't start. If you do smoke: please, if you possibly can, stop for the two weeks before your surgery. This is difficult—tobacco is truly addictive for many of us. If you can't stop for two weeks, *cut down* as much as you can.

Please don't smoke on the day of your surgery. Tobacco is bad for your whole body, but it is *terrible* for healing. Nicotine constricts blood vessels, reducing blood flow to many areas, including your skin. Smokers who have facelifts have at least a 15 percent risk of not healing in the area behind the ear, where the skin is stretched most. By reducing blood flow, nicotine decreases the skin's oxygen supply, so it can't heal. The stitches pull apart. A scab forms. You eventually heal with a wide, discolored scar.

Tobacco decreases your infection resistance. The tobacco damages your immune system and your lungs. Your lung power is further decreased during surgery by sedation and by lying still. Tobacco increases your risk of lower than normal levels of oxygen in your blood during surgery, *plus*:

- Coughs
- Pneumonia
- Wound infection
- Poor healing
- Just about anything else that you and your surgeon don't want you to have.

Your Blood Flow

All surgery increases your risk of phlebitis (inflammation of the blood vessels) and blood clots in your legs. The risk is small for most cosmetic surgery, because you are usually up and walking within hours after your surgery. However, poor blood flow in your legs can make your legs ache for days, even if nothing worse happens. Two weeks before your surgery, *think legs just before you go to sleep*:

- Point your toes down and then bend your ankles back so that your toes point up to your face.
- Do this *ten* times.
- Your legs should feel the stretch.

After surgery, starting in the Recovery Room (!), three times a day, do the same bending and stretching of your ankles ten times. Why? Your leg stretching makes your muscles pump the blood through your leg veins. The blood does not stagnate. Practicing before surgery gets you into the routine. You can stop leg stretches *on the tenth day after surgery* if you want to, although they are always a good idea.

Elastic Stockings. These stockings are not elegant. But if you have legs that ache or tire when you stand, have a pair of elastic stockings on hand. These are elastic knee-high hose, not support stockings or pantyhose. Buy these in any drugstore. Wear them to the operating room. Wear them while you're in bed after surgery. They will keep your legs from aching and swelling. A lot of surgeons (including me) routinely put elastic stockings on our patients and ourselves before long operations.

Blood Transfusions. Cosmetic surgery rarely requires blood transfusion. However, breast reductions and tummy-tucks can cause enough blood loss to make a transfusion necessary. You can get sick from a disease carried in a blood transfusion, although it's rare now to get AIDS that way. Hepatitis is a greater danger. You minimize your transfusion risks if you donate your own blood for your surgery.

Your body is constantly making new blood. Donated blood can be stored under refrigeration for 30 days, so you can donate one or two pints of your own blood for your own surgery. That way, if you need a transfusion, you get your own blood.

Your surgeon's office arranges such a blood donation. You have to donate the blood at the hospital where you will have your operation.

The hospital will order tests on the day of surgery to be sure that you get your own blood.

PREPARING PSYCHOLOGICALLY FOR SURGERY

Surgery depresses everyone—physically. You are inactive. The drugs slow down your body and brain. You lose sleep from worry before surgery. Your sleep is disrupted by drugs for days, even weeks, after surgery. You may wake up often at night or have bizarre dreams which tire you while you sleep. Your body will use all its energy to heal, leaving you none to spare.

Depression after surgery starts with *physical causes*. Your brain does not distinguish between a physical and a psychological "down." After an operation, you will feel that if only you had willpower, you would have energy, get moving, and feel better. You can't. This frustration leads to its own *psychological* depression. You can't stop the depressing effect of surgical and drug stress on your brain. However, you can prepare yourself to avoid psychological depression that feeds on your physical depression.

Consider Psychotherapy

If you are undergoing counseling, tell your therapist about your surgery. It helps to talk about any worries you might have. Equally important, your therapist should be warned that you will be "blue" after surgery and that it will partly be normal. Your therapist will be ready to give you support after surgery to stop the normal postsurgical depression from growing into a severe psychological depression.

Avoid Anything (or Anyone) That Makes You "Blue"

Convalescence is a time to avoid *all other stress*. Here's a list of things that might depress you and what you might do about them.

YOUR ANTI-"BLUES" CHECKLIST

Things That Cause the "Blues"	Ways to Fight the "Blues"
1. Reading about crime or watching the news on TV	1. Avoid the news for 10 days
2. Being alone	2. Have a friend stay with you
3. Talking with your "ex"	3. Have a machine answer your phone—don't call back unless you *want to*
4. Paying bills	4. Try to arrange to pay your monthly bills before surgery
5. Being cold	5. Buy a space heater for your bedroom
6. Worrying about work piling up at the office	6. Don't call the office—*you're out sick*
7. Worrying about your kids	7. Arrange ahead of time for your kids to be properly looked after
8. Pain	8. Have pain medicines handy at your bedside
9. The dark	9. Buy a nightlight
10. Fighting with your parents/in-laws/whomever	10. If confrontations seem unavoidable, curtail communications for a while
11. Feeling grimy or rumpled from having to lie in bed or not being able to bathe	11. Give yourself a sponge bath and change into fresh clothes

Is this irresponsible? No! It's only for ten days, for heaven's sake. You need to protect yourself if you want to get back to normal after surgery. It *is* irresponsible to take on stress when you are healing. Avoiding stress makes lots of us feel guilty—we "ought" to be involved, worrying, frantic. It's your choice. You can (1) pamper yourself for ten days *or* (2) call your surgeon in hysterics by Day 10.

Freida had cosmetic surgery on her breasts. Five days after surgery she called me at noon. She was crying uncontrollably. Her husband was at work. Freida hated being alone, and it was her fifth day at home alone. She was too tired to go out. She was going *crazy.*

Freida and I talked about her options. I reminded her that her reaction was a normal one after surgery. Freida ended up calling her next-door neighbor, who was happy to keep her company for the afternoon.

Not everyone has a neighbor, but everyone has a solution for the "blues." *Know your solution in advance.* You won't think clearly if you wait until you've cracked. And since your mood is not a surgical problem, a lot of surgeons will be baffled.

Do What Makes You Feel Good

Avoiding stress is good. You'll recover even faster if you do what makes you feel better. This box contains a list of "favorite things" and some ways to accomplish them. Use it to spark your own ideas.

A "FEELING GOOD" CHECKLIST

Some "Favorite Things"	Some Ways to Achieve Them
1. Not having to cook	1. Stock the freezer with frozen dinners
2. Watching sitcoms	2. Place a TV in the bedroom
3. Talking for hours to your best friend	3. Place a phone at your bedside and make daily, self-indulgent phone calls
4. Planning your next vacation	4. Stock up on maps and travel books galore
5. Doing jigsaw puzzles	5. Buy a *stack* of jigsaw puzzles
6. Seeing your family or other visitors	6. Let your family know that you'd like them to visit, or ask your church to spread the word that you'd like visitors for ten days
7. Long warm showers	7. Place a stool in your shower so you can sit and take long, warm showers once your surgeon permits
8. Buying fun things you don't need	8. Make a daily trip—once you're strong enough—to buy an inexpensive frivolity

---

Some "Favorite Things"	Some Ways to Achieve Them
9. Exercise	9. Take a daily walk, even if at first you don't get past the front door
10. Thinking how good you'll look soon	10. Put the mirrors away! You don't need to spend hours studying your swollen face and other "battle scars." Wait 'til you've healed!

Everyone's list and solutions are different. That doesn't matter. It *does* matter that you coddle your psyche until you are healed.

Don't Do What You KNOW You Shouldn't Do

Indulging yourself after surgery means indulging in a *relaxing, restful way.* I have had patients who just didn't listen and forged ahead: To paint the guest bedroom . . . to fix the roof . . . to drive 500 miles to see a friend. All of them took twice as long to recover as they should have.

MAKING PREPARATIONS FOR YOUR RECOVERY PERIOD

You don't go on a trip unless you have a ticket, money, and a suitcase—do you? You shouldn't go for cosmetic surgery without making the equivalent arrangements for some time off from work, your meals, medicine/bandages, post-op medical care and advice, means of concealing facial bruises, setting things up at home and last-minute preparations.

Your Job

You'll need *one week off from work, minimum.* With this, you will go back to work tired. If you must, that's fine, but be prepared. Arrange more than a week if you can. If you can't, make these adjustments:

- No social events for the first *two* weeks.
- No travel for the first *two* weeks.
- Go to work late, if you can.
- Call in sick, if you can.
- Don't drive if you can avoid it, for *two weeks*.
- Mentally prepare to feel exhausted at the end of the day for two weeks.

Your Meals

Preparing food is tiring. You don't want to cook after surgery. Your goal: two weeks of not more than 5 to 10 minutes per meal preparation time for you and your family. You may want to cook a week's worth of meals ahead of time and freeze them for later. (Better yet, have your family fix all the meals! Tell them this is their chance to have all their favorite foods!) *Buy* enough for two weeks of:

- Paper plates/cups
- Instant coffee
- Instant/frozen meals
- Vitamin pills
- Juice
- Frozen desserts
- Bread
- Prunes (if you may be constipated)
- Canned fruit
- Soup
- Flexible straws for drinking while reclining, or if facial movement is uncomfortable
- Yogurt, ice cream, custard, etc., if you can only eat soft food

Medicines/Bandages

- Refill all regular prescriptions before surgery.
- Buy acetaminophen (e.g., Tylenol) for minor pain.
- Have on hand these bandages:
  —1 box of gauze pads, 3 × 3 or 4 × 4
  —1 roll of tape (if you know you're skin is sensitive, buy the hypoallergenic kind)

—1 box of adhesive bandages
—2 boxes of facial tissues
—1 box of cotton swabs
—1 roll of paper towels
—1 small bottle of hydrogen peroxide (gets blood off skin/clothes)
• Stock cold pack or tea bags for ice compress, if you're having eye surgery.

Post-Op Medical Care and Advice

• Write your surgeon's phone number on a card and tape it to your phone.
• Schedule post-op appointments *before* surgery.
• Arrange rides (taxi/friends) to appointments in the first five days after surgery.
• Fill your surgeon's prescriptions for pain *before* surgery. Ask the office to mail them to you, if you forget to get them at an appointment.

Concealment (Facial Surgery Only)

Women	Men
1 large scarf	1 hat
1 pair tinted glasses	1 pair tinted glasses
Concealer cream (any makeup line)	Concealer cream (Clinique's men's line is best)
1 large hat (optional)	1 shirt/coat with collar that turns up
	1 scarf (optional)

Preparing Your Home

• Mouthwash/laxative in bathroom
• Cold cream/lip balm for dry lips at bedside
• Telephone at bedside

- Extra pillows for back support in bedroom
- Bottled water, juice, crackers, paper plates, paper napkins, pain medicine within reach of your bed
- Hard candy/cough drops within reach (your throat may be dry)
- Large bowl and old towel by bed, in case you feel sick.

You'll spend time in bed and time lounging in a chair or on a sofa. Ideally all the things you need should be duplicated—a set by the sofa or chair, as well as the bed. Of course, it's not always possible, but it's nicer for you.

Last-Minute Preparations Before Surgery

- Wash your hair the day before surgery (lying on the operating table makes it feel dirty).
- **Women:** Take off any nail polish before surgery. The color of the nails reflects blood oxygen, so it helps your surgeon to be able to see your nails. Also, polish will chip and crack before you feel ready to re-do it.
- Have a good snack just before bedtime the night before. You can't eat in the morning!
- Shower/shave/bathe morning of surgery.
- Put on clean bedding and turn down bed so it's ready for you to climb in when you get home.
- Floss/brush/use mouthwash morning of surgery. Your mouth will feel mousy after the operation.
- Coat your lips with Vaseline/cream/lip balm. Take some with you to the hospital. Dry lips will be a big problem for several days.
- Wear flat shoes and old sloppy clothes that are easy to get into for the trip home after surgery.

If you are staying in the hospital overnight, the hospital will usually send you a list of what to bring, but it should include:

- Pajamas/nightgowns/robe
- Toothbrush/paste/floss
- Makeup (women), razor (men)
- Extra underwear

- Books to read/crosswords/telephone numbers of friends
- Candy/snacks/gum for when you're allowed to eat
- Comb/hairbrush/shampoo/conditioner
- Small amount of change for newspaper, etc.
- Your own facial tissue
- Your own moisturizer, after-shave, cologne

All this seems like a lot to do. Actually one shopping trip and a couple of phone calls will get most of it done. You'll appreciate what you've done for yourself—after your operation.

Surgery Isn't the Time for Other BIG Decisions

Your recovery period is not the time for making other major decisions in your life. If you do, you may find you spend a lot more of your life *un*doing them.

> *Beth had cosmetic surgery when she was also negotiating her divorce settlement. She came in for a post-op appointment on the fifth day after surgery. She was upset because the final settlement was to be that afternoon. I suggested that she postpone the settlement. She said she wouldn't feel happy if she postponed it.*
> *Beth signed the agreement. Within a month she realized it had been a* big *mistake. Three years, a state Supreme Court appeal, and a new attorney later, she had undone the folly of the settlement.*

Be kind to yourself—and realistic too. You're not at your best after surgery. Let either the operation or the decision wait a while.

YOUR "SUPER PREPARATION" CHECKLIST

Physical

- Exercise.
- No dieting
- Take in extra protein, vitamins, and gelatin.

- No illegal drugs for at least two weeks prior to surgery
- Tell your surgeon about your prescriptions.
- Use no nonprescription drugs except acetaminophen for at least two weeks prior to surgery.
- Determine whether a medical checkup is necessary.
- Don't smoke—or at least cut down two weeks before surgery.
- Don't smoke for 24 hours before the operation—*please!*
- Do leg stretches at night to limber up your joints.
- Buy elastic stockings to improve your circulation.

Psychological

- Discuss the surgery with your therapist, if you have one.
- List, and plan to avoid, "downers."
- List, and plan to arrange, "uppers."
- *Accept fatigue* and physical depression as a temporary surgical side effect.

Recovery Period

- Get the maximum time off from work that you can.
- Stock up on two weeks' worth of quick food supplies.
- Stock up on medical supplies.
- Make post-op appointments.
- Buy post-op prescription(s).
- Buy "concealments" if needed.
- Arrange bedside comfort.
- Do last-minute preparations.

Then relax . . . you are ready!

CHAPTER   6

The Anesthesia
Experience

Your biggest risk in any cosmetic operation comes from the drugs you are given for anesthesia. Cosmetic surgery doesn't touch your vital organs—the brain, lungs, heart or liver. But *anesthesia affects every vital organ.*

What Your Surgeon May Not Tell You

Your surgeon probably won't have time to explain much about the anesthesia for your operation. There are hundreds of anesthetics and analgesics (drugs that sedate you or kill pain) and ways to use them. It would take your surgeon too long to explain it all—and he and you want the time to talk about your surgery. *Result:* You can end up confused about what drugs you were given or should have been given. You could be totally ignorant about your anesthesia.

Charles walked into my office and wanted a facelift. "I can't have any anesthesia," he explained to me. "It nearly killed me last time."

Charles had no idea what had "nearly killed" him. He assumed that all anesthetics are the same—if one nearly killed you, they all did.

Fortunately, I was able to reach Charles' surgeon. Charles had suffered from halothane hepatitis, a reaction to a specific anesthetic drug. This rare drug reaction had nearly killed him, but that drug wouldn't be needed for facelift surgery. The anesthetics I would be using for his cosmetic surgery would not be too risky for me to give him.

It isn't always easy—and is sometimes impossible—for you to get hospital records years after an operation. So, if you remember *what operation you had*, it's just as important to know *what anesthesia you had, too!*

KINDS OF ANESTHESIA

There are four basic kinds of anesthesia. I'll list them here and then discuss the ones that are used in cosmetic surgery so that you will know what to expect from them.

- Local anesthesia: Only the surgical area is numbed. A needle is used to inject the numbing liquid into the area that the surgeon will operate on.
- Local anesthesia with sedation: The surgical area is numbed for local anesthesia *and* you are given drugs (pill or injection) to relax your body and mind. *You are not fully asleep.* Most cosmetic surgery is done using local anesthesia with sedation. The fact that it can be done this way does not necessarily mean that "local/sedation" is best for you.
- Anesthetic block: A needle is used to inject a numbing solution around one or more large nerves. *Result:* one large area, such as your arm, has no feeling. You remain fully awake. Block anesthesia is rarely used in cosmetic surgery, so I won't be giving you more details.
- General anesthesia: Your mind is put fully to sleep. Injections and/or gases you breathe are used to do this.

There are also two uncommon ways of blocking awareness of pain during surgery: acupuncture and hypnosis. Some acupuncturists swear that their technique is as effective as any anesthetic. I have seen movies of, and read reports of, patients in China undergoing major surgery with no anesthetic except acupuncture. It works in ways we don't understand. It is *not* generally accepted by American doctors. But if you think acupuncture will be an effective anesthetic for you, an open-minded cosmetic surgeon may be willing to work with the acupuncturist of your choice.

Hypnosis works by putting you in a trance. Again, it is *not* generally accepted as an anesthetic. But if hyponosis works for you, a surgeon *might* be willing to try working with your hypnotist.

LOCAL ANESTHESIA

Operations in which local anesthesia is usually used include:

- Removal of moles
- Correction of small scars
- (Some) upper-lid "tucks"
- (Some) chin implants

Your surgeon may call this "straight local." The drugs used to numb the pain are usually a combination of (1) a "-caine" drug, (2) the hormone epinephrine, and (3) a preservative.

Xylocaine®, Novocaine®, and Marcaine® are the commonest "-caine" drugs. All these drugs are synthetic compounds that are chemically related to cocaine, which is a powerful local anesthetic itself. Cocaine has dangerous side effects, so the synthetic "-caines" are safer to use.

Epinephrine is a natural body hormone better known as adrenaline. One of the actions of "epi" is to tighten the muscle fibers in your blood vessels. The effect: *much* less bleeding.

Virtually all medical drugs have preservatives so that the drugs don't alter into less effective or toxic breakdown products. Common preservatives include citric acid, sodium chloride, sodium metabisulfite, methylparaben, and sodium hydroxide.

Typical Example of Local Anesthesia

Dot had a large hairy mole in the middle of her cheek and wanted me to remove it. My nurse brought Dot into the minor operating room in my office, where she lay down on the operating table and my nurse put a paper drape over her clothes.

I marked where I would cut around the mole, using a surgical indelible purple marking pen. My nurse cleaned Dot's face with a surgical soap. I washed my hands and put on surgical gloves.

My nurse held Dot's hand and turned up the music to distract her. I covered Dot's eyes with moist gauze pads so that her eyes were protected from the surgical light. This also kept Dot from trying to watch, which would only make her more nervous.

I inserted a #30 needle (smaller than most fine pins) near, but not into, the mole and injected a drop of xylocaine. This immediately numbed the injection site. Then I slowly injected more xylocaine mixed with epinephrine. Xylocaine works virtually immediately.

I took a fine scalpel, cut out the mole, and sewed the incision closed.

Dot could feel pressure but she felt no pain. It took about two hours for the anesthesia to wear off. When it did, Dot felt an irksome ache but no pain in the surgical area.

Drug Allergies

True allergic symptoms include a skin rash, hives, and asthma. If you are prone to *severe* allergies, ask your allergist to check that you aren't sensitive to any of the drugs you will get at surgery. *This includes the preservatives.* A number of people are sulfite allergic, and sulfites are used to preserve medical drugs.

The "Impending Doom" Reaction

Many patients are wrongly convinced that they are allergic to epinephrine. This drug, which chemically resembles caffeine, protects against anaphylaxis, which is shock and asthma from a drug allergy. Epinephrine opens up lung passages and is used to *treat* allergies. However, epinephrine does cause side effects, which become noticeable in 30 seconds to a few minutes after it is injected. Thus you would become aware of a side effect shortly before, or soon after, surgery began:

- A thumping heart
- Nervousness
- Restlessness
- A feeling of impending doom
- Feeling "about to die"

Some people get the same reaction from coffee. One patient of mine had such severe "epi" reactions that he was convinced that he had had a heart attack each time he had local anesthesia. (He had *not*. His heart was fine.) He was unusually sensitive to epinephrine and was relieved to find that he had no ill effects when the epinephrine was used in a very weak strength.

Can "Epi" Be Dangerous?

Yes. It stimulates the heart and raises your blood pressure. This can lead to heart malfunction or high blood pressure if you are given too much epinephrine, if you have heart disease or high blood pressure, or if you are taking prescription blood-pressure drugs that make you supersensitive to epinephrine.

In Chapter 5, I told you how to minimize the risk of an unexpected reaction between a prescription drug and your anesthetics. Best of all, have your *surgeon and your prescribing doctor talk to each other, so that each knows what the other is planning to give you.*

LOCAL ANESTHESIA WITH SEDATION

Operations in which local/sedation is usually used include:

- Facelift
- Upper- and lower-lid "tucks"
- Nose "jobs"
- Ear setbacks
- Breast *enlargement*
- Dermabrasion

- (Some) breast lifts
- (Most) chin and cheek implants
- (Some) armlifts
- Browlifts
- Eyeliner tattooing
- (Some) male breast reduction

Your surgeon may also call this a "local/general." It is a combination: local anesthesia and sedation. The pain of the surgery is stopped by local anesthesia. But your anxiety and your pain from the local anesthesia injections is blocked by sedation. The sedation also makes you relaxed, sleepy, less anxious, and more forgetful, so that a long operation passes quickly. The drugs that may be used to sedate you include narcotics, true sedatives, or barbiturates in combination with special-purpose drugs such as anti-nausea compounds.

Narcotics. Demerol (meperidine) and morphine are the two most common. Demerol is a man-made drug. Morphine is a poppy-derived drug. Their good and bad effects are similar. For surgery, they are given through an intravenous (IV) injection or by injection into a muscle (IM) such as the hip. They commonly cause nausea and vomiting, so a drug to stop nausea is usually given. Antihistamine-derived drugs and Compazine are the two most common anti-nausea drugs used.

Diazepam (Valium, etc.) and Related Drugs. These are true *sedatives*—they relax you. Unlike morphine and Demerol, they *don't* kill pain. Valium and Versid are the most commonly used. These drugs put some people to sleep. Other people can take *huge* doses of these drugs and get little sedation. The effective dosage tends to vary with your weight, your body fat/muscle ratio and your liver function—people who drink fairly heavily get rid of Valium as well as alcohol at high speed. (Variation can be extreme. I have had one patient sleep for hours after 10 milligrams of Valium, and another was wide awake after 100 milligrams!)

If you have had diazepam-type sedatives before, *tell your surgeon how you have reacted*, so he can judge how much you may need. These sedatives are usually given by intravenous injection or by mouth. Injections into muscle are painful and are no more effective than pills.

Barbiturates. These drugs, which you may think of as "sleeping pills," are also used as sedatives. The new ultra-short-acting barbiturates are increasingly popular. "Short-acting" pentothal (also used in general anesthesia) is used much less, because the diazepams are safer for local/sedation.

Sedative Hangover

All sedatives will leave you hung over. These drugs may get you comfortably through surgery and then take *days* to get out of your body. Do not expect to be wide awake after local/sedation anesthesia. I have had a very few patients who said they felt no effect after two days. You should plan on *five days* of gradually improving fuzziness in the head and *another five days* of residual fatigue. *Exception:* A low dose of sedation by mouth will leave most people hung over for only two days, at most.

Is Sedation Dangerous?

Of course it can be. All these sedatives make you breathe less deeply and less often. The goal of local/sedation is to have you awake enough to talk to your surgeon if he speaks to you, but relaxed enough so that you rest comfortably during surgery. Don't count on local/sedation to put you "out."

Typical Example of Local/Sedation

Lawrence was in his midtwenties when he decided to have me change the appearance of his humped nose and his protruding ears. I did this surgery on Lawrence as an outpatient in a surgery center.

On the day of his surgery, Lawrence checked in to the surgery center at 7:00 A.M., an hour before the operation. He had had nothing to eat or drink since midnight the night before.

He changed into a cotton gown, and his clothes were put in a locker.

Lawrence was then taken to a pre-op room. Here he lay on a stretcher and a nurse put an intravenous needle in his arm. His pulse and blood pressure were checked.

I instructed the nurse to give Lawrence a small dose of Demerol and an anti-emetic (anti-nausea drug) a half hour before his surgery. These were injected into his hip.

At 8:00 the nurse and I wheeled Lawrence into the operating room, and helped him onto the operating table. A "seat-belt" strap was placed across his hips.

Sticky pads were placed on his chest, and these were attached to the heart monitor. A pillow was put under his head and another under his knees, so that his neck and back were not stretched.

Next, I gave Lawrence a small test dose of Valium through the intravenous tubing, so there was no painful needle injection, to see how he reacted to the Valium. Within a minute Lawrence felt much less nervous but was otherwise awake.

I washed my hands and was assisted into my surgical gown and gloves by the scrub nurse, while the circulating nurse washed Lawrence's face with surgical soap.

The scrub nurse and I put surgical drapes around Lawrence and I covered his eyes, explaining step by step what I was doing.

Then the circulating nurse, under my directions and while I watched her, gave Lawrence more Valium, slowly, while I talked to him. Lawrence's speech became slurred. When he dozed but would still take a deep breath when I asked him to do so, the Valium was stopped.

During this phase of maximum sedation, I injected local anesthetic into Lawrence's ears. He slept through the injections.

I did the ear surgery. By the end of the ear surgery, Lawrence felt quite awake. I had the nurse give Lawrence additional Valium.

When he was sedated for the second time, I injected local anesthetic into his nose. He took a deep breath during the first few injections, in response to the pain of the injections.

I made the incision into the nose and worked on the soft tissues. Toward the end of the nose surgery, Lawrence was awake again. For the final step of the nose surgery—when I chiseled the bone—Lawrence was sedated with a final small dose of Valium to help him relax.

Lawrence was awake and talking by the time I taped the bandage on his nose.

In the recovery room, Lawrence slept for about 45 minutes. He woke up thirsty.

Lawrence said that he remembered all of his surgery. However, he remembered no pain *and* no needle injections. *In fact, all he remembered were snatches at the end of the ear surgery and again at the end of the nose surgery.*

He was not nauseated.

Two hours later Lawrence was not dizzy when he walked. His standing pulse and blood pressure were normal.

He was assisted to his car. His wife drove him home, where he went to bed, and slept on and off for the rest of the day.

He was very tired for two days. He felt groggy for another three days. He felt back to normal five days after that.

Teenagers: Beware of Local/Sedation

Local/sedation is unpredictable in teenagers. Some cosmetic surgeons insist that *all* of their teenage patients have general anesthesia. Most of us are not so rigid. We don't really know why, but some teenagers become *excited* when they are given sedation! I think people tend to become excited from sedation when they are very nervous, and most teenagers are more nervous about their surgery than adults. This excitement usually subsides in 15 to 20 minutes. But during that time, you may move wildly and have to be held onto the operating table. Such excitement reactions are very upsetting—while you have them and afterwards. If you are really afraid of the surgery, you should probably choose general anesthesia. If you aren't sure, sometimes talking about your anxiety with your surgeon will be all you need to feel reassured.

Who Remembers What After Local/Sedation?

About 30 percent of my patients *do not remember the injections* after surgery, but react to the pain—for instance, by breathing deeply.

About 35 percent of my patients *don't react to the injections at all*, and do not remember them.

About 15 percent of my patients *say that the injections hurt them while I am injecting, but afterwards do not remember pain, even if they remember the injection.* This may seem nonsensical. If you remember an injection from a needle, you ought to recall the pain. But sedation changes how you feel pain.

A very few patients have told me that they remember some pain but that nevertheless they preferred sedation to general anesthesia and would choose it again.

Where Is Most Local/Sedation Surgery Done?

Local/sedation is done anywhere that a surgeon has the help and the equipment to give intravenous drugs and to resuscitate you if something goes wrong. This could include:

- Hospital operating rooms
- Surgery center operating rooms
- Office operating rooms
- Cosmetic surgery clinics
- Hotel suites converted to cosmetic surgery clinics

To be safe, local/sedation needs more equipment and staff than local anesthesia does. It needs less than general anesthesia. It's safety lies in your being sedated but not so deeply asleep that you don't breathe properly. It's obvious that you need to breathe to live. This makes it equally obvious that any surgeon giving sedation must be prepared to use mechanical means to breathe for you in the rare event that your breathing stops from the sedation.

GENERAL ANESTHESIA

Operations in which general anesthesia is usually used include:

- Breast reduction
- Suction lipectomy
- Tummy tucks
- (Some) nose surgery
- Cosmetic surgery in little children, for example, ear setbacks
- (Some) breast lifts
- Any operation for which the patient—for medical *or* psychological reasons—shouldn't have local/sedation.

General anesthesia means "put to sleep." You remember nothing about the surgery *at all*. Hundreds of drugs are used for general anesthesia. The commonest groups are pentothal and other sedatives, gases, e.g., "laughing gas" (nitrous oxide), and curare.

Pentothal and Other Sedatives. These are used to begin your anesthesia. They do not keep you asleep but will be the last thing you remember.

"Laughing Gas" and Other Inhaled Gases. These keep you asleep. "Laughing gas" (nitrous oxide) is used together with morphine for some general anesthesia, but laughing gas alone won't keep you asleep. In most general anesthesia, you are given gases such as halothane, ethrane, and fluothane.

Curare and Other Muscle-Paralyzing Drugs. These are used if your surgery requires completely relaxed muscles and the gas you are breathing doesn't also relax your muscles. Muscle relaxants are *rarely* needed for cosmetic surgery.

Oxygen is given with all general anesthetics, of course! Since your face is covered by a mask to give you the anesthetic gas, you can't breathe in the oxygen from the air around you.

Is General Anesthesia Dangerous?

Of course it *can* be. Complications of general anesthesia in healthy patients having elective surgery (99 percent plus of cosmetic surgery patients) are extraordinarily rare. Serious complications are *less than one chance in 100,000*. People are at increased risk if they are severely overweight, have angina or other heart disease, and are extremely heavy (two packs a day or more) smokers, or have lung disease. General anesthesia can still be *safely* done, but it requires consultation before surgery with your internist and usually with an anesthesiologist to decide exactly how your anesthesia should be given.

Typical Example of General Anesthesia

Mandy, a teenager with greatly enlarged breasts, needed a breast reduction. This is always *done with general anesthesia. Mandy had her laboratory tests (a blood test and a urine test) the day before her surgery. She did* not *spend that night in the hospital but went home after the testing.*

Mandy had nothing to eat or drink after midnight.

She returned to the hospital at 6:30 A.M. to check in for her 8:00 A.M. surgery. She changed into a hospital cotton gown. Because she would stay in the hospital to recuperate, her valuables were given to her mother to take home.

She was taken to the preoperative area, and her laboratory test results were checked.

Mandy got on a stretcher, and I came in to check her. A nurse anesthetist interviewed Mandy and checked her heart and lungs, then placed an intravenous needle in Mandy's arm. She was given light sedation through the intravenous tubing.

Mandy was wheeled back into the operating room by the circulating nurse and the anesthetist.

I helped Mandy onto the operating table, from the stretcher. Sticky pads were placed on Mandy to monitor her heart. The anesthetist checked Mandy's blood pressure and pulse and called in the anesthesiologist for the beginning of anesthesia. (The difference between an anesthetist and an anesthesiologist is explained shortly.)

I held Mandy's hand while the anesthetist injected pentothal. In 30 seconds Mandy was asleep: her eyes were closed and did not flicker when her eyelashes were touched. (Some anesthetists will ask you to count backwards, say the alphabet, etc., to help them tell when you are asleep.)

The anesthetist put a tube down Mandy's throat to give her anesthetic gas and oxygen. A tube is necessary to secure oxygen flow to your lungs during long operations; short ones lasting 30 to 60 minutes can be done using only a mask over the mouth.

After the surgery was done, the nurse anesthetist removed the breathing tube. Mandy was moved, asleep, from the operating table to the stretcher and wheeled to the recovery room.

Mandy began to wake up in the recovery room 15 minutes later. When she woke up she felt cold and shivered. (This happened because anesthesia dilates your blood vessels and lets you lose body heat.) She spent one hour in the recovery room, and then was wheeled back to her hospital room.

Mandy felt nauseated about four hours later. She threw up once that afternoon and felt better. This was from the effects of the anesthesia. She had nothing to eat or drink that day but was given fluids through her intravenous tube.

Mandy was able to eat light food the next day. The intravenous needle was removed. She felt very tired and weak. The next day she felt stronger, although sore.

She had surgery on a Tuesday and went home on Friday, the third day after her surgery. The fatigue and grogginess took ten days *to go away.*

Mandy went back to school after two weeks. She still felt weary. She didn't have her usual energy for six weeks after the anesthesia.

WHO GIVES WHAT ANESTHESIA?

An *anesthesiologist* is a doctor specializing in anesthesia. He usually supervises one or more anesthetists. An *anesthetist* is a nurse trained in anesthesia.

Neither an anesthetist nor an anesthesiologist is needed to give straight local anesthesia.

An anesthetist or anesthesiologist always gives general anesthesia. In a hospital or clinic, an anesthetist is always supervised by an anesthesiologist. Depending on state law and local regulations, anesthetists may give general anesthesia and/or heavy sedation in a doctor's office.

Local/sedation is *usually* given by your *surgeon* and not an anesthetist. Local/sedation is so safe that an anesthetist is rarely needed. If an emergency arises, your surgeon must either manage alone or call in an anesthetist or anesthesiologist for help.

An anesthetist/anesthesiologist is a *must* with local/sedation if:

- You have a serious illness that makes anesthesia *extra risky*—for example, heart disease, lung malfunction, liver malfunction.
- The hospital where you are having surgery *requires* an anesthetist for your surgery. This is rare.
- You are having *major* cosmetic surgery in your surgeon's *office.* An office operating room is not staffed with extra help. An anesthetist is usually present in case an emergency arises.

- You are super-anxious and don't know if you can "take" local/ sedation. If the sedation does *not* work, the anesthetist can put you to sleep with general anesthesia while your surgeon continues to operate.

Anesthetists/Anesthesiologists Are Very Expensive!

Ideally, an anesthetist would be present whenever you get sedation, but most people can't pay the usually unnecessary $1,000 to $3,000 that an anesthetist or anesthesiologist will charge. The cost depends on the length of your surgery and where it is done. For instance, the charge for an anesthetist or anesthesiologist may be more at a major general hospital and less at an outpatient surgery center or cosmetic surgery clinic. Any cosmetic surgeon would prefer the luxury of an anesthetist giving the local/sedation. It would make it easier for us, but it is often neither practical nor necessary for your safety.

YOUR "KNOW-YOUR-ANESTHESIA" CHECKLIST

- Do you know what anesthesia you are having: local, local/sedation, general?
- If you've had a previous reaction to anesthesia, have you informed your surgeon?
- Do you know if you will go home after surgery or stay overnight?
- Do you have serious medical problems? If so, do you *know* that an anesthetist will be present?
- Where will your surgery be done? If it is the doctor's office, have you actually *looked at the operating room*? Do you know how it will be staffed for your operation?
- Do you know the cost of the operating room and anesthesia?
- Is your surgery strictly cosmetic? If not, check with your insurance company. *Most insurance will not pay for the cost of any nonaccredited operating room.*
- If worry about the pain of surgery is making you too anxious, don't panic. Your surgeon can prescribe a sedative dose for you for the night before the operation.

CHAPTER 7

The Three Phases of Healing

We have a dictum in cosmetic surgery: "The unhappiest person has the best result." You would think that if you have a complication, your result will disappoint you, and that if you heal properly, you'll be pleased. Not necessarily.

Jean had a breast enlargement. She developed internal scarring (a capsule) around her breast implants. Her breasts became round and firm —almost hard. Such capsules are a fairly common complication of breast enlargements. Often, exercise or massage will prevent them. Treatment varies—from "popping" the capsule in the office by putting pressure on the implant to replacing the implant. However, Jean was thrilled with her capsules and wouldn't hear of any treatment. *"They're like the way I looked and felt when I was pregnant. That was the happiest time of my life. I love it!"*

Daniel consulted me after another surgeon pinned back his protruding "Dumbo" ears. This operation is called an otoplasty. *Daniel told me, "It infuriates me that I spent all this money for such a poor result."*

I examined Daniel's ears—front, back, sides. His scars were perfect. His ear shape was perfect. His ears were nicely placed, close to his head but not squashed against the scalp. He had a great surgical result.

"I'm not quite sure what is bothering you," I said.

Daniel was amazed. "The tops of my ears stick out from my scalp more than the lower part. Can't you see?"

"Only a millimeter at most, and that's normal," I explained. I showed him my ears and pictures from textbooks. Daniel had a perfect surgical result, but it wasn't what he wanted. *He had been teased about his ears as a teenager. He wanted his ears squashed as flat against his head as possible. Daniel was too embarrassed to return to his first surgeon, so I agreed to re-operate to try to do this for him. I explained to Daniel that by re-operating, he ran a risk of having his ears stick out more, not less. The risk was worth it to him. At surgery, I overcorrected his ears so that they lay absolutely flat against his head. This squashed look is an undesirable complication of otoplasty. Daniel was thrilled. His ears were "right" at last.*

We would all like a perfect surgical result. But by "perfect" we usually don't mean that the surgery was done properly. It means that we look exactly the way we dreamed of looking. Most people are thrilled with their cosmetic surgery, because the result pleases them, even if it is different—sometimes better—than what they imagined. But to understand your result you need to understand your healing.

You may look terrible at first after surgery and end up with a perfect result. Or, you may look great, and, as the months go by and the swelling subsides, you may find that your result is poor or disappointing. This chapter tells you how to interpret your healing. It will show you:

- How to tell if your healing is on target
- How to deal with complications
- When and how to have "touch-up" surgery
- How to deal with your surgeon if he proves to be difficult

Healing has three phases: (1) an acute phase, the first two weeks after surgery, (2) a plateau phase, from weeks three to six, and (3) a scar remodeling phase, which lasts from week seven to forever. Each phase does something different to the way you look.

Acute-Phase Healing: The First Two Weeks

When your bandage comes off, you are probably prepared to look either "hideous" (swollen, bruised, repulsive) or "perfect"—an instant gorgeous result. *You won't see either.* You will look somewhere in between having a bad case of the flu (for facial surgery) and having been in a moderately bad car accident, escaping with minor injuries.

Surgery is controlled trauma. You won't look as though you've been assaulted with a hammer unless you had a serious complication (bleeding, infection). But you *will* look and feel injured. The area of your operation is sore, red, puffy, and numb for two weeks. You'll see daily improvement as the pain, soreness, swelling, and bruising subside. In the acute phase, it is almost impossible to tell how good (or bad) your final result will be, unless your surgeon put something in the wrong place.

Paula had a breast enlargement. When her surgeon took off her bandages, Paula could see that she was lopsided. Her left breast was fine. Her right breast was almost under her arm. Paula's surgeon assured her that the lopsidedness was a temporary result of swelling. Of course it was more than that. He had lost his bearings during the operation, and the pocket for the breast implant had ended up too far over on the side. This was not a disaster, but time alone wasn't going to fix it. Paula needed a touch-up operation to reshape the pocket and replace the implant. She knew it the moment that the bandages came off and probably her surgeon knew it too—he wasn't ready to admit it. However, one week later he and she agreed her right side wouldn't improve and needed some repair work. She had recovered enough from surgery and her initial disappointment to be ready to go ahead and have the correction surgery done.

On the rare occasion that you do look good when the bandages come off, don't rejoice too quickly. You *could* see your good result gradually fade away as the swelling subsides. Figures 7-1 through 7-3 illustrate this point.

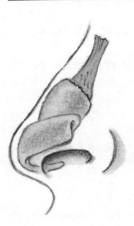

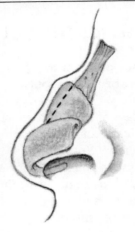

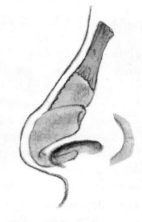

Figure 7-1.

Soon after nose surgery, swelling in the skin can conceal any irregularities along the top.

Figure 7-2.

With the swelling now gone, the irregularity (remaining bump) is clearly visible. (Dots show where surgeon must carve down excess.)

Figure 7-3.

The final result, after further surgery—even with the swelling gone, top of the nose is now smooth.

Bill had a nose operation. When his surgeon took the bandages off, Bill was thrilled. His nose looked perfect. Alas, a perfect nose five days after surgery is almost destined to be too small once the swelling is gone. (Swelling from nose surgery takes six to twelve months, or longer, to subside.) During the eighteen months after Bill's surgery, he gradually saw his new, final nose show itself to be tiny, sunken in at the top, and fat at the tip. Bill needed his nose re-done. In the meantime, Bill had moved. So, he came to me to have his nose redone.

What You Can Reasonably Expect When the Bandage Comes Off

The accompanying table lists some problems, the ultimate goal of surgery, the surgical method, and what you can expect to see during the acute phase of healing.

Table 1: Common Problems and Acute-Phase Appearance

Original Problem	Surgical Goal	Surgical Method	Acute-Phase Appearance
Eye bags	Bags gone	Fat out	Lids puffy
Tiny breasts	Breasts larger	Implants in	Big, swollen
Big breasts	Breasts smaller	Excess removed	Big, swollen
Nose hump	Hump gone	Bone out	Nose looks fat
"Dumbo" ears	Ears flat	Tissue cut	Ears red, puffy
Small chin	Chin larger	Implant in	Chin big, swollen
Fat neck	Neck thin	Fat out	Neck lumpy
Saggy lids	No sags	Sags tightened	Puffy, swollen
Bulgy thighs	Bulge gone	Fat out	Thighs swollen
Fat nose tip	Tip fat gone	Tissue out	Tip appears fat

As you can see, no matter what your surgery, there will be a major change in your anatomy, but it will be unshaped and too big. The "fat nose tip" listed in the "Problem" column is a perfect example of how swelling (edema) can hide your result. (Karl Malden's nose is a prime example of such a nose.) Here, the excess fat and cartilage in the tip of your nose are removed, but the swelling from the surgical trauma promptly fills up the space where the cartilage and fat used to be. Your nose doesn't look bad—it just doesn't look better. Your nose may feel softer, since swelling is not as hard as cartilage. Gradually, over six to twelve months, your "new" nose tip appears. However, no one but you and your surgeon will notice. After the first week or two, you can go out in public without feeling like a circus clown. You will *not* have "I have just had a nose job" written all over your face. These changes from swelling are *not* obvious—but what is virtually invisible to a friend can be very noticeable to *you*.

How to Handle an *Acute Phase* Problem

If something is obviously in the wrong place or is very painful or unusually swollen, it can be corrected in the acute healing phase.

Anything else usually waits. Here are some examples of serious problems that would require immediate attention:

- One breast looks to be in the wrong place.
- One side of your face doesn't move.
- Your ears *still stick out!*
- Your new chin is *under* your jaw.
- You *really hurt.*
- It's not merely puffy—there are *big lumps of swelling.*
- You have a fever above 100 degrees.
- What you see is getting *worse, not better.*

If any of these problems occur, call or see your surgeon. Explain and/or show him the problem.

What to Expect From Your Doctor

- That he listen to your questions and worries.
- That he (not just his nurse) examine you or arranges to do so.
- That he tell you what caused the problem.
- That he tell you what he plans to do about it.
- That he be totally honest with you.

Herbert called me a week after nose surgery. He had a horrible taste in his mouth. He couldn't breathe out of one side of his nose. He had a headache that was killing him. His nose throbbed on the side that was stopped up. I had seen him two days earlier and removed his nose packing. He was fine then. Herbert wanted to know—what is the problem? I didn't know.

What did I do? I asked him to come in to see me immediately.

What did I find? I had overlooked a fragment of packing in the back of his nose. It was causing an infection.

How did I treat the problem? I removed the packing and prescribed antibiotics for the infection.

What did I tell him? Exactly what I found and how it happened.

Should he have waited? No.

Did he get better? Yes. The horrible taste, the throbbing, and the trouble breathing improved right away. The headache was better within hours.

If your surgeon doesn't know what your problem is, expect him to say what the possibilities are and how he is going to find out and treat you. It's okay if he says "wait," so long as he can tell you why you and he are waiting and what he is looking for in the waiting period.

Diane had severe pain in both breasts after surgical breast enlargement. She had no fever, and her breasts were not swollen more than usual after surgery. I thought her pain was nerve pain, in which case it would get better by itself. It could have been an early sign of inside bleeding or a bad infection.

I would have expected abnormal swelling if she were bleeding inside. I would have expected redness and fever if she had an infection. We waited for twelve hours. She didn't get better or worse. We waited some more. Her pain began to go away and finally disappeared. But at first I didn't know it was nerve pain. I was prepared for it to be something worse.

Your surgeon should be able to tell you what bad things could be happening. He should be ready to detect a disaster, even if everything is probably fine.

When to Worry

You are sure there is something wrong, but your surgeon pats your hand, telling you that you're imagining it and not to worry. If you can see and feel a problem, either you are suffering hallucinations (unlikely) or *he should have some idea of what it is*. He should be able to tell you *why* what you see and feel is not worrying him. If he can't tell you that, he hasn't thought about your problem.

What to Do About It

If you think your surgeon is truly out of touch with your problem, you should make it clear that you are worried. Ask him to send you to someone for a second opinion, and if he won't, *go to another plastic surgeon for his opinion anyway*. You don't need permission.

If something is really wrong and you can't reach your doctor, or he won't listen, *go to an emergency room*.

Who Pays for It?

Your surgical fee includes all your surgeon's care for six weeks after surgery, except for fees if you need more surgery (more on this later, in Chapter 9). So, there is no charge if your surgeon treats you in his office. *You* pay for a second opinion from another surgeon. *You* pay for an emergency room visit.

Standard insurance will often (not always) reimburse you for an emergency room trip or hospital care for complications, such as bleeding or infection, that arise after cosmetic surgery (even if they won't pay for the cosmetic surgery itself). Prepaid health plans (HMO, PPO, IPO) won't pay for care by a nonmember physician but will usually treat you if you are a member and go to one of their enrolled doctors for care of the complication.

PLATEAU HEALING PHASE:
Weeks Three Through Six

In this four-week period, your improvement in appearance will seem to be stuck. You have recovered, in that your bruising, redness, and obvious swelling are gone. You think you are healed, and you're unhappy because you don't see day-to-day improvement. The surgery doesn't *feel* right, and your scars may get worse. They look thick and pink. You are convinced that something is wrong—but it's not. This is normal healing.

This is the phase when your body is depositing protein in the surgical area. To your body, this is like any other kind of wound. You plateau because your body is removing water and body fluid from the surgery area while it replaces them with a healing protein gel. Your body is working like crazy to heal: constantly putting in new protein, taking it out, rearranging it, waiting to see what will happen next. Your body doesn't know that the surgery wasn't an injury. It doesn't know that it was a onetime, intentional action. So your body is waiting to see if you are going to get "hurt" again.

Healing Has Its Own Priorities

This plateau phase of healing has its own inner time clock. For most people it is four weeks. It may be shorter or longer, depending on your physiology and general state of health. Some people know that they are fast or slow healers. I had one astonishing patient who had a breast enlargement and reached the *end* of her plateau phase in two weeks. I have had a few patients in whom the plateau lasted seven or eight weeks. This can be discouraging. If you've had surgery before, you may remember how your inner time clock is set. Regardless, *you can't speed it up.*

What controls your plateau? It's almost certainly hormones and chemicals released by your brain and nerves during healing.

Roger, on whom I performed a facelift, already had a permanent nerve injury to one side of his face, the result of internal brain hemorrhage twenty years earlier. On his nerve-injured side, the facelift scars took years to fade and flatten. On his normal side, the plateau ended after the usual month, and the facelift scars looked perfect six months after his surgery.

Stress Prolongs Your Plateau Phase

Even minor stresses can prolong the plateau a day, even a week. For example:

- A cold
- A minor blow to the operated area
- Too much exercise
- Overwork
- Too little sleep
- Anxiety or anger

Your surgical area will react to almost any real but usually insignificant stress with pain, aching, swelling, redness, and numbness all getting temporarily worse. The worse the stress, the greater your setback. What to do? First, do your best to avoid any stress in this plateau phase. Second, wait.

Overnight, It's Over!

Ninety percent of people notice that the end of their plateau phase comes *overnight*. You go to sleep with the same old puffy face, nose, or whatever that you've seen for the past month. You wake up in the morning and feel and see an improvement. You wonder if it's only imagination. It's not. For a few unlucky people, the plateau does not end overnight but draws to a close in tiny steps over a week or so. The change ends up being as great as, but it is less dramatic than, the overnight improvement.

Plateau Phase Problems

Many problems that arise during the plateau period have to do with unevenness of healing or the previously unnoticed asymmetry of all faces and bodies—including yours.

The Body "Split." You may notice that one side of your body will heal faster than the other. This makes sense. Our bodies are not symmetrical. Each of us has a *dominant side*. Usually our right hand and foot and the right side of our face are larger and better coordinated than the left. Your dominant side may heal faster, but you are unlikely to notice this except after breast and nose surgery. If your nose swelling subsides faster on one side, as it often does, your nose will look slightly crooked until the plateau phase of the other side ends. As for the breasts, most women notice that their dominant-side breast hurts less and feels normal days before the other breast.

Lopsided Complications. Many minor complications develop on only one side. For instance, an infection around a stitch may leave your left eye swollen and the right eye fine. A small blood clot below one ear after a facelift may leave that side of the neck swollen.

Such minor complications may lead to prolonged swelling because your tissues are inflamed. The extra swelling from a tiny complication may last up to 12 weeks after surgery—twice as long as your plateau phase would otherwise be. This swelling after a minor complication is rarely visible to anyone except you and your surgeon. Still, you will find it bothersome until it goes away.

The Mirage. Your body is asymmetrical, but you may never have noticed the details of your natural asymmetry until after your cosmetic surgery. Then, you may see features that you blame on your surgery but which you have had all your life. As a result, you think your plateau is lasting forever, when in fact it is long gone.

Tina consulted me for eye surgery. I took photographs during her consultation. Tina moved and had her eye surgery done in her new hometown. She returned to see me a year later, in distress. Two weeks after her eye surgery, once the swelling subsided, Tina saw that her left eyebrow was higher than the right one, her left eye was wider than the right eye, and her left lower lid sagged, compared with the right.

Tina was not imagining what she saw. Her surgery *could* have caused all three of these changes. I examined Tina and rephotographed her eyes to compare the new photos to the ones from a year earlier. To Tina's surprise, all these "new" features had been present before her surgery. All three features were unchanged. Her eyes had looked this way all her life. It wasn't a healing problem—she had never noticed the fine points of her face until she studied herself after surgery.

How to Handle the Plateau Phase

Wait. No matter how great your dissatisfaction, this is rarely a good time for your surgeon to re-operate on you. Why? Your problem may be from swelling, which will correct itself. If not, the swelling will make re-operation difficult, so that you are less likely to get a good result.

There is, however, one exception to this policy. Toward the end of the plateau phase, if a problem is evident and re-operation is inevitable, *and* there is a reason not to wait any longer, your surgeon may agree to, or even suggest, an early re-operation. For example:

As a resident I was taught that no plastic surgeon ever re-operated until six months after the first operation. One afternoon I was with a great plastic surgeon, now retired. Together, we went to see a patient of his from Iran, on whom he had done cosmetic nose surgery a month before. She said to him: "Doctor, my husband gave me the money for this surgery. I go back to Isfahan in ten days. The nose is not right. I understand about the swelling but my nose is still too big. I cannot go back to my husband with my nose too big."

The surgeon looked at her nose, listened, and said, "Surgery Monday. Bandage off Friday. Isfahan Tuesday." She asked, "You will make it perfect?" He replied, "Nothing is perfect. I will make it smaller."

I was shocked. Didn't he know he was supposed to wait six months before he re-operated? Finally I asked him about it. "It's simple," he explained. "Her nose is still too big. It's not all swelling. She'd get a better result if we waited, and if she lived here I'd tell her to wait. But do you want me to tell her to travel 10,000 miles next year to have an operation that I can do adequately now?"

I have no idea if this surgeon billed his patient for the second surgery. (Many cosmetic surgeons, including me, would not.) But it does point out the unpredictability of cosmetic surgery, even in the finest hands. Nose surgery is especially complicated. We operate largely by feel. The nose swells. It is disastrous to make a nose too small. This lady had a delicate nose. Too small a nose would have been catastrophic. Result—the tedium of a second operation to get the result that she and her surgeon wanted.

When to Worry About Plateau Phase Problems

Even when things go wrong, they are *rarely* urgent. For example,

- Your new enlarged breasts have numb patches but are also sensitive, so that you put on a bra gingerly.
- Your nose feels stuffy and forms hard crusts inside that feel sore.
- Your eyes tear easily and you can't wear contacts yet.
- Your facelift scars behind the ears are slow to heal.
- Your new smaller breasts have a patch in the crease underneath that is slow to heal.
- Your scars are itchy, lumpy, red.

Don't keep your worries to yourself. If your surgeon does not know about your problem already, call and have him check you. If he knows, but the complication seems to be getting worse, not better, call him to have him check you. And if he already knows and it's not worse, call to be checked in a week or so.

What to Expect From Your Doctor

- To be reassured when he looks as though he has seen this a million times before.
- That he or his nurse will care for the wound, if necessary.
- That he or his nurse will tell you how to care for the wound, if needed.
- That he should explain what's going on if you ask him.

Rosa was a heavy smoker. She had a facelift. Two weeks after her surgery, a quarter-sized patch of skin behind both ears had not healed. I told her that it would be at least another week, probably more, until it healed, and that healing would be much *faster if she stopped smoking.*

One week later Rosa called my office in a panic. She had looked in a mirror for the first time. "My face is infected! It's falling apart!"

Rosa came in to see me. Her wound was much better, but she had not seen it before. I explained that what she was seeing was what I meant by "not healed." Rosa was very relieved. "Oh, so that's what it looks like. Okay."

Rosa was not experienced in surgical healing. Neither are you. Your surgeon is. Ninety percent of plateau phase problems are part of normal healing or minor delays. They need only patience and office care. *Even an unpredicted, untreatable, uncontrollable plateau phase problem can still turn out fine,* needing only minor care.

Erica had cosmetic surgery, and, unknown to anyone, was allergic to the inside sutures. She could feel every inside stitch. They itched. From the second to the sixth week after her surgery, every stitch was expelled (spat out) by her body through the scars. A tiny white speck of stitch would appear in the scar. I would pull it out with forceps. No allergy medication helped. There was nothing to do but wait until her body rejected all the stitches, which it finally did.

When to Worry

- If you get steadily worse instead of better.
- If you are sure your surgeon is wrong. About 10 percent of the time, you and not your surgeon will know the cause of a plateau

phase problem and/or what to do about it. If he doesn't listen the first time you tell him, *keep on telling him what you think.*

Sometimes the doctor is right.

Carol had nose surgery. She was sure that I had removed too little bone from her nose and that her hump was still there. I was equally sure that I had removed enough bone and that the ridge on her nose was from swelling. Carol practically ground her teeth at me in frustration, because I didn't believe her. Suddenly, overnight, six weeks after surgery at the end of the "plateau," the ridge disappeared. I had been right after all— it was swelling!

Sometimes the patient is right.

Thea had suction lipectomy (fat suction) of her heavy hips. She hated the elastic garment I told her to wear after surgery. She wouldn't wear it. Her swelling would not go down. I was sure that the best solution was the elastic support tights. Thea was sure that the best answer was exercise. We negotiated a truce. I let her swim for 15 minutes for three days in a row. She agreed that if her swelling was not much better, she would wear the elastic tights. Thea was right. After three days of swimming, her swelling was almost gone.

SCAR REMODELING PHASE:
Week Seven to Forever

After six weeks, you are healed from your surgery. You don't need bandages. Your incisions won't fall apart if you pull. You can do anything you want without hurting your surgery. The surgery feels like part of you and you feel back to normal.

Your Body Never Stops Healing

But there is still *lots* for your body to do, especially for scars, nerves, and skin discoloration. After six weeks any skin discoloration that has occurred will only begin to fade. Bruised nerves may signal their recovery by tingling in areas that previously were numb from surgery.

Your scars will just begin to soften. They are still stiff or lumpy. Your skin may be irregular or ridged where scar protein (collagen) has been deposited below the skin. In this phase, your body will remodel skin and internal scar tissue. Scar protein, six weeks after surgery, looks under the microscope like a jumbled, tangled heap of spaghetti (Figure 7-4). Your body will proceed to line up the scar protein fibers, removing some and rearranging some until over the months the "spaghetti jumble" evolves into fewer, thinner, straight protein fibers lying side by side, all going in the same direction (Figure 7-5).

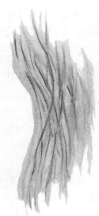

Figure 7-4.

Six weeks after surgery, scar tissue seen under a microscope looks like tangled spaghetti.

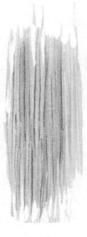

Figure 7-5.

Over time, the protein fibers that form the scar tissue arrange themselves more neatly.

This scar rearrangement and improvement will go on for the rest of your life.

A plateau pattern occurs during this lifelong remodeling. You may see or feel a sudden improvement in a scar about every three months. *After six to twelve months, remodeling is 70 percent complete.* Re-operation now, if you need it, is reasonable. But there is no end to your healing. You can still have surprises—both good and bad—long after you think you have healed.

Terry had low thyroid function, which was treated. She also had a patch of knee numbness from a bruised leg nerve. Her feeling returned suddenly seven years later. Although her low thyroid may have explained a small delay in healing, it couldn't explain seven years of it! Her injured nerve took all that time to heal.

How to Handle the Scar Remodeling Phase

If you need a retouching operation, or a major re-operation, it can now be done during this phase, at about six months. If you aren't sure what to do, don't worry. This phase lasts for the rest of your life. You lose nothing by waiting until you see clearly what the right decision will be for you.

If your result bothers you a lot, six months after surgery may have been a long time to live with it. Your re-operation can proceed.

If you feel "iffy"—you like the result but a little more time might turn "good" into "perfect"—it might be better to wait.

Healing from surgery is stressful. The rare disasters tend to occur within the first two weeks. If you survive them, then you need patience to wait for your result to appear.

Once the plateau phase of healing is over (about six weeks after surgery), and you can see that the swelling *will* go down and you *will* improve, you are over the worst. Some snags lie ahead, but you are usually happy that your operation is over, happy that you had it, happy not to have to return to your surgeon for six months or so. Your result may be so good that it's goodbye to the cosmetic surgeon, until you decide to have more surgery!

Even if something major or minor has left you less than happy, time and/or another operation (usually minor) should set things right within a year. Then, if you still aren't pleased, the next chapter tells you what to do.

CHAPTER   8

Your Final Result: Good, Great, or Poor?

After your cosmetic surgery is completely healed, you might feel that something could be improved, and that your final result is disappointing. Such a "not right" result could be as (relatively) minor as a scar that won't lie flat, or as important as trouble breathing after cosmetic nose surgery. Regardless of how "insignificant" your dissatisfaction may be, you can be in anguish.

HOW SERIOUS ARE THE FLAWS?

Surgery is not guaranteed. Your result is not mass-produced like a car rolling off an assembly line. Your result is more akin to the work of an artist—and everyone knows that even the great Monet painted some pictures that are better than others. He didn't—and couldn't—guarantee a patron a great work of art. Your surgeon cannot guarantee your result, either. Assuming that you understand this, the question remains: *How do you judge your result, and what should you do about it, if you are not satisfied?*

Minor Flaws

These include minor problems that are easy to fix or honestly not noticeable. Often my super-critical eye will see a minor flaw that is invisible to my patient. For example:

- A breast reduction scar is slightly ruffled.
- A nose is a *millimeter* too long.
- A tiny bulge of fat shows in one lower lid.
- A hair punch graft is a shade out of place.

Minor flaws are common, and almost all are easy to correct with minor office surgery. If a minor flaw can't be fixed, it can be psychologically accepted. An example of a problem that can't be fixed is a hair transplant that is slightly out of place. By removing the graft and shifting it to a better position, you may leave an obvious scar behind, which may be worse than the slightly out-of-place graft. Or, a residual bulge of fat in your lower lid may be uncorrectable because your eyelid muscle is too weak to hold in the fat in that area. These are minor problems. You may not like them, but when no one else notices, after a while you will stop seeing them, too.

Moderate Flaws

Moderate problems are readily noticeable to you and your surgeon, though others may not see them. (You will be surprised by how much other people don't notice.) They are more complicated to correct. The corrective surgery may require sedation. Further surgery may only improve, not fully correct the problem. For instance:

- A fatty bulge in the middle of your neck after a facelift
- A navel too small after a tummy tuck
- One breast implant a half-inch lower, even an inch, compared with the other side
- One hip with a residual bulge after fat suction

These problems rank as *complications*, minor to moderate. Even though the result could devastate you, most people look so much better after cosmetic surgery that they are still pleased. Often, the bother of further surgery to correct such flaws may not seem worthwhile.

Major Flaws

Now we're discussing serious problems. The surgery may need to be redone completely. In some cases, you might even decide that the surgery made you worse, not better, and you clench your fists saying, "If only I had known!"

- Your ears stick out, just as they did before.
- Your neck is sagging, badly.
- Your nose is tiny and crooked, and you have trouble breathing through it.
- One upper lid droops badly.
- Your scar(s) are red and lumpy, itch, and look terrible, a year after surgery.

Such results are *usually* from unavoidable complications—bleeding, infection, severe swelling or poor healing. They may also be the result of an inappropriate technique. They are always unsightly and virtually always warrant further surgery. Depending on exactly what the problem is, you may need to wait six months to have it corrected, or you may benefit from earlier re-operation.

Really Bad Complications

The *rarest* of cosmetic surgery flaws are such problems as:

- Massive infection or bleeding requiring hospitalization and antibiotics, transfusions, or both
- Massive loss of skin requiring extensive skin grafting
- Extensive nerve damage requiring microsurgery and nerve grafting

These kinds of complications are usually apparent immediately after, or shortly after, your surgery and often require intensive treatment and/or one or more major operations. Even so, your end result is likely to be disappointing. Such severe complications may be more likely to occur in the hands of a careless surgeon *but by no means always.* An utterly unforeseen infection or a nerve lying in an abnormal position can cause a disaster no matter how skilled the surgeon is.

Putting Flaws Into Proportion

As a rule, the minor flaws are an inevitable part of healing. The "moderates" may result from a fine surgical judgment that was short of perfection or a problem such as a tendency to bleed that is no one's fault, but part of the way you heal. The "majors" tend to be either a rare, unforeseen complication, result from an oversight or a misjudgment, or reflect a previously undetected problem in your body. For example, a serious allergy to a drug you are given can cause a terrible rash and resultant infection that neither you nor your surgeon could have known about in advance. The really major problems may be a "bolt-from-the-blue" complication, perhaps even the first of its kind, or they may be caused by a careless judgment.

UNDERSTANDING YOUR OPTIONS

What are you going to do? Do you suffer? Does your surgeon have to try to fix it for you? There is no right or wrong. Much depends on your surgeon's policy and personality. These are the possibilities:

- Your surgeon re-operates without charge.
- Your surgeon re-operates and charges you a full fee.
- Your surgeon has a flexible "No Policy" Policy. He charges you a full fee, unless you and he agree that for some reason he ought not to charge you.

Let's take these possibilities one at a time.

Your Surgeon Re-operates for Free

A lot of surgeons, including myself, take pride in having patients with good psychological as well as surgical results. We want our patients happy. If I think I can make a scar better . . . if just trying will help satisfy you that it's your best result . . . if it bothers you enough to make more surgery tolerable . . . and if it can be done in an office operating room, within a year after surgery, then I don't ask my patients to pay. Ninety percent of all problems, including minor, moderate, and some major flaws, can be handled in this manner.

If your insurance will pay for the corrective surgery, your insurance is billed. If you need more than minor surgery—for example, if the "neck part" of your facelift must be re-done—then you still don't pay the surgeon, but you *will* pay for the cost of the operating room and/or a new implant, if needed.

I understand that this may seem unfair to you. Why should you pay anything at all, if it wasn't done right? I can only repeat: *Surgery comes with no guarantee.* Even a severe complication is part of the risk of surgery. Re-operating without charging you a surgical fee is the surgeon's effort to help you without subsidizing your surgery—which would be impractical.

This policy *can* at times pose a problem for the surgeon. A few patients will inevitably demand, as a "right," free treatment to which they aren't entitled. For instance, I had one patient on whom I did a breast enlargement. When it didn't lift her breasts (I had warned her that it wouldn't), she demanded that I do a breast lift for free. I explained why I would not do this: Her surgical result was fine. She had decided against a breast lift because of the scars involved. It had been *her* decision to have a breast enlargement, knowing its limited result for her. Unpleasant encounters with more than a few such patients could make a surgeon stop doing anything for free!

Your Surgeon Re-operates and Charges You the Full Fee

Many cosmetic surgeons charge for any re-operation. Their reasoning is that cosmetic surgery is a luxury. No one promised perfection. It's not funded by the government, and it's not funded by cosmetic surgeons. You got the best your surgeon could give. If you don't like the result and want more surgery, you pay for it.

You may not think this is fair, but it is certainly clear, simple and understandable. Unfortunately, a policy such as this makes it impossible for your surgeon to re-operate for free—even if you have a problem he would like to take care of that way. If his *policy* is to charge for all of his surgery, then when he makes an exception, it could be argued on legal grounds that he had thereby admitted that he was negligent—whether or not he actually was. If this is your surgeon's policy, you and he may be obliged to abide by it, so it helps to ask *before* your surgery about what might happen.

Your Surgeon Has a "No Policy" Policy

Surgeons with this policy mean well and want to stay flexible for their patients. They take the stand that if you really have a complication, they will fix it without charge. But they will charge you if they feel you ought to be satisfied, but are just a complainer. Needless to say, this policy can lead to ill feeling and arguments between you and your surgeon as to whether a fold of skin or a scar cyst is a complaint or a complication. Your surgeon may label you a perfectionist complainer; you may label your surgeon totally unreasonable. It would drive me frantic to have this kind of "no policy" policy. Some surgeons manage it well. If this is your surgeon's policy, *it's up to you and him to come to an agreement. Clarify ahead of time, exactly what he considers to be a complication and what he is prepared to re-do for free.*

Keep Cool As Long As You Can

What if your doctor insists on charging you, and you are convinced that you should not pay? Try to stay calm and reach a friendly agreement. It's unlikely that he will change his mind once you both get angry. Ask him to go over with you, step by step, what he said, and what you understood him to say, during the original consultation(s). He may realize he unintentionally misled you to expect a certain outcome, and therefore may now agree not to charge you for minor additional surgery. If your finances make the additional surgery unaffordable, explain your dilemma. Try to show him that you would pay if you could, but you can't.

If after exhausting every reasonable means of discussion, you cannot come to a mutual agreement with your doctor, you may feel that you want to sue him, to get even. For most problems, finding yourself another surgeon—and paying for a re-operation—may be infinitely better for *you*. (More about the pitfalls of lawsuits later in this chapter.)

What You Will Never Get

You will not find a surgeon who re-operates, for free, on another surgeon's poor result. For instance, if you had cheek implants put in that were much too big, you would want them changed. Your surgeon might offer to re-operate without charging you. But since you think he erred the first time, you don't trust him to re-operate. Yet, you don't have the money to pay a new surgeon.

You have to decide whether to take the risk of having it done for free, to find the money for a new surgeon, or to live with the poor result.

DISAPPOINTMENT, COMPLICATION, OR MALPRACTICE?

You should have some idea of where your disappointing result lies on the spectrum of dissatisfaction. At one end is the small "ugly" scar, the result of poor healing, that will improve with time. At the other end would be extensive facial scarring and nerve damage after a disastrous facelift. You will react emotionally to any poor result. You can help yourself to determine where you stand, objectively, with these three steps:

1. Get a second or third opinion.
2. Wait six months.
3. Try to be fair.

Get a Second Opinion

Have another cosmetic surgeon examine you and advise you whether or not you were properly treated and what to expect. Be wary if this doctor is too ready to condemn your surgeon. Personal animosity or professional jealousy may be at work. Also, be wary if he is too prompt in defending your surgeon. He may want to protect a colleague, and so be less than open with you. To avoid this, you might seek your second opinion from a well-qualified surgeon out of your community, perhaps in the next nearest city.

Wait Six Months

Give yourself six months at least, from the date of your surgery, before judging your result. It may take as long as a year. Your disappointment may fade when time corrects the problem. You could find yourself in the embarrassing position of having complained vigorously about a bad result that disappeared.

A model had a facelift. She didn't like her scars. She did not work for six months to deliberately establish a record of "loss of employment" to bolster her malpractice lawsuit. When her case came near to trial a year later, her lawyer asked me to examine her. She had looked terrible to him a year ago, but now she looked fine. I examined her. Her scars had faded and blended. Her swelling was gone—and so was her claim of malpractice.

Try to Be Fair

Studies show that you remember about 20 percent of what your surgeon tells you before surgery. This is not surprising. Your surgeon knows it all, but it's new to you. If you had a class in biology in school or college, and tried to remember the details six months later, it wouldn't be crystal clear in your mind. The same is true of your surgical consultation.

The studies also show that we tend to forget the unpleasant aspect of a consultation—the talk about complications. A good surgeon will have discussed with you many common (usually minor) and serious (usually rare) complications. He will never guarantee a result, any more than a lawyer guarantees the outcome of a lawsuit.

Before you decide it is your surgeon's fault, try to be sure if your result is consistent with what he told you might happen.

In general, bad scars, swelling, and less-than-hoped-for results are not complications, but individual variations of healing. Bleeding, infection, and slow healing are complications, but they are *largely unavoidable*. A poorly executed, even wrong operation, done by an unqualified, incompetent surgeon and leaving you with extensive permanent damage, is undeniable negligence.

KNOWING WHEN TO SUE

It is my (very biased) opinion that the pain and suffering that you bring on yourself with a lawsuit are worse than virtually all surgical complications. So from a purely selfish point of view, I would not file a lawsuit unless I were forced to do it. I've seen too many people who ought to win lose—and vice versa.

At the same time, you might consider a lawsuit to draw attention to an irresponsible surgeon. Or your result may be so devastating in itself that you feel you have to sue, even though you may know or suspect that it wasn't your surgeon's fault.

A patient had surgery for baggy lower lids. Six hours after the surgery, she developed unexpected internal bleeding around her retinal nerve. As a result, her vision was permanently damaged, despite immediate and proper care.

As a doctor, I know that the damage to her vision could not have been either predicted or prevented. It is one of the extraordinarily rare risks of such surgery. But if I were sitting on a jury, even if I knew the doctor was not at fault, I might award damages to help the injured patient, financially. So might you.

This is an example of a devastating complication that was no one's fault.

Strict Liability in Malpractice

The legal doctrine of strict liability means that fault is irrelevant. Only your result is what is considered in the case. The law has trends. The trend in medical malpractice is toward *strict liability*: Your damage, not the doctor's care, is the issue. Nevertheless, most malpractice still depends on whether or not your doctor was negligent. My personal opinion is that we need a national insurance that you can take out to protect yourself against the unavoidable hazards of surgery, including elective cosmetic surgery. If you don't want a bad scar (who does?) and you get one, the insurance would reimburse you a set amount. Then, malpractice could do the job it was meant to do—to control negligent, irresponsible doctors.

In the meantime, if your problem can't or won't be resolved between you and your surgeon, should you sue? These are three instances of patients who did, and did not, sue and why.

Gregory was someone who should have sued but didn't. While performing surgery on his stomach, Gregory's surgeon left a large metal instrument in his abdomen! This caused Gregory to undergo three more operations to remove the instrument and treat the scarring and infection it caused. Gregory knew his surgeon had made a mistake and yet, he did not sue.

Ridiculous? You might think so. Gregory didn't. He had been involved in a major lawsuit before and had seen a person whom he knew was in the right lose the case. Between his insurance and his surgeon's not billing him, Gregory was not ruined financially. He didn't want to hassle himself with a lawsuit. He didn't have the time (five years), the money ($10,000), or the interest (he hated fights) and he genuinely liked his doctor who, having admitted his mistake, took care of all of Gregory's complications with sincere dedication. He wanted to forget all about it and get on with his life.

This is not a one-of-a-kind instance. I have seen many patients make similar decisions.

Albert was a patient who sued, but had no case. He had a leg mole that might have been cancerous, so his surgeon removed the mole with a lot of surrounding normal tissue, in case it proved to be a cancer. It was not cancer. Albert didn't like the leg scar. He sued for his anxiety, when he thought he might have cancer, and for the ugly scar. Two years and ten thousand dollars later, Albert lost his case.

Why had he sued? He thought his surgeon was cold, callous, uncaring. Albert had plenty of money, and he felt that the $10,000 he had spent hassling his surgeon had been worth it, for the satisfaction of giving him "a hard time."

(This kind of conduct can be risky. A few surgeons have successfully countersued people who sued them without adequate cause.)

As for a patient who rightfully sued and won—Lucy had a breast lump and no family history of cancer. A plastic surgeon removed the tissue from both her breasts (an operation called a subcutaneous mastectomy) and reconstructed her breasts. The patient had various complications, including one implant that ended up far out of position, with a very hard capsule. She also had chronic shoulder pain from damage to a nerve during surgery. She contended that she should not have had the surgery and that her doctor had intentionally misled her about what to expect. He contended that based on his exam and what she had told him, the operation was warranted and her poor result unavoidable. She sued and she won. The surgeon appealed the decision. Since appeals take one or more years to be heard, and the decision can lead to an entirely new trial, she settled with the surgeon's insurance company rather than fight the appeal.

Lawsuits are easy to file and hard to win. If you believe you have no recourse except a lawsuit, there are certain things you should know before you begin.

Don't Sue When You Are Angry

You probably will, anyhow. You may feel that you have been so mistreated that you ought to be angry and that you must sue. But, when you are angry you tend not to think clearly. Your lawsuit will be a claim for money, and in filing the suit you are putting your own money at risk. Decide right away if your chief reason is anger. If so, try to make peace with your surgeon or at least wait to file your suit until the heat of your anger is past. Even if this takes months, the statute of limitations (the time past which you can't sue) is long enough to let you wait a while. *A lawsuit is a business decision: it is a two- to five-year investment of your time, and ten to fifty thousand dollars of your money,* on the possibility that you might win enough to justify your loss of time and reimburse you for your loss of money. Keep a cool head for this decision.

Know How to Resolve Your Anger With Your Surgeon

I think that the best way to resolve your anger is to go to your surgeon and tell him that you are upset with the way he is treating you. Tell him that you don't think he cares. Tell him why. Or, if you can't bring yourself to do that, go to another cosmetic surgeon for a second opinion. See if he can explain your result to you. Ask him to contact your surgeon to let him know how you feel and to help you settle your differences. If your surgery was done by a reputable plastic surgeon, he almost certainly wanted to help you. Besides, we are more aware of your psychological needs than most surgeons, because cosmetic surgery affects you psychologically. Nevertheless, surgeons are human. There is a human tendency for a surgeon to get angry with you if he thinks you are angry with him. Sometimes a surgeon knows that things didn't turn out the way you wanted, expects you to be angry, and gets angry with you before you get angry with him. You don't have to like him for this. It is in your interest to resolve your anger and his, if your other choice is to risk hurting yourself with a lawsuit merely to get even with him.

Be Prepared for Your Surgeon's Response to the Threat of a Lawsuit

An exceptionally decent, honest, and kind plastic surgeon can see your point of view when you are upset and can admit a mistake.

Dr. Jones, a colleague of mine, had a patient who was angry with her result and wanted to sue. He explained to her why her surgery had turned out so poorly, despite the best he could do. He then said: "But I understand why you are upset. My only concern is that you go to a good lawyer. There are a lot of lawyers who either don't know the malpractice field, or who are going to take advantage of you."

Few surgeons have the confidence to be so forthright. If your surgeon is this straightforward with you, you can be sure that he is good, because he has the ability to admit a mistake and cares enough about you not to hide it from you. You can't *expect* this to happen, but you should know that Dr. Jones exists and is your ideal standard of reference to judge how your surgeon treats you when a problem occurs.

A more typical reaction would be for your surgeon to be angry and/or upset with you. Regardless of whether you or he are "in the right" your best approach is to explain your dissatisfaction and your intention of filing a lawsuit. He should listen to you. You should listen to his reply. Then your conversation is best ended. If you start to argue with him it is unlikely to be helpful. It will probably make you both even more upset. Your surgeon may contact you a day or a week later, when he has thought over your complaint, with a suggestion as to how he can help you. But you can't expect him to be supportive of you right after you explain that you may sue him. Your surgeon's dismay at such a time is just as human as your dismay with your result.

Most Lawyers Don't Like Cosmetic Lawsuits

Believe it or not, there are relatively few lawsuits stemming from cosmetic surgery. Most people heal well and are delighted with the results. Complications are rarely severe or uncorrectable. But even if you have a valid case, a malpractice lawyer may be reluctant to file suit for you. The legal reasoning goes like this:

1. You had cosmetic surgery because you didn't like the way you looked.
2. You disliked your looks enough to have surgery.
3. The surgery came with no guarantee.
4. You still don't like the way you look.
5. So, why blame the surgeon? You are no worse off than when you started.

You think it obvious that you are much worse off: You spent time and money on the surgery, you had the mental strain of the recovery and the disappointment of failure. The law may not see it your way. First you have to show your present physical and mental damage. Next, you usually have to show that the doctor was at fault. Only then can the jury consider loss of income and medical bills as a basis for how much money to award you. Anxiety and worry don't count unless you can show how it harmed you—and it's hard to show that kind of harm.

Know How to Choose a Good Lawyer

Do you know how to find a lawyer who is right for you? Here are some questions to ask yourself:

Is your lawyer a member of the Association of Trial Lawyers? Many lawyers never go to court. A malpractice suit requires a *litigation lawyer*. Your local Trial Lawyers association will confirm your lawyer's membership.

The address of the Association of Trial Lawyers of America is 1050 31st Street, N.W., Washington, DC 20007. The phone number is (202) 965-3500. They may confirm that your lawyer is a member of their association. Also, they may refer you to a "big name" outside of your area, if that is what you think you need.

Has your lawyer been a public prosecutor? Most trial lawyers get their basic training as prosecutors for city, county, state, or federal government. A litigation lawyer without experience as a prosecutor ought to have some other important litigation experience, such as extensive experience in a litigation firm working as an associate with seasoned trial lawyers.

What is your lawyer's reputation? A publicity-hungry trial lawyer is unlikely to serve you well unless you have lots of money and/or a high-profile, publicity-worthy case. Even then his need for publicity may outweigh his dedication to you. However, a successful litigator may be mentioned in the newspaper when he wins a case. Ask your lawyer about his experience in winning cases. If you have the opportunity, go to the courtroom and see how he fares.

Make Sure You Have All the Facts

If you made such a poor choice of a doctor that you are now suing him, be extra careful in choosing your lawyer. Thousands of new lawyers are graduated from law school every year. They don't come with board certification in medical malpractice—there is no such thing. You need to ask, or be told about:

- Your lawyer's credentials
- Cost
- Time
- How to fight, and chances of winning
- Trial preparation

Lawsuits Are Expensive. Most lawyers take malpractice cases "on contingency." This means that they do not charge you by the hour. Instead, they take a percentage of the settlement awarded to you by the jury—if any. This percentage is usually 25 to 30 percent. The highest I have heard is 50 percent.

You still pay for expenses, which include travel for your lawyer, copying and messenger fees, cost of court reporters for depositions, and cost of transcripts and expert witnesses. Depending on the complexity of your lawsuit, expenses may total from $5,000 to $50,000 that *you* pay, win or lose. Ask your lawyer to estimate your costs. To be safe, double the estimate! Lawsuits tend to be more, not less, difficult than expected.

Lawsuits Take Time. If you want to win a lawsuit, you can't leave it to your lawyer. He didn't have the operation. He doesn't have your knowledge of what was said and done. You have to be prepared to spend hours and days for one to three years in depositions, reading medical records, thinking of and tracking down information and witnesses to help your case.

This time is taken from your job, your family, and your rest. You will lose sleep, perhaps even a job, a spouse or a friend. You could gain an ulcer or a therapist. It may all be justified by the damage you have suffered and the likelihood that you will win. However, if a lawyer tells you that you "have an easy case," you "won't need to get involved," or that he'll "take care of it all," then he is either woefully inexperienced or misleading you (probably unintentionally in an attempt to reassure you). Nevertheless, don't be misled. *Winning a lawsuit is hard work for you and your lawyer.*

Lawsuits Are Warfare. To win a lawsuit, you must fight. If you don't like to fight, you will probably regret intensely that you ever sued. A lawsuit is not a matter of data weighed dispassionately for justice. Your lawyer will attack your doctor. Your doctor—through his lawyer—will attack you. There is no middle ground.

The law talks a lot about "amicable" relationships between lawyers and the litigants (you and your doctor). This is like saying that professional football is amicable compared to mayhem between barbarians. It is still a fight. Feelings run high. There is a saying about the prosecution of criminals for rape: "First the victim is raped by the criminal, then by the courts." This statement, albeit extreme, represents the feelings of many people who have been in court, knowing that they are right, only to find that *our legal system rewards the person who wins the fight, not the person in the right.*

Ideally, you should be in the right *and* win. But if you are not a fighter, unless you have an extraordinarily winnable case and/or an experienced fighting lawyer, stay out of the courtroom. You are likely to get hurt again.

Preparation Wins a Case. If your lawyer does not prepare, you are unlikely to win. The first things a trial lawyer will almost certainly do is to organize your case into a trial notebook and to start summarizing all the evidence *for use at the trial.* He will prepare you and your witnesses carefully. He will learn all he can about your operation.

An unprepared or sloppy lawyer who is confident of winning is like a coach telling you it's okay to be out of shape for the game: sheer foolishness.

YOUR "SHOULD-I-SUE?" QUESTIONNAIRE

If you answer "no" to any of the following questions, you should definitely rethink your intention to sue.

- Are you damaged?
- Is the damage permanent and visible?
- Is your damage the result of negligence, or so incapacitating as to make negligence irrelevant?
- Are you sure you are not suing on a burst of anger, and that it is the right business decision for you?
- Do you have twice the money your lawyer says you will need for expenses?
- Are you a fighter by nature?
- Is your lawyer a seasoned litigator and fighter?
- Are you prepared to be in the right and still lose, even though you hope it won't turn out that way?

It is your legal right to sue anyone for anything, whether or not a judge throws out your case, a jury finds against you, or you get countersued. It may be easier, cheaper, and less painful to have time or another surgeon put you to rights, rather than resorting to legal warfare.

At the same time, if you have been dreadfully harmed by a negligent and incompetent doctor who took advantage of you, you are entitled to seek compensation. Most doctors, even though we loathe the present malpractice system, would sympathize. Fortunately, it is a rare cosmetic patient whose situation is so extreme!

CHAPTER 9

To Cancel or Not to Cancel:
Second Thoughts and Financial Worries

ARE YOU HAVING SECOND THOUGHTS?

Most people aren't really hesitant about cosmetic surgery, once they've made the decision to have it done. Still, you can find yourself in an awkward situation if you're having second thoughts. There are a lot of good reasons to have cosmetic surgery. There are a few reasons to postpone or cancel surgery. The reasons vary from deciding that you are actually comfortable with the physical flaw, to deciding that you aren't financially able to pay for surgery. Here, I'll discuss the six most usual causes of hesitation and how you should assess them.

Hesitation Cause #1: Indecision

My most indecisive patient was Kate. She had already had a breast enlargement when she came to see me. She wasn't sure, but she thought the surgeon had made her too big. She was a full B cup. I thought her size was right. She was not sure she agreed with me.

"I can remove your implants," I offered.

"Then I might be too small," Kate replied anxiously.

133

"Or I could take out your implants and replace them with smaller ones," I said.

"Then I might be too big." Kate hesitated. "Will you decide for me and promise that I'll be happy with the result?"

I shook my head. "I can't. I can help you decide what is right, but this is your body. You should make the final decision. I can't promise how you will feel about it."

Kate got quite annoyed. She insisted that she didn't make decisions. "I can't," she protested. "I'm like that."

At last Kate decided to have the implants replaced with smaller ones. But the next day she couldn't decide if the decision was right. I did make a decision then—to do no surgery. Kate's surgical result was fine. She was such an anxious person that she couldn't cope with *any* decision, before or after she made it! Having another operation would only give her more decisions to worry her. *Moral:* If you can't decide about surgery, the message to yourself is "Don't do it!"

Hesitation Cause #2: Guilt

Almost 100 percent of cosmetic surgery patients feel guilt at some point—guilt about spending the money on something that makes them feel vain or extravagant. Guilt is not a good reason to hesitate over cosmetic surgery. If the surgery is going to *help* you, there is no place for guilt.

Hesitation Cause #3: Embarrassment

Again, almost 100 percent of people hesitate at some point because the thought of having the surgery makes them feel awkward or embarrassed. It is reasonable to feel this way. Surgery is private. Discretion is all you need to avoid further feelings of embarrassment. In Chapter 10 you can read more about whom to tell and how to parry nosy questions.

Hesitation Cause #4: Timing

Timing can be an excellent reason to hesitate over your surgery. Cosmetic surgery can be scheduled around time-gaps in your life: vacations, sick leave, in between school or job changes, or just before or after you move. No time? Surgery can't be squeezed in when there is *no* time.

Hesitation Cause #5: Pride

Let us say that you have a physical flaw that you *know* could be improved by cosmetic surgery. But you have a reason to take pride in the way your "flaw" looks. This can be a fine reason *not* to have the surgery.

Paula, a mother of five children, wanted her baggy eyes "done," but she wanted to be sure that I would leave her wrinkles *alone. She said, "I earned every line in my face from raising my children. My kids and my wrinkles mean a lot to me."*

Joan was 14 and had a scar on her face from an injury from playing basketball on her school team. Joan's mother brought her in to see me and wanted the scar "fixed." Joan's scar reminded her of how she helped win the school championship. She loved her scar and wanted it left alone. I agreed with her. It wouldn't help Joan to change her scar.

Hesitation Cause #6: Money

A compelling reason to hesitate over surgery is if you can't afford to pay for it. "Afford" can be a complex decision.

Ellen was a teenager who had decided to have a cosmetic chin implant and cosmetic nose surgery during the spring break of her senior year in high school. Although she had applied to an expensive private college, she didn't expect to get in. Psychologically and financially she was set for her local community college.

Between the time of her consultation and her surgery, Ellen—much to her surprise—was accepted by her first choice, the private college. Thrilled? Actually, she felt torn. She thought she was obliged to have her cosmetic nose surgery, but she needed the money for college tuition.

Ellen's choices were:

- To go ahead with surgery and not go to the expensive private college.
- To just not pay for the surgery and place the responsibility of what to do in my hands.
- To call my office, explain, and cancel surgery.

Ellen felt trapped. Her mother called me at home to see how much I would "mind" Ellen's canceling her surgery. There was obviously *one right solution*: cancel the surgery. Not only did Ellen need the money for her education, her top priority, but now that she had been accepted by the private college she felt more confident. Her surgery was *much less necessary, psychologically.*

It can be awkward for you if you reach the point where you aren't sure about having surgery or that you *don't* want to have it done. Here are some thoughts to help you cope with the situation.

You *Can* Cancel Your Surgery

Most patients like their plastic surgeons. It isn't uncommon to feel that you will be disappointing your surgeon if you cancel. But remember that your surgeon's mission is to help you. *It's not your duty to help your surgeon.*

A good surgeon will be happy if you realize, in advance, that you don't want surgery. There is nothing more discouraging for a surgeon than to have a patient say, afterwards, "I wish I hadn't done this." That really makes us feel like failures. So if you decide to cancel your surgery:

1. Call your surgeon's office.
2. Explain that you want to cancel surgery. If you don't want to give a reason, say, "It's not the right time."
3. Explain that you feel awkward, and that it's not the surgeon's fault. That makes you and him feel better.
4. If you find you are being pushed to give reasons or to reschedule, repeat what you said. Say "thank you" and "goodbye."
5. Remember, scheduling surgery does *not oblige you legally to have the surgery*. But if you cancel, it is more considerate to cancel immediately and not wait until the night before. Your surgeon will probably lose money if you cancel less than a week or so ahead.

What If I'm Not Sure? If you're not sure, you should *cancel*. Indecision is a psychological sign that the time is not right.

What if you are sure you want surgery, but you aren't sure if you should have it for financial reasons? Cosmetic surgery is as much a financial investment as buying 100 shares of stock.

THE COSMETIC SURGERY—WISE INVESTMENT GUIDE

If you have a *yearly income of $100,000*, then five or ten thousand dollars for cosmetic surgery may not be a problem. The 99 percent of us to whom five thousand dollars is serious may need the answers to these questions:

- Should your surgeon advise you on finances?
- Will your surgeon let you pay in installments?
- Is your surgeon too expensive?
- Can your surgery be done free?
- Should you wait to save more money?
- If you don't have the money—must you cancel?

Should My Surgeon Advise Me Financially?

No. Your surgeon has a personal interest in having you spend your money on his surgery. He may not mind if you cancel, but it's not reasonable to ask him to decide if you *should* cancel. Naturally his inclination will be to advise you not to cancel. Besides, even if he is totally objective, your surgeon's financial judgment may not be any better than yours.

Will My Surgeon Let Me Pay in Installments?

Some cosmetic surgeons will make financing agreements with you. For instance, you can pay 20 percent down and the rest in monthly installments. I don't think this is wise. Here's why.

Ralph, a patient of mine, had cosmetic surgery. Two months later, quite unexpectedly, he needed *emergency heart surgery*.

What if I had financed Ralph's cosmetic surgery with time payments and he couldn't afford to pay me, now that he was sick? I would have felt compelled to cancel his debt to me. Many surgeons would feel the same. I wouldn't be happy thinking that the debt he owed me was adding to his heart stress and diminishing his chance of recovery.

But what if I didn't feel that way and went after Ralph's money? While he was sick in hospital, a lien could be placed on his house or his car could be repossessed, depending on how his cosmetic surgery loan was secured. In the end, Ralph would not have benefitted from our financing agreement.

Financial institutions are in the business of lending money. They do it right and they do it all the time. Refinancing a loan could benefit a bank as well as you. You wouldn't let a loan officer operate on your nose. I think it is poor judgment to let your doctor be your bank.

Is Your Surgeon Too Expensive?

Cosmetic surgeons' fees are much the same across the country. They tend to be higher in the cities. In Manhattan, in fashionable New York suburbs, in Beverly Hills and in fashionable Los Angeles suburbs, you can pay two or three times as much for your surgery as elsewhere. Here's why:

- Rent and all other expenses in these fashionable areas are higher.
- Incomes tend to be higher, so people are willing to pay more for cosmetic surgery.
- For the wealthy, a high price may not be bothersome—it may be a status symbol; the difference between five and fifteen thousand dollars may seem negligible.

In general, you will pay more for a "fashionable" surgeon. He may be fashionable because he is particularly good. The higher cost may in fact be good value. But if you think the price is too high, comparison shop this way:

- Get out your phone book.
- Find the *least fashionable county within about 20 miles of you.*
- Call that county's Medical Society.
- Ask for the names of three Board Certified plastic surgeons.
- Call all three offices and ask the fees for your surgery.

If these surgeons are much cheaper, it may be worth the trip to talk with one or more of them. However, if a lower price is the *only* thing going for them, don't choose one solely on that basis. Don't go further for a consultation than you would travel for surgery. Keep it practical.

Can I Get Cosmetic Surgery Done for Free?

Yes. A few major teaching hospitals have plastic surgery residency programs in which you pay *no surgical fee, only the hospital cost.* In exchange, *you are operated on by a resident,* who may have *0* to *2* years' experience in cosmetic surgery. In other words, you are agreeing to be a "guinea pig."

What You Get Is:

- Free surgery
- Some, perhaps much, supervision by a plastic surgery professor
- Surgery done by a resident who will probably, in four years or so, be Board Certified.

What You Give Up Is:

- The personal attention which comes from having your own doctor
- Continuity—residents come and go and you may not be looked after by the same one from start to finish.
- High expectations: studies show that surgical residents (in any field) have a higher rate of complications than physicians who have completed their training. If this weren't the case, there would be no need to have a resident training program.

Some patients are happy with this compromise. Your resident may be destined to become a great surgeon. Or, he may be destined to be thrown out of the residency program (although this is extraordinarily rare). You will have a somewhat higher rate of complications and a somewhat higher rate of annoyance with the way you are treated.

Ophelia was a middle-aged woman who had her facelift and brow lift done for free by the resident staff at an excellent teaching hospital. One month later, she came to see me. A large area on her scalp had not healed, and she had a bald patch above one ear. This is what she told me:

"They operated on both sides of my face at the same time. The senior resident told the junior resident that he was doing it all wrong. I never saw the professor. I think he came in for a minute. When I went back for my follow-up appointments, the senior resident wasn't there anymore. No one had time for me. I demanded to see the professor. He acted like I was crazy, told me I was doing fine, and asked me what I expected when I had surgery done for free."

Ophelia healed in another six weeks. Her hair grew back in the bald patch, but it took a year. The poor healing had resulted from the residents' pulling too hard and being a bit rough with her skin. Still, Ophelia looked better after her facial surgery than she had before. Nevertheless, she felt she would go to a private plastic surgeon if she had the option of starting over again.

In my residency training program, we assisted the professors when they operated on their own patients. This meant that we were present from start to finish, and that the cosmetic patient knew us. It means that we prepared the patient before surgery and helped the professor throughout surgery. Only with the patient's knowledge and consent, and when the professor felt we were knowledgeable enough, did we actually hold the scalpel or scissors. However, we had our own resident clinics. Patients in our clinics were operated on by us, with the professor supervising. These patients always knew they had the option of being the professor's private patient, if they wished. The hospital charged them for the residents' care. It saved the patients some money (not much), but most preferred us residents, because of the convenient location of the clinic.

Residents are learning new skills all the time. Very few cosmetic surgeons will let residents operate on their private patients. When they do, the supervision is constant and intense. The patient would be told ahead of time that a resident would be assisting. The resident is likely to do only a small part of the surgery, unless he is near the end of his training and is experienced. Free cosmetic surgery is not the same as having a plastic surgery professor for your private doctor.

Other Financial Considerations

Even if you have the money for surgery, you might want to ask yourself how the surgery might affect your finances. Do you have a secure income? You will lose time from work. Will you be paid for that time? If not, can you afford not to be paid?

Is there a risk that taking time off for surgery could lose you your job? If so, would that be a disaster? Or are you thinking of a job change, anyhow?

The cases below are a few practical examples of Financial Do's and Don'ts.

Clara, a mother on welfare, was saving her child support money so that she could have cosmetic breast enlargement. The money was given to her, but not to use on herself. Her children suffered, as did the public. This is a clear Don't.

Sally and her husband had money in a joint savings account. Sally wanted to use it for cosmetic eye surgery. Sally didn't work. Her husband had been saving the money to help pay for his mother's cancer treatment. Again, this was a clear Don't. *It wasn't Sally's money.*

Matthew had inherited some money and saved more. He had planned to buy his wife a fur coat. He changed his mind and bought himself a facelift. Regardless of whether you like what Matthew did, the money was his to spend as he chose. Financially, this is a Do.

Suzannah was paid alimony. She paid for her cosmetic surgery, using her alimony. Her "ex" was furious, but it wasn't his money. Suzannah was legally entitled to the money and could spend it as she pleased. Financially this was a Do.

Financially, your surgery is a "Do" *if*:

- The money you spend does not endanger your means of support.
- The money is *yours to spend*.
- Neither you nor a dependent *needs* that money for basics.

If I Don't Have the Money—Must I Cancel?

There are three ways to "afford" surgery, if you don't have the money. You can have someone give you money for the surgery, you can borrow the money from family or good friends, or you can borrow the money commercially.

Tracy had lost over 50 pounds and had a large fold of excess skin hanging down from her abdomen. It was ugly, irritated her skin, and made her feel deformed and dirty. Her insurance would not agree to pay for surgery. Tracy was divorced, supported herself and her children, and knew that she could not afford surgery. Her parents gave her the money for surgery for a birthday gift.

This is fine if you have parents who can afford it. Remember that such large gifts may be a burden. Who pays if you have a complication? Will you resent having to be grateful for the gift? Is it not a real gift but barter—will you be expected to pay back the gift by doing something in return? If so, be clear what the exchange is, and that you will be happy to do it.

A Wise Family Loan

Jean, who was 19, wanted cosmetic nose surgery. Her mother disapproved. Her father didn't object but didn't have money to pay for the surgery. He was saving for Jean's college costs. Jean got a restaurant job. She saved up half of the money for her surgery. Her parents and grandmother were so impressed that they gave her birthday money to help toward the surgery. Jean borrowed the balance of the cost from her parents. She had the surgery. She continued the job and repaid the loan.

Problems With Family Loans

Len was 17 and wanted his parents to pay to fix his "Dumbo" ears. They wouldn't. He persuaded them to "lend" him the money. He promised that he would pay it back, but he knew he wasn't going to do it. He thought it would serve his parents right when he refused to repay them. This wasn't a happy family. Len's parents were not fooled. They planned to use his financial irresponsibility to excuse them from paying for his college tuition. Solution: Len realized he was asking for trouble by taking the loan and got a second job to pay for his surgery. That, or canceling his surgery, were his only honest choices.

A family loan is as much a legal loan as a bank loan. Whoever lends you the money may in fact need the loan to be repaid. For instance, there are laws about how much money a parent can give a child each year. The IRS will tax, as income, gifts over $10,000 from a parent to a child.

Equally—or more—important is not taking advantage of a position of trust. A family loan is not a gift for the taking.

Finally, for families in a state of perpetual strife like Len's, a family loan that is not repaid can become yet another bone of contention, leading to more harm and ill feeling than any surgery would justify.

Don't Ask Your Surgeon to Help Fool Your Family

Tara was separated from her husband. She told him that she needed to borrow money from him for surgery. She knew he didn't approve of cosmetic surgery, so she asked me to help her by preparing for him a false statement saying that her surgery was not cosmetic.

Tara felt that this deception was justified. She wanted the surgery to help her start over, now that she and her husband were separated. I declined her request.

Your surgeon isn't going to help you get money from anyone under false pretenses. It is a form of fraud. If you want cosmetic surgery to help you, *it isn't a wise investment to get the money improperly.*

The Five Rules for a Family Loan

1. Write out how much you are borrowing, how much the interest will be, and how the principal will be paid back—monthly, quarterly, etc.
2. Have the written agreement signed in front of a notary and keep a copy for yourself.
3. The interest rate *should* be lower than high bank rates. Family loans should make the loan more affordable.
4. Pay the money back as agreed.
5. If you can't repay the money on time, *make another written agreement, just as a bank would.* It should state the new conditions—when it will be repaid, how much, to whom.

Commercial Loans Are Your Last Resort

For many people the decision is clear: If cosmetic surgery requires a bank loan, then it must wait. Other people reason that if you can finance a Mercedes, why not a tummy tuck?

If you are sure that the money to repay the loan will be yours in a short time, a commercial loan may make financial sense. For instance,

- You know you'll be getting a salary bonus in three months.
- You're divorced and your house has been sold. When settlement is made, you'll have more than enough money for the surgery. But you want surgery now because your new career starts next month.
- Your appearance is such—baggy eyes, sagging neck—that you don't look as good as you should on the job. There is plenty of room for advancement. You are certain that your income will rise once you look better.

A commercial loan is a mistake if you live on a fixed income, if you will need loans in the near future for other purposes besides surgery, or if you have no insurance or savings to turn to for unexpected events such as a car accident. After all, *you* schedule surgery. Accidents schedule themselves!

What If I Have Already Paid My Surgeon— and Decide to Cancel?

Go right ahead. It's not too late, unless the surgery has actually begun. I have never heard of a surgeon not refunding the money of a patient who paid in advance, then canceled. He should do it automatically. Don't be embarrassed to remind his office. If you are worried, call your bank and stop the check. If for some extraordinary reason your surgeon keeps your money, the County Medical Society will help resolve your dispute. It is hypothetically possible for you to end up filing a small claims suit to get your money back, but to the best of my knowledge, it has never happened. Most of the time it's the other way around: A patient wants me to keep the money because she's sure she'll have the surgery . . . sometime. But I don't feel comfortable keeping her money indefinitely and insist on returning it to her. You'll find most cosmetic surgeons respect your finances.

CHAPTER 10

Whom to Tell About Your Cosmetic Surgery— and How

Cosmetic surgery is a personal decision. Inevitably you need to decide how you will deal with it in public. Whom should you tell before surgery, and what should you tell them? Afterwards, how do you handle questions?

Should I Tell My Children?

Children may not understand that *any* adult can be embarrassed. If you have children, it's safe to tell them that you need medical treatment for a problem—and it may be best not to tell them much more. Judge your own children. One patient told her teenagers about her cosmetic breast surgery. The next day the neighborhood knew all about it!

Should I Tell My Friends?

Of course you have to tell the trusted family member(s) or friend(s) who will help take care of you after your operation. If you have friends who have had, or plan to have, cosmetic surgery, they may be your best and safest confidants. They are more likely to respect your privacy. However, if you confide in others than your *closest* friends, you should assume that your surgery will be discussed openly by the people you tell.

If I'm a Teenager, Should I Tell My Parents?

Parents have a legal right and duty to know about their minor children (those under 18). Also, chances are it's the parents who are paying for the surgery. If your parents are divorced, your *custodial* parent is the one who needs to know. Most surgeons will—and should—insist on meeting one parent before your surgery, even if *you* are paying for the operation.

If your parents seem violently opposed to your cosmetic surgery, it may be because they are afraid that something will go wrong, or that you will be disappointed. They may think that you aren't old enough to make a decision that could affect you for the rest of your life. And some parents may object because they consider your surgery to be an unnecessary expense for them.

If any of these reasons apply to you, it is very important that you sit down with your parents, explain to them why the surgery is so important for you, and reach a happy agreement about it. Sometimes, though, you and a parent are so at odds with each other that such a discussion might only lead to yet another fight.

Trisha was 17. She wanted to reduce the size of her extremely enlarged breasts, which were constantly sore and constantly embarrassing. I met with her first. Later I met with her mother, who was uncertain at first but at the end understood the operation and agreed that Trisha should have it and that she and her husband would pay for it. But her husband fought constantly with Trisha. He was "too busy" even to discuss the surgery over the telephone with me.

The day before Trisha's surgery, her father insisted that I meet with him. He came in with Trisha and her mother, very upset and angry. He said he was going to cancel Trisha's surgery and wanted to tell me why. He began with severe criticism of Trisha's "immaturity," and she left the room on the verge of tears.

I listened to the father. Then I told him that he ought to know what operation he was canceling. I explained everything: What the surgery did, why Trisha wanted it, and what it would do for her. After an hour and a half, Trisha's father understood the operation and Trisha's desire to have it done. He agreed that Trisha should have it done. She had the surgery, and not only did it make her look and feel normal for the first time since puberty, but it became possible for Trisha to take part in sports.

If you are experiencing a problem convincing your parents that having cosmetic surgery is important to you, I suggest:

- You find a surgeon you like and have a first consultation. Expect the doctor to request a meeting with at least one of your parents.
- If one parent is sympathetic, have him/her come with you to the surgeon for a second meeting.
- Ask this parent to sit down and tell the other what the surgeon suggested.
- Finally, if one agrees to your surgery and the other doesn't, get *both* parents to meet with the surgeon.

If your parents still don't agree with you? You probably have no choice except to save your money and have the surgery after you turn 18.

Should I Consult My Young Child Before Arranging His/Her Surgery?

Yes! A number of parents want to compel their child to have a cosmetic operation, for the child's sake, even when the child is *opposed* to the surgery, or isn't sure he wants it.

A mother came in with her 13-year-old daughter, Laura. When she met me, Laura did not know that I was a plastic surgeon, nor why her mother had brought her to see me. Her mother did all the talking. "Laura has a horrible nose, Dr. Morgan. It is just like her Dad's. It spoils her face. Without it, she could be pretty. She needs her nose done just to get on in life. Look at it! Tell her to have it done. For her own good."

Laura, who was pretty, was sitting on the exam table looking miserable and mulish.

"What do you want, Laura?" I asked.

"I want to be left alone. I like my nose."

Of course I wouldn't operate. No good cosmetic surgeon would operate on someone opposed to having surgery. If your child doesn't want it done, don't argue. Let the child say no. After all, Barbra Streisand was told that she would never succeed until she had cosmetic nose surgery. She refused and still managed to attain "a little success." It was the right decision for her. So, what your child wants is what counts.

Handling Negative Reactions

Your cosmetic surgery will seem reasonable to you and your surgeon, but you *can* get some peculiar reactions from other people. Sometimes you get negative reactions when you *least* expect them.

Dr. Smith was a well-known and thoughtful surgeon. However, he considered cosmetic surgery to be a disgrace to the dignity of medicine. He considered anyone who "chopped themselves up" for vanity to be a lunatic or a fool. It was not until his teenage daughter wanted her nose changed—and it really helped her—that he changed his attitude. If you had been Dr. Smith's patient, you would have felt criminal if you had confided in him about your cosmetic surgery *before* he changed his opinion.

Cosmetic surgery is like taking a trip. If you plan ahead, you can sail through calm waters. If you don't, you can have a bumpy ride. It can be truly depressing to get the wrong reaction from people around you, after you've invested time and effort in improving yourself through surgery. It helps a lot to know what has happened to other people, so you can decide how best you can prepare, and so that you know there's nothing wrong with you, if you get a reaction you don't like.

Elsie was an attractive, self-confident mother of two children. She decided to have cosmetic breast surgery. Her breasts had shrunk and drooped from pregnancy. She wanted them uplifted and a little larger. She didn't tell anyone except her husband and her best friend, who lived hundreds of miles away.

Elsie had no trouble with her operation which was done on an out-patient basis. Six weeks later she left for a long weekend to visit her best friend. "Darling," her best friend said as she picked her up at the airport. "You're coming to lunch at my club. I've arranged for you to be the guest of honor."

Elsie was flattered—until she arrived at the luncheon. "This is Elsie," announced her best friend, "Elsie, I knew you wouldn't mind telling all of us about your breast surgery."

"We're dying to see your scars!" said one lady.

"We just want to take a peek," said another.

This really happened. "I nearly died," Elsie told me, confiding this nightmare to me at her follow-up visit. "I wanted to sink right through the floor. I walked out the door and took the first plane home. How can a friend do something like that?"

The answer is—easily. People are inquisitive. If someone knows that you have had surgery, you're considered fair game for all inquiries about it. We ask strangers in elevators how they got a bruise on their face or a cast on their leg. Cosmetic surgery is even more fascinating, and it makes many people forget their manners. It doesn't matter who you are.

Marsha, a socially prominent, wealthy widow in her sixties, was in bed, sleeping. It was the middle of the night. Her telephone rang.

"Hello," said Marsha, groggily.

"Hello? Marsha?" asked a woman's voice.

"Yes. Who is this?"

"Oh, you don't know me, but I'm thinking about having a nose job. I was talking to Dennis Smith. Do you know him?"

"No."

"Well, he is a friend of Doris Brown. You know Doris?"

"Yes."

"Well, Dennis remembered Doris telling him years ago that you had cosmetic surgery at the _____ General Hospital. I'm thinking of doing that and I was wondering what operation you had, and how much it cost, and your surgeon, and so on. Did you have a nose job or a facelift?"

"I was speechless," Marsha told me later. "I was so surprised I almost began to answer the woman's questions! It's the shock of it. After I realized it was none of her business, I told her so and hung up."

Does this just happen to women, because we're more vulnerable? No. Men are not immune.

Albert was a middle-aged professional man. I treated him for acne scars. He was grocery shopping after work one day when a strange man accosted him in the cereal aisle, saying loudly: "Aren't you the guy my brother told me about who had the dermabrasion for his acne? I've always wondered why a guy would have that done!"

What would you have said? Albert said, "Wrong guy. Sorry," and moved on.

Interestingly, teenagers seem to be more tolerant of each other's desire to improve and need for privacy.

Sam was 18. He had a cosmetic nose operation done during Christmas vacation. He was standing in the school cafeteria line in January when someone in the group behind him whispered loudly: "Sam had schnoz surgery during vacation. He claims it was for a deviated septum but I bet it was cosmetic." This remark was greeted with shrugs, a couple of blank stares at the speaker and a bored, "So what?"

Rudeness from friends can be well intentioned. Rudeness from strangers can be mere curiosity. However, bad reactions from fellow workers often result from envy or jealousy.

Should I Tell My Co-workers?

Bea had lower-lid surgery to smooth out some bulges, and she confided in a friend at work. A few days later another employee accosted her in a hallway saying: "How can you justify wasting your money on doing your eyes? Don't you have anything better to spend your money on? I think that's dreadful. Aren't you ashamed?"

Bea felt angry and humiliated, but she was sensible enough to realize that this woman's outrageous behavior was most likely due to her resentment toward Bea for having been promoted over her some months before.

What should you do? A lot depends on your personality. First, remember that having cosmetic surgery doesn't make you vain. It's nothing to be ashamed of. In fact, you should be proud to be taking steps to solve a personal problem.

Men Aren't Immune to Comments

Men, just like women, can be harassed at work if it is known that they have had cosmetic surgery. A man can be even more self-conscious than a woman, because it is more accepted for women to spend money on their looks. However, studies show that men, like women, are hired or promoted on the basis of looks *as well as* competency. One study involved showing employers two sets of photographs: the first were of middle-aged men *before* cosmetic surgery and the second showed the same men *after* cosmetic surgery had corrected baggy eyelids, jowly faces, and prominent ears. The employers marked the "afters" as people they would hire and the "befores" as people they would not. In 1986 the *Wall Street Journal* printed an extensive article about the benefits of cosmetic surgery for corporate executives. A large number of middle-management executives have found that their stalled careers are followed by promotion after cosmetic surgery. For a lot of men, cosmetic surgery becomes a business decision.

A man who has had a facelift and looks much better should be as proud of that as a woman. Teasing by other men usually reflects jealousy. Getting ahead in your career is not a vain or frivolous reason for cosmetic surgery—provided that you already possess all the other qualifications for getting ahead. Looking better through surgery will *not* make up for a lack of other professional assets.

Tom, an executive in a large corporation, was beginning to feel the pressure of competing with some of the younger up-and-coming salesmen in his department. He decided to have a facelift. Some weeks later after he'd healed sufficiently, he was at a business lunch. A rival sitting across the table from him whispered loudly: "Hey, did you get a load of Tom? I heard he spent five thou on a facelift just to look a little younger! Talk about being vain . . ."

Tom was embarrassed, but he knew he couldn't ignore this man without looking as though he were ashamed of his surgery. Fortunately, he'd planned ahead for such comments. "Jealous, aren't you, Mack?" he retorted, with a smile. "My surgeon said he couldn't do a damn thing for your face."

Laughing, the group got down to work.

How to Handle "Nosybodies"

You may love the results of your surgery and want to tell the world. You may not be the least self-conscious about it. You may be as proud of your surgery as you would to be making capital improvements in your house. Go right ahead—tell the world! However, if you no more want to reveal the fact of your surgery than you would publish your bank account or your love letters, or if you are not sure what to do —keep it private. You can always talk later on. You *do* need to plan how to keep your surgery private, though. Here are some suggestions:

- Tell only the person who will care for you after surgery.
- Know how you will respond to nosy questions.
- Don't lie about your surgery unless you can be convincing.

There are four ways I know of to contend with intrusive questions about your cosmetic surgery. I call them the aristocrat's approach, answering a question with a question, answering with humor, and answering evasively.

The Aristocrat's Approach. This approach was used on me once. I was in an English hotel. I saw a man in the lobby with a dog. "What a nice dog," I said, cheerfully American. I got hit with a stare so blank and icy that it hurt. The man was the Duke of Something, and he didn't speak to anyone who hadn't been formally introduced. His look was so cold it would have stopped a baboon, and it made me feel like one. If you can handle people's questions this way—and you don't care if you offend them—give it a shot!

Answering a Question With a Question. This approach is more "American"—it will make your interrogator uncomfortable but will probably seem less offensive than the English method of "sending them to Coventry"—i.e., ignoring their existence. Consider this interchange:

Them: Didn't you just have a facelift?
  You: Where did you hear that?
Them: Someone told me you were out of work, having cosmetic surgery.

You: Why do you want to know?
Them: I'm just interested. Well, did you?
You: I'm sorry. I'm not interested in having this conversation.
Them: There's no need to be rude.
You: You don't think your *questions* are rude?

This method challenges a snoopy question with a forthright question that puts inquisitors on notice that they have overstepped their bounds.

Answering With Humor. This approach does not challenge your questioner. It is less likely to lead to ruffled feathers—if you care to avoid them.

Them: Didn't you just have a nose job?
You: Are you kidding? Why mess with a work of art?
Them: Your nose looks swollen.
You: So maybe I'm allergic to you!

Answering Evasively. If you can't freeze out rudeness or parry it with questions or humor, you can tell *part of the truth*. The risk is that further questioning will press you into a reluctant admission that you had cosmetic surgery. Decide what you will say. My patients have found these useful:

- Say you were treated. Do not use the words "surgery" or "operation."
- Do not identify the area treated.
- Make your treatment sound boring.

The following statement applies to any kind of surgery: "I required medical treatment for a very painful condition." This is *always true* because you received sedation for the pain of surgery.

Here are some more evasive but true descriptions of cosmetic surgery:

- If you were born with it: "I was treated for a congenital anomaly."
- If it was for acne: "I was treated for a minor infection."
- If it was for aging: "I was treated for muscular weakness."
- If it was breast surgery: "I was treated for a glandular condition."

You may prefer to lie. If you do, be careful not to make things worse for yourself. One patient explained her nose surgery as "sinusitis" on Monday and as "a fall at home" on Tuesday. A co-worker assumed that she had had a fall when drunk! An evasive answer would have worked better than the inconsistent lies.

Dealing With Official Snoopers

You have a *legal* right to privacy. You might not want your work file or school record to include details of your cosmetic surgery. It need not. People in authority may try to insist that you tell them, simply because they are inquisitive and use their authority to snoop.

> *Vera was a teenage patient with a rapidly growing breast tumor that needed urgent surgical removal. Vera was in tears the night before her surgery. A teacher had threatened Vera with a failing grade unless she "confessed" the details of her medical problem to justify her school absence. "As soon as I tell her, it will be all over the school," sobbed Vera.*
>
> *The teacher had a right to know only that Vera was absent from school for a compelling medical reason. I wrote to Vera's teacher, offering to provide Vera's medical details if the teacher first supplied me with a copy of the state statute allowing her access to Vera's medical records. This put the teacher on notice that she was attempting something illegal. She left Vera alone.*

If someone in authority pressures you to reveal private medical information, that person may be entitled to confirm that you have a reason for your absence. If they insist on knowing, you can ask your surgeon to write to the authority on stationery that does not reveal that the surgeon is a cosmetic or plastic surgeon. The letter can say:

> Mr./Ms. Blank will not be able to work (attend class, whatever) for about _____ days, from _____ to _____ for medical reasons.

An employer may also have a right to know whether your absence is for an emergency or treatment of a life-threatening condition. Your surgeon will not lie.

If an authority presses you for details to which you think that person is not entitled, you can ask your doctor to write, as I wrote to Vera's teacher:

> Medical information is confidential. If you believe that you have a right to this privileged information, please write to me stating the basis of your belief and provide me with a copy of the pertinent statute giving you legal access to the information.

Who Has a Right to Know?

If you submit a claim to your insurance company, the insurance company has a right to know the details of your surgery, so they can decide how to pay.

If your surgery is, for instance, scar revision for an injury at work, then workmen's compensation (a form of insurance) is entitled to the medical details. Surgery done to repair work-related injuries is usually reconstructive, not cosmetic.

How to Know What to Camouflage

Humans are inquisitive. Friends may want to know if you had surgery because they want information before *their* surgery. Or they may be merely curious. It helps to know what other people look for, so that *you* can know how best to hide it. Resign yourself to questions . . . you can't control the curiosity of others. Chances are, if you're clever, they won't be able to tell you had surgery.

> *I operated on Wally, doing a facelift, nose "job," acne surgery, upper-lid tuck, lower-lid tuck, and hair transplants. Two weeks after surgery, the scars and every telltale sign were gone. It unnerved me. I knew I had operated, but I couldn't see where!*

However, if you know in advance what people will be looking for, you will know in advance how to foil the detection. For instance, if you are going to change your hairstyle after surgery, why not change it a few weeks *before*? If you might wear a scarf tied dashingly around your neck to hide bruising from a facelift, buy one and wear one *before* you go in for surgery. If you don't normally wear makeup and would consider using it after surgery, buy the makeup and even have a consultation with a makeup specialist (your surgeon can recommend one) so that you have and wear your new makeup in advance. When you start using camouflage *before* you have anything to conceal, you'll get used to using it and no one will associate your "time out" with any detectable outward change in makeup, clothes, hairstyle, and so on.

Some Telltale Signs

Here's how people *might* be able to tell you had cosmetic surgery—if they knew what to look for:

Telltale Scars
- Lower-lid tuck: A white or red line just below the lashes of the lower lid
- Facelift: A white or pink scar all along the front of the ear

Telltale Skin Changes
- Fat suction of the thighs: Rough irregular skin on the sides of the thighs, usually with brown spots
- Dermabrasion: A perpetual blush on the cheeks
- Facelift: White patches behind the ears from inflammation or infection while healing

Telltale Makeup and Hairstyles
- Upper-lid tuck: Upper-lid eye shadow that shows, when it never did before
- Face or brow lift: a new hairstyle with the hair longer, combed in front of and behind the ear

Telltale Clothing Changes
- Fat suction of thighs: Suddenly wearing pants and looking good in them
- Breast enlargement reduction: Suddenly wearing loose blouses and sweaters that conceal breast size *or* suddenly wearing form-fitting tops to show off breast size

If You Are Having Surgery—Relax

I was in an elevator in a New York store with a friend. In the elevator were six other people. I could tell that: Two of them had had cosmetic nose surgery in the 1950s (very squashed piggy noses); two had had nose surgery in the 1960s (better noses, but much too small); and one had had cosmetic nose surgery in the late 1970s (I saw the faint shadow where nose tip cartilage had been carved away).

Off the elevator and out of earshot, I asked my friend, "Did you notice the noses of the people in the elevator?"

"Sure. They all looked normal to me."

What I can see as a plastic surgeon is invisible to other people. Rest assured that not only can cosmetic surgery help you psychologically, but once you're healed, the surgery will not be obvious to others!

P A R T

The
Procedures

T
W
O

INTRODUCTION

This part of my book explains each major cosmetic surgery procedure in detail, including:

- What surgeons call it
- What it will do
- What it won't do
- When to have it
- Where to have it
- Conditions that increase your risk
- How much it costs
- Insurance coverage
- Usual anesthesia
- How long it takes
- The operation: before, during, and after
- Bandages
- What to do about pain
- The healing process
- Taking care of your wound
- Stitches
- Scars
- My assessment of the procedure
- Side effects and complications

I've also included special tips for each procedure; tips on when and how to resume work, parties, sports, and sex; and candid comments from patients who may have had the operation.

Although you may want to read about every procedure, it's more likely that you'll want to skip around, learning about the operation or operations that you're especially interested in having. For that reason, I've included *all* the pertinent information for *every* procedure, even though it may seem repetitious to those of you who read every one.

Time and again, I've found that patients want to know *exactly* what I'm going to do. That's reasonable—the more you know, the better you're able to make an informed choice about whether to have the surgery. For many patients, a verbal explanation isn't enough. That's reasonable, too. When I was in medical school, I found that telling me "a muscle is tightened" didn't give me a clear idea of what happens to the patient's skin and tissue. I had to *see* it happening.

Since I can't take you into the operating room with me, I've included illustrations to help you understand each operation. Graphic pictures like these don't usually appear in books for what doctors call the "lay public." If you find them "too much," just flip past them.

On the other hand, if you want to know still more, you can consult some professional texts. They're expensive, so try to get them through a library. Try dipping into *Plastic and Reconstructive Surgery*, second edition, by Converse (W. B. Saunders, 1980) or *Aesthetic Plastic Surgery*, second edition, by Rees (W. B. Saunders, 1980).

Part II of this book has more information about the details of cosmetic operations than you'll find in any other book written for the general public. It should make your surgical experience easier and less confusing. If you think that after reading about one of the procedures you're ready to *do* it, not just *have* it done—there's a little more to it than that. But I've taught you as best I can until you join me in the operating room.

CHAPTER   11

Procedures for the Face and Head

Face and Neck Lift— Facelift Surgery

What Surgeons Call It

Surgeons call this operation a rhytidectomy, a rhytidoplasty, a face-neck lift, or a face-neck lift with SMAS flap and platysma flap, depending on what is done. "SMAS" is surgical shorthand for submusculoaponeurotic system, which is the deep tissue of the face that blends with the platysma muscle of the neck.

What It Will Do

A facelift should make you look great for your age and *may* even make you look years younger. It will tighten loose skin and muscle and remove bulges of fat in your neck, and it will tighten the loose tissues in your face.

What It Won't Do

A facelift will *not* stop aging. It can't turn the clock back 20 years or *any* set number of years. It can't guarantee any practical changes in your life such as a new job or a new love. Nor can it remove wrinkles (see Chemical Peel).

How Long It Will Last

Until modern techniques were developed, a facelift merely tightened the skin and lasted two to five years, at best. Today's facelift surgery corrects age-related changes in many tissues—fat, muscle, and deep tissue layers in the face and neck—as well as tightening the skin. For many people, the results may be permanent, to the extent that the fat does not return and the muscles do not loosen. The skin will loosen again with time, though, and the muscles *may* loosen to some degree. A reasonable best estimate of "how long it will last" for the techniques we use now is 5 to 10 years.

When to Have It

The right age may be any time from 35 to 75. You should consider having a facelift when the changes of age bother *you*, not someone else in your life. You should not believe claims that the operation will stop aging, but a facelift that is done early (before age 50) may prevent you from developing the hanging folds of neck skin that are a "trademark" of aging in some families. If you are over 65 and considering your *first* facelift, you may need a "re-do," less extensive than the first operation, within 18 months for a good result.

This operation is best *not* done in the middle of a personal life crisis—the unavoidable ups and downs of facelift recovery make this *the hardest cosmetic operation to handle, psychologically.* Save this operation until the crisis is behind you.

Where to Have It

Your facelift may be done on an outpatient basis in a doctor's office operating room *or* an outpatient surgery center *or* a hospital outpatient operating room. Sometimes a facelift is done on an inpatient basis, with a hospital stay of one or two nights. The doctor may advise doing the surgery this way if you have a medical problem like high blood pressure or angina (chest pain) which requires in-hospital supervision after surgery. Some patients prefer to stay in the hospital because there is no one at home to take care of them or because they don't *want* their spouse/kids/friends hovering over them. Sometimes in-hospital care simply seems easier.

Conditions That Increase Your Risk

If you have a **tendency to bleed** or are taking a medicine that thins your blood, your risk of bleeding during facelift surgery is considerably increased. The surgery lifts up the skin of the lower face and upper neck, and if you are bleeding prone, every tiny blood vessel in the skin can ooze more than usual, causing a hematoma (a blood clot that needs to be drained). **High blood pressure** also increases your risk of excessive bleeding, especially if it is above 150/100. **Smoking** increases your risk of poor healing after any surgery, but *especially* after a facelift. Studies have shown that men and women who smoke and who have facelift surgery are *10 to 20 times more likely to have the incision behind the ear heal slowly*, leaving a wide scar and patches of discoloration. Smoking reduces the flow of blood and oxygen to your skin, and this may be why smoking is strongly linked to poor healing.

Usual Anesthesia

Facelift operations are usually done under local anesthesia with sedation.

How Long It Takes

Facelift surgery usually takes 3 to 3½ hours. But it may be an hour shorter or longer, depending on how much your skin bleeds and what has to be done. Men tend to bleed more because each beard-hair follicle has blood vessels around it. So, a male patient's facelift may take longer, simply to stop all the bleeding. A person with much fat in his or her neck will have a longer operation, since it takes time to remove the fat.

The Operation

(Figures 11-1 through 11-5)

Before

You will arrive for your surgery about an hour before it is scheduled, having had nothing to eat or drink since midnight the night before. You will change into a hospital gown and be taken to a preoperative area, where an IV will be placed in your arm so you can be given a solution of dextrose and/or saline to prevent dehydration during your surgery. You will probably also receive a dose of antibiotic through the IV to help keep down infection after surgery. Probably you'll also be given some sedation at this time.

Your surgeon or a nurse will prepare your face for surgery by marking the incisions on your face and fastening your hair back with rubber bands or tape to keep it out of the way during surgery. (Sometimes these steps are done in the operating room.)

You will then be taken to the operating room and assisted onto the operating table. A safety strap is put across your hips. Sticky pads are put on your chest to monitor your heart and a sticky pad is put on your hip, under your gown. This is a grounding pad, to make surgical cautery safe for you. (Surgical cautery means using an electrical instrument to seal off blood vessels and stop bleeding.) Your blood pressure will be checked and you may be given some oxygen to breathe through a little tube near your nose or mouth. A little gauze pack will be put in each ear to keep surgical soap from dripping in. Your face is then washed with surgical soap, and sterile drapes are put over your body and around your face. You will then be given more sedation until you are dozing.

During

Note: Not every person needs every step done as described here. For instance, if you have no excess fat in your neck, then fat is not removed. Working on one side of your face at a time, your surgeon injects the side with local anesthetic to numb the skin and the nerves near the skin. (When he does the other side, you will be given additional sedation.) Once your facial skin is numb, your surgeon will cut through it from above the ear, in front of the ear, and behind the ear, back into the hair to free the skin from the face and neck. He will suction or cut out the fat deposits that lie under the skin of the neck. Reaching under the skin, he will then free up the deep layer of tissue in the face (the SMAS), trimming any excess, and will also free up the platysma muscle in the neck (the looseness of this muscle is what makes the neck sag). Then he will pull the muscle layers in the face and neck up and back and use stitches behind and above the ears to secure these tissues in their new positions. It is these stitches that do the major work in lifting your face—the skin does not hold your face tight. After the muscles have been secured, the surgeon will pull the outer layer of facial skin up and back, securing it with stitches above and behind the ear and trimming the excess skin.

If the center of the neck also needs work, the surgeon will make a short incision under the chin and cut out or suction excess fat and tighten the neck muscle. (He may do this step first, before lifting up the facial skin, depending on how he works and on what your face needs.)

At this point in the operation, you are a little more than half-way through. You will be beginning to wake up and may feel restless. You'll be given further sedation before the surgeon injects the local anesthetic into the other side of your face.

If your face needs drains for bleeding, your surgeon may put the drain tube in on the operated side now, or he may wait until he finishes both sides, in which case he will leave all stitching of the outer skin to the end of the operation.

Since much of the surgery is done *under* your skin, you may feel pulling as your surgeon gently lifts the skin of the face away so that he can put in the muscle or SMAS stitches, or find tiny areas of bleeding that he needs to cauterize. This pulling is not uncomfortable; it's a faint sensation if you feel it at all.

There are many nerves in the face. Most of them will be numbed. However, any one of several nerves low in the neck may not be completely numbed and may need an additional injection of local anesthetic during the operation.

Once both sides of your face and the work under the chin is done, your surgeon will remove the packs from your ears, wash your face, and probably wash your hair to keep soap and/ or bloody drainage from irritating your scalp under the bandage. Once your hair is patted dry, he will wrap your face with a bulky dressing.

If you were having more surgery than a facelift—for instance upper and lower lid surgery, a brow lift, a chin enlargement—these steps may be done before or after the facelift, depending on your surgeon's way of working.

After

When all of your surgery is over, you will go to the recovery room. You'll probably be ready to go home in about 2 hours, although if you are nauseated or fall asleep, it may be longer. Once you're home, you'll go to bed and rest and/or sleep.

Face and Neck Lift

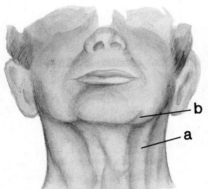

Figure 11-1.

Before face-neck lift surgery, the bands in the front of the neck (a) are from the platysma neck muscle. The face-neck lift will tighten and trim these. The face-neck lift reduces looseness (b) along the jawline (jowls) by tightening the deep (SMAS) layer of the face.

Figure 11-2.

The face-neck lift incision (a) starts above the ear, then goes in front of and behind the ear and back into the hair. The platysma neck muscle is lifted and tightened to firm up the neck. This muscle is cut at (b) or at the back below (c) so that your neck does not feel too tight after the muscle is pulled snug. Stitches (c) sew the platysma neck muscle in place after it is tightened. The fat that lies between the skin and muscle will then be cut or suctioned away.

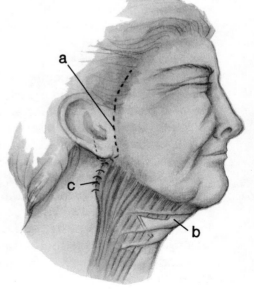

Figure 11-3.

The skin is pulled up and
back to tighten it (a) after the
deep tissues have been
pulled snug. Notice that there
is enough excess skin to
overlap the ear.

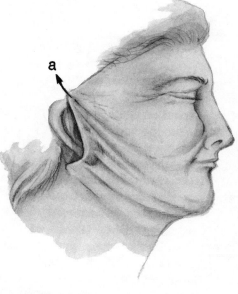

Figure 11-4.

After the face-neck lift the
jawline is tighter (a), the neck
is smoother (b), and the
facelift incision is largely
hidden by hair (in front) and
by the ear (behind) (c).

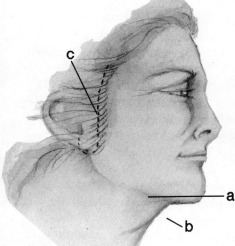

Figure 11-5.

After the face-neck lift the
looseness from the platysma
muscle and excess fat is
gone (a). The line at (b) is
from muscle deep in the neck
and is not changed by a
face-neck lift.

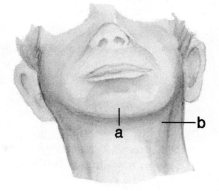

The Process of Recovery

What to Do About Pain

You should have little or *no* pain after a facelift. You'd expect a lot of aching or throbbing, but your skin will be numb from the surgery because tiny nerves going to the skin are cut. So long as you don't talk a lot, you should be comfortable. If you do have pain, *you should report it to your surgeon immediately,* because he'll need to see you sooner than usual. The cause of the pain may be bleeding under your skin (a hematoma), or your bandage may be too tight. If you develop pain *inside* either ear, it usually means that soap trickled down your ear during surgery. It may irritate your ear and need to be washed out, or you may even need eardrops to control infection and relieve pain.

Bandages

Your face and neck will be wrapped up "space helmet" style, with bandages going around your scalp and neck and around your face, framing but not covering it. You will have padding around your ears so you won't hear well when you talk on the phone. This bandage is usually removed after 2 days.

Your surgeon may have put one drain under your skin on each side of your face, especially if you bled more than usual at surgery, or if a medication or your blood pressure put you at a high risk for bleeding. These drains are little plastic tubes (the shape of a long, flexible straw) that are under your skin and come out behind your ear. They may be attached to little plastic bottles (the size and shape of a large lemon) to collect the fluid that gathers beneath your skin. These drains are removed when your bandage is removed. If it is left in for longer than 2 days, a drain may irritate the skin over it, leaving a little thickening or ridge of swelling along the path of the drain for 8 to 12 weeks after it has been removed. You don't feel the drain when it is in place, but you do feel a tug when it is pulled out.

Taking Care of Your Wound

I let my patients shower the same day that the bandages are taken off, unless they had drains that were removed at the same time. In that case, they can shower the day *after.* I permit my patients to get their hair wet at the same time, but not to use shampoo until three days later. You can use a *cool* blow-dry after you rinse or shampoo your hair, but your skin won't feel heat, so don't risk hot curlers or a curling iron near your face for 2 weeks. You could burn your skin and not even feel it.

You can have your hair professionally washed and set 2 to 3 weeks after your operation. Your hair can be tinted or colored 3 weeks after surgery, *if* you have completely healed. Otherwise, if a patch of skin remains open, you must wait until that is sealed. You can have a permanent 6 weeks after surgery, unless it is a no-ammonia permanent. These gentle permanent solutions can be used 3 weeks after surgery or 1 week after every open area is healed, if that occurs later than 3 weeks.

Men as well as women can wear concealer cream or pancake makeup to cover the bruising as soon as the bandage comes off—pat it on with a sponge and pat it off with makeup remover. You can pat your face with a cool washcloth, if you don't like the creamy feel of makeup remover on your skin. At the end of a week women can put on regular makeup instead of, or as well as, the makeup you used to cover bruises. At the end of 2 weeks, men and women can return to their usual face-cleansing regimen, if it is more vigorous than what I've just described. Until then, no scrubbing with rough washcloths.

You should not sunbathe for 6 weeks. The surgical trauma to your skin will make you much more prone to a sunburn, or to brown discoloration in patches. When you do sunbathe, you should use at least a #15 sunscreen for the first summer after your facelift. (It will still allow you to tan.)

The Healing Process

Your face will look strange to you when the bandage first comes off. You will look pale from the surgery and sedation, yellow/green from the bruising, puffy, and without your normal expression. Don't be alarmed. You will end up looking like yourself—an improved version—as the bruising and swelling go down.

Your face will be noticeably swollen for 5 days, and it will be puffy for another 2 weeks. The swelling in your face will make you feel a little unnatural when you smile and talk. This will abate in the first 2 weeks after surgery, but you may have some feeling of stiffness for as long as 6 weeks. Since the facelift tightens the outer layer of muscle in your neck, your neck may feel quite

Facelift Surgery: Recovery-at-a-Glance

This chart represents the *average* recovery times for this cosmetic operation.

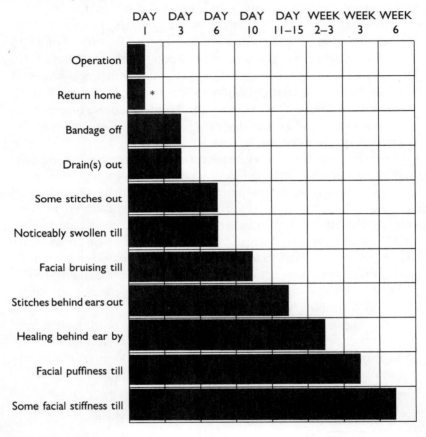

	DAY 1	DAY 3	DAY 6	DAY 10	DAY 11–15	WEEK 2–3	WEEK 3	WEEK 6
Operation								
Return home	*							
Bandage off								
Drain(s) out								
Some stitches out								
Noticeably swollen till								
Facial bruising till								
Stitches behind ears out								
Healing behind ear by								
Facial puffiness till								
Some facial stiffness till								

*Unless hospital stay is required.

tight—all the time, or just when you talk or eat. This can last for 5 to 15 days, and some feeling of pulling may last a few weeks longer.

You should be prepared for your neck and lower face to look bruised because of staining from blood in your deep tissues. You'll probably first notice bruising on your lower cheeks the day that your bandage is removed. However, by the end of 10 days you will have little or no facial bruising, but your mid or lower neck may be bruised purple, even though your surgery does not go to the bottom of the neck. (Remember, bruising tends to work its way downward because of gravity.) You may have a faint tinge of yellow in your skin up to 21 days if you have sallow skin. This may not be bruising, but temporary skin discoloration from the surgery. You may notice that healing behind your ear seems particularly slow. It may be crusted or a sore may persist for 3 or even 4 weeks, especially if you are smoking during your healing period, or if you slept with a pillow after surgery.

Your hair may thin temporarily at the temples. This is because the trauma of surgery can cause a number of hair follicles to go into a resting state and shed, all at the same time. It may take hair 6 months to grow back in.

Stitches

You will have stitches in front of your ears and under your chin. These are removed about 5 days after your surgery (3 days after the bandages are removed). You will have stitches, staples, or both in the incisions behind your ears. These stay in longer, because this area is slow to heal. They will not be removed until 7 to 14 days after surgery.

Your stitches may pull or even hurt when they come out. Take an acetaminophen product such as Tylenol before you go to your stitch-removal appointments and carry some with you as well, in case you need them afterwards.

Scars

You will have one *long* scar around each ear. It starts above the ear, goes down right in front of your ear, then, staying close to the earlobe, it goes behind the ear up to the hairline and then back through the hair toward the back of the neck.

The scar in front of your ear lies in a natural crease, so it is hardly noticeable even right after your surgery. The scar above your ear is completely covered by your hair. It is the scar behind your ear that may pose a problem. This one may be pink and lumpy for months, and, if you are slow to heal, it may leave patches of red and brown, around a stretched (½ inch) scar. This is the likely trouble spot for your facelift scars, but it can usually be covered completely by your hair.

You will often have a very short scar just under your chin as well, because an incision here is needed to remove fat under the chin and to tighten the muscles in the middle of the neck.

Tips

- A facelift is often combined with upper and/or lower eyelid surgery, but if your facelift is done by itself, you may have little, if any bruising around your eyes. So you don't need to invest in tinted glasses or large sunglasses.
- If your hair is very short, you should let it grow out a little before your surgery to hide the facelift scars, especially the one behind your ears. You needn't change your hairstyle permanently—the scars will fade and improve with time. Even so, you may want to avoid super-short hairstyles if the scars are visible. However, remember what is visible to you may *not* be noticeable to others.
- Having a permanent a few weeks before surgery will fluff out your hair around the facelift scars and hide any temporary thinning in the hair above or behind your ears.
- Cold weather is a good time to have a facelift. The cold *won't* make your recovery more uncomfortable, and wrapping your face with a scarf to hide the bandages or bruising will seem perfectly natural.
- *Men:* Since the surgery will make your lower cheeks and jawline skin numb for weeks, and in patches for up to a year, invest in an electric razor if you don't already have one. The gentleness of the electric razor will eliminate the skin nicks that are inevitable if you shave your numb skin with a safety razor after surgery.
- Use a neck roll instead of a pillow to sleep on while you're bandaged. Recent studies show that using a pillow may increase your risk of poor healing behind your ears, because the pillow puts pressure on the bandage, compressing delicate skin around the stitches. Don't go completely without anything, or you may have a stiff neck as well as a facelift to recover from.
- Buy a small bottle of baby shampoo so that you can wash your hair soon after surgery. A stronger shampoo may irritate your healing skin.
- If you don't have a blow dryer, buy a small one so that you can wash your hair at home and blow it dry. A brisk towel-dry won't

be possible, and you won't feel up to having a beauty-shop shampoo for 2 to 3 weeks.

- In the second week after surgery, your bruising may have worked down to your *chest* before it fades. (Gravity pulls it down.) Be sure to have a few high-necked dresses, shirts, blouses, or sweaters and perhaps even a scarf to tie around your neck to conceal this last stage of bruising.

Back to Work

About a quarter of my patients go back to work at the end of a week. Their bandages are off and they cover the bruises with makeup. If you go back this early, though, you'll feel quite tired. Also, be prepared for other people to comment on your facial appearance. They may not have the slightest idea that you had a facelift, but they'll see that you don't "look yourself," that your face is quite puffy, and that your lower face or upper neck are bruised.

The majority—75 percent—of patients go back to work after 2 weeks or a little longer. At this point, the obvious swelling is down, and makeup and combing your hair over the behind-the-ear scars will conceal the telltale facelift surgery signs. You may *feel* conspicuous, but you won't actually *be* conspicuous.

Back to Sports

You should do *no* sports for 2 weeks, except some stretches to keep your joints and muscles loose. You can begin stretching (*at a slow pace*) after a week. Exercise—swimming, jogging, Nautilus—will make your face swell and will delay your return to looking and feeling normal.

Back to Sex

Sex greatly increases your facial blood flow and will therefore increase your risk of bleeding for the first week after surgery. So abstain. In the second week, you will still have stitches in and your face will be swollen. Although increased facial blood flow is not likely to cause internal bleeding, it can cause renewed swelling in your tissue or lead to pulling on the remaining stitches. So it is best by far to abstain from sex for a full 2 weeks.

Back to Parties

More than any other operation, you have a facelift to look your facial best. So going to a party too early is likely to make you feel uncomfortably self-conscious. Unless you heal faster than usual and are more self-possessed than most people, stay away from parties for a month. Your face will ache if you are out late during the first 3 weeks after surgery.

How Much It Costs

Your surgeon's fee will be from $3500 to $5000. The cost of the operating room and anesthesia will be from a minimum of $1000 for local/sedation to a maximum of $3500 or more if you have general anesthesia and stay in the hospital for 2 or 3 days.

Insurance Coverage

Your insurance will *not* pay for or reimburse you for this operation, even if your facial loosening is the result of an injury or from radiation skin damage. The *only* exception is the insurance reimbursement plans available to some corporate executives in which their company will pay them for *any* medical or surgical treatment. Unless you have this kind of coverage, no amount of reports, photographs, or presurgery argument will make your insurance pay for this operation.

My Assessment of This Procedure

This operation can be surprisingly easy for you. Major complications are *rare*. You will be pleased by the lack of pain involved, but you will be irked by the time it takes for the bruises to fade and the swelling to go down. There are also a considerable number of temporary problems: bumpy scars behind the ears; jaw numbness lasting 6 months or more; and the thickening of your skin that may develop under the jaw or where a drain was placed—with faint traces of residual skin thickening persisting 6 months. Even if it doesn't show, a lumpy scar behind the ear can catch on a brush or comb until it flattens over 3 to 6 months.

It does help to be realistic, though. A patient complained to me after a facelift that the corners of her mouth still drooped. They did this because she never smiled! A facelift will *not* change your expression or make you look happy. You have to do that for yourself.

Side Effects and Complications

Side Effects

Minor side effects are legion after a facelift, as you would expect. After all, your face has been dramatically tightened in many layers and areas. You may have firm, lumpy scars behind your ear or in your back hairline for as long as 3, 6, or even 12 months. Scars can usually be hidden by your hair—but you will *feel* them, and that will be bothersome. Your neck may feel tight. Your face and neck skin will be numb, with most of the feeling back by 6 weeks, but sometimes numb patches on or close to the ear remaining for a year. Occasionally, feeling will not return to a numb patch. Your temple hair may shed so much hair at once after surgery that it will be noticeably thinner, and the full thickness of your hair may not return for as long as a year. The skin on your face will feel dry. If your surgery is done in winter, you may find that you need moisturizer on your face when you have never needed it before, or—if you don't want to use moisturizer—that you need to run a humidifier in your room at night to keep your skin from feeling dry in the morning. People who live in hot but *dry* climates may notice the same problem as those who live in heated buildings. Because surgery irritates your skin and makes it swell, the texture of your skin may feel firm or tough to you, noticeably for 6 weeks, but not returning to its normal softness for 3 to 6 months. You may feel—or even see—ridges or cords of swelling in your neck and lower face until the swelling is completely gone, around 6 months after surgery. The sideburn area of hair in front of your ears will be narrower after surgery, and set closer to your ear from being pulled taut. The scar under your chin may indent slightly, creating a little valley just behind your chin that shows up on profile. This may bother you, and if it does not soften after 6 or 12 months, it may need minor surgery to correct it. A very tight pull in your upper face may give round eyes a faint almond shape for up to a year, until all the swelling is gone. Even perfect scars may be noticeable in some people—a thin white or pink line can show by contrast in people with ruddy, sallow, or tanned skin. Behind your ears, the scars may widen or move lower, becoming visible at certain angles or with certain hairstyles. These side effects are the reason that facelift recovery takes emotional stamina. Many patients who think it would be preposterous to be bothered by a scar you can only feel, not see, find that after surgery, to their surprise, they are like other people and rub and worry about that lumpy scar even though they *know* they were told it might occur and would flatten in time. Most people nevertheless find that these annoying side effects are a small price to pay for the results. As time goes by, the results show more and the side effects bother you less, as they diminish.

Complications

The complications of facelift surgery are similar in kind to the side effects, except that they are unusually severe or leave permanent or prolonged traces. For instance, instead of just numbness from bruised nerves in your facial skin, you may have bruising around the nerve to your lower lip. This nerve *moves* your lower lip, and when it is bruised, your lower lip on that side will not move with the other side when you smile. The nerve virtually always recovers, but it can take two years for lip motion to return.

Another complication would be postsurgical bleeding that leaves not only bruising but a tablespoon-sized blood clot, as well. This might require three or four extra visits to your surgeon so that he could draw off the blood clot with a small needle as it became liquid. (Fortunately, your skin is usually numb, so the needles don't hurt.) If the blood is not drawn off, you may have a thick lump of scar where the clot formed for a year or even two. Even if the clot is drawn off, thicker skin will tend to persist where the blood collected.

The complications that your surgeon worries most about are major bleeding, nerve damage, or poor healing. The bleeding problem would require re-operation to drain the blood and to stop the bleeding. The poor healing could require re-operation if a large (inch or more) area of skin would not heal. The nerve injury might require re-operation if the muscles of your face did not move properly and showed no sign of recovery. All of these occur rarely, unpredictably, and unavoidably. Although it seems evident that bleeding or poor healing might be uncontrollable, most people think that nerve damage would obviously be the surgeon's *fault*—but not necessarily so. We know where the nerves are supposed to lie, but some nerves travel in unusual places or are unusually sensitive to bruising. Thus, in 50 people a nerve bruised from nearby surgery would still work perfectly, but in the 51st person a nerve malfunction might develop after exactly the same operation.

These serious major complications are intimidating if you are considering surgery, but that is true if you look into the rare, potential problems of doing almost anything at all.

John: No Longer His Wife's "Father"

John, a businessman of 50, decided to have his face lifted and his upper and lower lids done at the same time. Divorced some years ago and recently remarried, he seemed uncomfortable talking about his new wife. She did not come with him to my office. John's surgery went well, except for an infection behind one ear which probably started when he scratched under his bandage with a pencil to soothe an itching stitch. The infection only needed local care and was healed in 2 weeks. Before his surgery, John looked much older than 50. Afterwards, he looked quite good for his age. John's wife came along for his six-week visit. She was not much younger than he was, but she was extremely beautiful and looked much younger than her age. At this visit, John was content and relaxed for the first time that he had seen me. He and his wife told me—jokingly, but it was clearly important to John—that at a recent convention, she and John had gone together, as usual, but this time no new acquaintance had asked to be introduced to John's "daughter"!

Georgina: A Psychological Lift

Georgina, a guidance counselor, had been married and had children, but she had been divorced for a number of years. As a young woman, she had had a double chin, even when she was thin. But by the time Georgina was in her early forties, that double chin, combined with the early skin-loosening that ran in her family, made her look faded, worn, and nondescript. She had a facelift combined with upper lid surgery to correct excess skin drooping across her lids.

After her surgery, Georgina had a minor complication—a blood clot formed on one side in her upper neck below her ear. It delayed her return to work for 3 days, and it also required several office visits to draw off the blood, so that it would not leave a lumpy scar. Despite this, Georgina arranged interviews for a new job—and got a good job offer 2 weeks after her surgery. Even before the swelling and bruising were gone, I could tell that the surgery had done something for her, psychologically as well as physically. Georgina was delighted with what her operation had done for her: she had a nice profile for the first time in her life and looked attractive and youthful for her age. She told me after she healed that the surgery not only helped her feel "worthy" of her new boyfriend, but it put to rest, for good, her feelings of ugliness and worthlessness that had been traced back, during therapy, to episodes of sexual abuse she suffered as a child. For her, the surgery was not only correction of her physical appearance but also the last stage in her recovery from emotional trauma.

Sue-Ann: A Bothersome Scar

Sue-Ann was a 59-year-old retired government employee who had been widowed several years before. She asked me if she was too "plain" to have a facelift. She said that she had always been plain, but time and widowhood had made her look even worse. After studying her face together, she and I agreed that besides a facelift, she would benefit from having her lower lid bags removed and her broad, bumpy nose made smaller and straight. (Her upper lids were fine.)

Sue-Ann had her surgery and recovered easily. She was bothered by the scar behind one ear, which shrank, pulling her earlobe slightly to one side. I did minor scar revision in the office 3 months after her surgery to correct this. Sue-Ann was honest about herself—she was unusually plain. Even so, surgery made a big difference in the way she looked. Besides having her bags smoothed, her nose improved, and her face looking good for 59, she also began to walk straight instead of stooped over. I didn't ask her about this, but she volunteered that she no longer felt that she had to hide her face. "I can enjoy kids again," she told me. "I don't feel too old to play with them, anymore."

Norman: A New Outlook

Norman, in his midforties, was engaged to be married for the second time. He decided to have surgery before his marriage—and it turned out to be fairly extensive. In addition to his facelift, he had hair transplants, upper and lower lid surgery, and nose surgery. He was a very fast healer and had no complications—not even the usual annoying side effects. He was very pleased. In fact, he was so pleased with the way he looked that he decided not to get married. He discovered after his surgery that he had been looking for his fiancée to be his reassurance that he was still attractive. Looking so good after surgery, he didn't "need" her anymore—a discovery that came in time to save both of them a lot of emotional pain from an unsuitable marriage.

Nina: A Necklift Was Enough

Nina was in her late thirties when she came to me for her facelift. She had married in her teens, and her first child was about to go on to college. Nina had been very fat 20 years earlier but had lost the weight. The weight loss, combined with time, had made her face skin loosen much earlier than most people's. She told me that her husband thought she was "nuts" to have surgery but that she couldn't stand looking "so blah" at such a young age.

Nina only wanted a necklift—and that was all she needed. The rest of her face had not been stretched by her teenage obesity and had retained its elasticity. Her necklift surgery was quite extensive: she had a thick residual layer of fat in her neck and the skin was very lax.

Nina was very bruised after her surgery and had two ridges in her upper neck from swelling where the skin had been lifted and the fat trimmed away. She could feel them—and sometimes see them —and they took 6 months to flatten. Even so, she seemed happy and less bothered about the temporary ridging than many patients are. She looked her age instead of 10 years older. A month after her final visit, Nina's father called me. He said that he wanted me to know that Nina's husband had always been good to her, and faithful, but that since Nina's surgery, he was looking at Nina "like he's seeing a new person—a woman, not just a wife, if you know what I mean."

What Other Patients Say

- **Grandmother, 62:** "The drains shocked me, really. I've never had anything under my skin before. I took time to heal. Six months was on the short side for me, but that was four years ago and I still look great, so I have no complaints about the end result."

- **Salesman, 46:** "My kids laughed at me. I had the facelift for my job. The younger guys made me nervous. I look better, but it wasn't like day or night for me. But now I don't worry about the younger guys. I guess that got cut out along with the rest of my face."

- **Grandmother, 75:** "I needed two operations. I hadn't had facial surgery before. It was a lot to go through and it couldn't work miracles, but I like what it did for me."
- **Executive, 60:** "My wife and I had this done at the same time, so we wouldn't be jealous of each other. My skin took a year to get all the feeling back, but it took ten years off me by fixing my neck."
- **Male scientist, 40:** "I knew I wanted this done, and I had to push for it because I was on the young side for a facelift. It didn't take a year off my face but I look great and I'm signing up for another the minute I turn 50, whether I need it or not."
- **Housewife, 50:** "I looked terrible before the surgery, I thought, and my husband thought I was just silly to have this done, but I look good now. I can dress up and feel my face doesn't clash with my clothes and my husband is simply green with envy and now he's talking about having one done, as though no one in the family thought of it before!"
- **Male space engineer, 43:** "Overall—good. I rate my neck an A—no loose skin. I rate my face a B to B+—it wasn't so bad to begin with and the change isn't so great. I rate my scars a B. They get red when I work out or if I take a hot shower. I can't see behind my ears, so I don't know how to grade the scars back there. No one else looks behind my ears either, so I don't see that it matters."
- **Actress, 49:** "It worked! People *believe* me now when I lie about my age."

Cosmetic Upper Eyelid Surgery

What Surgeons Call It

This procedure is called an upper lid blepharoplasty, from the Greek words for "eyelid" and "to mold or shape."

What It Will Do

Upper lid surgery will make your eyes look brighter, larger, and more rested by removing loose skin, stretched muscle, and excess fat. It should give you visible eyelid above the lashes, so that eyeshadow will show. Your eyes will look more youthful, because loosened skin and muscle are associated in people's minds with old age.

What It Won't Do

Upper lid surgery will *not* erase, remove, or change the wrinkles and crow's feet at the corners of your eyes. Also, it won't lift your brow. (If your eyebrows are heavy and hang down over your eyes, see Brow Lift.) It won't make your eyes symmetrical, and with the excess skin gone, you may notice asymmetry in your upper lids that you didn't see before.

How Long It Will Last

The results tend to be long lasting. Over time—10 years or more—the skin *may* become loose again and you may need a re-operation. On the other hand, your results may be virtually permanent.

When to Have It

You can need upper eyelid surgery in your teens, if droopy upper lids appear. This may run in your family. However, most drooping lids tend to occur with age. Thus it is most common to have the surgery between 38 and 50. Often the surgery is done at the same time as a facelift; however, about half the people who have their upper lids done require this operation 5 to 10 years before they need a face-neck lift.

Where to Have It

Upper eyelid surgery is usually done on an outpatient basis in a doctor's office operating room *or* an outpatient surgery center *or* a hospital outpatient operating room. An overnight hospital stay is rarely needed.

Conditions That Increase Your Risk

Note: All three of these factors are important because they can lead to irritation of or pressure on the nerve of vision (the optic nerve).

Any **underlying eye disease** increases your risk because a surgical complication might worsen the eye disease. If you have any **bleeding tendency**, your risk is slightly raised, because bleeding around the eye after surgery can injure the nerve of vision, causing a temporary, or even permanent, change in vision. **High blood pressure increases** your risk because you are more likely to bleed if your pressure is high. This happens because high blood pressure can dislodge tiny blood clots, leading to renewed bleeding or more extensive bruising.

Usual Anesthesia

A local with sedation, given by your surgeon, is usually used for upper eyelid surgery. Even though you will be fairly heavily sedated, and the area will be numbed with local anesthesia, you may feel a pull, or even a sharp pain, when the excess fat is cut away. The nerves around the fat may still be able to detect the pulling as painful. This pain, if it occurs, is very brief.

How Long It Takes

Upper eyelid operations usually take 1 to 1½ hours. The most important factor is bleeding. If the blood vessels in your tissues are tiny and therefore don't bleed much, surgery can proceed rapidly. However, *all* bleeding around the eye must be stopped. So your surgery could be prolonged, if you have large veins.

The Operation

(Figures 11-6 through 11-9)

If you are having *only* eyelid surgery, it will almost certainly be done under local anesthesia with sedation. Since it is fairly easy to numb your upper lids, this procedure can even be done in a minor operating room—if your sedation is light so your recovery time is short.

Before

You will arrive about an hour before your surgery is scheduled. Usually, you will have had nothing to eat or drink after midnight the night before. If your sedation is to be light and your surgery is scheduled for the afternoon, you may have been allowed to have a light breakfast. You will change into a hospital gown, then go to a preoperative area or directly to the operating room.

In the operating room, you will be helped onto the operating table, and a safety strap will be placed across your hips. Your surgeon may make surgical markings in purple surgical ink now, or he may wait until just before your surgery, since these marks can smudge when you open and close your eyes. An IV will be placed in your arm so that you can be given a solution of sugar and/or saline to prevent dehydration during surgery. Your sedation may be given through the IV, or you may be given sedation by mouth if that is what you and your surgeon decided was right for you. Sticky pads will be put on your chest to monitor your heart. (They may not be used if you are having light sedation by mouth.) A sticky pad will also be put on your hip (under your gown) to serve as a ground so that surgical cautery can be safely used. (Surgical cautery means using an electrical instrument to seal off blood vessels and stop bleeding.)

Your face will be washed with surgical soap, and sterile drapes will be put around your face and over your body. If your sedation is light, you can talk and your surgeon and his nurses will talk to you to reassure you.

Next, your surgeon will cover one eye while he does the markings on the other, if he has not already done them. This will feel scratchy on your upper lids but won't hurt.

If you are having intravenous sedation, you will now be given enough sedation to make you relax—or even doze off, depending on what is best for you. Next, your surgeon will take a tiny needle and inject a drop of local anesthetic at the corner of either lid. Then, working from this one numb dot, he will slowly inject more anesthetic until your lids are numb. One eye is covered while your surgeon works on the other one. If you are lightly sedated you may feel faint pressure or pulling.

During

Following the curve of your eye, the surgeon will remove the stretched muscle and excess skin, starting from the inner corner and ending at the outer corner or just beyond. Under these muscle fibers lie the fat deposits at the inner and middle upper lid. Your surgeon will gently coax the bulging fat out and remove the excess. He *won't* try to remove all the fat, since it is needed as a shock absorber for your eye. Also, removing too much fat can make your eye look sunken.

The fat at the middle of the eyelid is easier to remove because it lies right under the muscle. If you are lightly sedated you may feel pressure as your surgeon works on the inner fat, which is deeper and a little harder to reach. The fat is numbed with local anesthetic before it is removed; even so, you may feel stinging as it is trimmed.

There are little variations in upper eyelid surgery that your surgeon may or may not do. If your brows are heavy, he may put a stitch or two in the muscle behind the eyebrow to give it a little lift. If the weight of the tear gland at the outer part of your eye is helping to make your eyelids sag, he may put in a stitch to support the tear gland. These are technical variations.

The next step is to be sure that all the bleeding has stopped. Finally, your surgeon will sew the incision closed with fine thread (sutures) of silk or nylon. A cold compress of gauze soaked in ice water is put over that eye, and your surgeon does the other upper lid.

After

You will be in the recovery room for about an hour—perhaps more if you were heavily sedated. You are then allowed to go home—to go to bed, keeping ice or cold compresses over your eyes.

Cosmetic Upper Eyelid Surgery

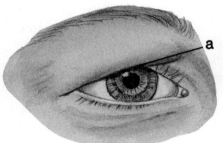

Figure 11-6.

Before upper eyelid surgery, the excess skin hangs over the lids (a), sometimes concealing much of the eyelash line.

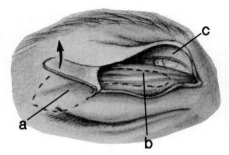

Figure 11-7.

The first step of surgery is to remove the excess skin (a). The stretched muscle fibers under the skin (b) are also removed. Under the muscle you can see the inner (medial) area (c) of excess fat.

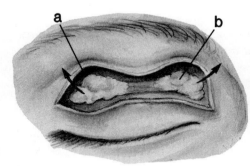

Figure 11-8.

The largest amount of excess fat usually is seen in the outer eyelid (a). The inner, or medial, area (b) tends to have less fat, but it can form a noticeable bulge at the inner corner of the eyelid.

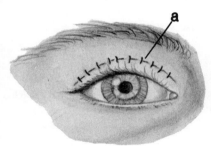

Figure 11-9.

After surgery the scar lies in the natural crease line of the upper lid—virtually invisible (a).

The Process of Recovery

What to Do About Pain

Your upper lids may ache, starting an hour or so after surgery. Bending over may make them throb. Severe pain or intense throbbing is very rare, and *you should call your doctor* to alert him if this occurs. Possible reasons for severe pain include a bandage that is too snug, a stitch that has come out, or unexpected bleeding.

The Healing Process

Your upper lids will be swollen and sore for about 5 days. Bruising varies greatly, from minor (gone in 7 days) in one person to major (traces lasting up to 1 month) in another. Your eyes will be sensitive to light, wind, and dust for 2 to 4 weeks. Your upper lids may be irritated and teary for about 14 days. Because your eyes will be irritated easily, and to avoid pulling on the surgical incision, you will not be able to wear contact lenses for about 10 to 14 days. Usually, you see your surgeon again on days 3 and 6 and then 2 weeks and 4 weeks after the operation.

Bandages

Bandaging is usually tape or a little strip of gauze over your stitches. Some surgeons will bandage your upper face with an Ace bandage and keep you in bed for the first 24 hours after surgery to rest your eyes. However, the trend is away from this, because it seems to be unnecessary.

Taking Care of Your Wound

You will want to avoid anything that could irritate your eyes. You should not use eye makeup for 7 to 10 days. Eyedrops such as Natural Tears may be soothing if your eyes burn, itch, or feel gritty. This usually improves once the stitches are removed (day 3-5). If your eyes tend to be dry, use a lubricant such as Lacrilube at night. If your eyes are dry, their natural secretions will be thicker than usual, and you'll wake up with gummy eyes. The lubricant helps prevent this. If your lashes or your incisions build up crusts in the first week or so after surgery, you can cleanse them three or four times a day with water, eye makeup remover, or Lacrilube. Simply put a drop on a cotton swab and gently coat the crust. With each application crusts soften, loosen, and fewer will form.

Using cold packs on your eyes in the first 24 hours after surgery will reduce bruising (see Tips), but you may want to use cold packs for a week or two, in the evenings, for an hour or so. Your eyes will feel sore by the end of the day.

Stitches

Your stitches will be removed by your surgeon, or his nurse, 2 to 5 days after the operation, depending on the kind of stitches used. This will sting a bit.

Scars

The scar from an upper lid operation will be a fine line that lies in your upper lid crease. It may extend slightly beyond the outer corner of your eye.

Tips

- To keep your eyes cold after surgery, you can use tea bags, small plastic bags, or commercial eye packs.
- **Tea bags:** Before going for your surgery freeze a supply of wet tea bags. Tannin, a natural chemical in tea, helps combat swelling. A tea bag is just the right size to fit over one eye. When it melts, refreeze or discard it and apply another set. If tea bags feel *too* cold, put gauze pads between your eyes and the tea bags.
- **Plastic bags:** Buy a box of the smallest Ziploc plastic bags. Like tea bags, they're the right size to lie comfortably over an eye. Half-fill the bags with water and freeze. After surgery, place a frozen Ziploc bag over each eye to keep the surgical area cold. When the ice melts, discard the bag or refreeze to use later. If the bag feels *too* cold, place a layer of gauze between your eyelid and the bag.
- **Commercial packs:** Commercial packs are more expensive than tea bags or plastic bags, but they don't involve work for you. You will need to buy at least two sets—one to use and one to freeze.
- You will want to conceal, as much as possible, the telltale signs of surgery:

- *Lightly* tinted glasses conceal your eyes without looking stagey. You can use them if you *don't* normally wear glasses. Besides, your eyes will be slightly light-sensitive after surgery, and lightly tinted glasses will make them more comfortable.
- If bruises appear on your cheeks, you can camouflage them with pancake makeup or concealer cream. Virtually all makeup lines now make an opaque concealer cream or concealer stick. Most men don't mind using this technique.

Back to Work

Most people feel and look ready to work about 1 week after surgery. However, if you're extensively bruised or more than normally self-conscious about the surgery, you may decide to stay out of the public view for a few days longer—as about one-quarter of patients do. Even after 2 weeks, you may find that, although you are *much better than you were,* your upper lids still feel stiff and sore.

Cosmetic Upper Eyelid Surgery: Recovery-at-a-Glance

This chart represents the *average* recovery times for this cosmetic operation.

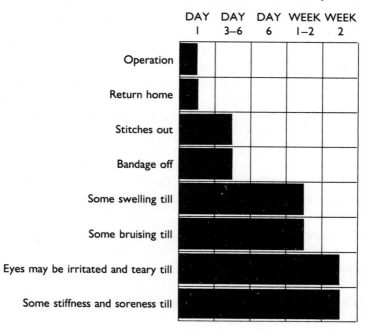

Back to Parties

You can usually count on looking and feeling right for a party 2 weeks after upper lid surgery. If you aren't self-conscious and don't mind people noticing and commenting on your surgery, you *might* feel like a party as early as 1 week, but the late night (and alcohol) may leave you tired and may make your eyes swell the next day. If you want to be *absolutely* safe, postpone parties for 3 weeks.

Back to Sex

Your sutures are removed within a few days, so even a minor blow to your face could pull the fragile eyelid skin apart. This would give you a wide or thick scar. Postpone sex for at least 10 days.

Back to Sports

You can begin stretching exercises at the end of a week, but don't do bending or lifting. It will make your eyes ache and swell. After 2 weeks you can resume swimming, aerobics, and other sports—but not ball sports. (An exception is tennis. You can play a baseline game, but you should not play at net yet.) After 3 weeks you can resume all sports, but start slowly and build up. You will not have your presurgery endurance at first.

How Much It Costs

Your estimated cost for upper lid surgery will be $1000 to $2000 for the *surgeon's fee* and $500 to $1000 for the operating room and anesthesia. Remember, prices vary, being higher in large cities, lower in rural areas, and rising every year.

Insurance Coverage

Insurance will *rarely* pay for eyelid surgery, but it *might* if you can show that your eyelid skin droops so much that it blocks your vision. If your excess skin droops to the lashes and beyond the edge of your eye, it's reasonable to pursue insurance, but if it doesn't even come to your lashes, don't waste your time. Your insurance company is unlikely to take your word that your vision is blocked, so have an ophthalmologist (eye doctor) test the visual fields of your eyes. This testing—done in his office with you looking at a chart—will show if your vision is hampered. His results plus a photograph of your eyes should be submitted to your insurance company *before* your surgery. Request a written reply as to how much you're insurance will pay, if they say they will "cover" your surgery. It may take 4 to 6 weeks to get your answer.

My Assessment of This Procedure

Eyelid surgery is one of the easiest operations for you to undergo: your recovery is fast. Even with the swelling, you can see the improvement a week after surgery. You will have little or no pain. The telltale signs of surgery are easily hidden. The operation is well designed to correct the tissues that are directly causing the problem.

Side Effects and Complications

Side Effects

A number of surprising or annoying side effects can result from upper eyelid surgery. Your upper lid may be numb for about 6 weeks, so that you can't put on makeup without looking in the mirror. Also, your eyelid scars feel firm and stiff. These scars soften quickly, but it will be about 6 weeks before they feel normal. Tiny white dots called milia may appear where one or more stitches were placed. These may take 2 weeks to appear and another 6 weeks to absorb. One eye may seem to heal faster, with less bruising and swelling, and you will be impatient with the slowness of the other side. Also, swelling at the inner corner of your eye, where the scar ends, may take 6 weeks or longer to smooth out completely. In the meantime, you have a faint fullness in the inner corner of your lid that no one comments on but that *you* don't like. I have seen several "glamour" photographs of celebrities in which I can spot the same telltale fullness—but when I've pointed it out to patients, they've had trouble seeing what I'm talking about. However, when it is on *your* face, you will see it.

Complications

Complications include red, swollen, or visible scars. These are unusual but distressing and usually fade within 3 months. Bleeding, poor healing, and infection are extraordinarily rare. Your tear glands may temporarily produce fewer tears, leaving you with dry or irritated eyes. This effect may last several *months* or in a few cases, may make eye lubricants necessary, indefinitely.

Perhaps 5 to 10 percent of the time, a scar does not lie completely flat. Minor correction can usually be done in the doctor's office, but in about 1 percent of cases, poor healing makes more extensive surgery necessary.

There is a rare possibility after *any* eye surgery or treatment that bleeding will irritate your nerve of vision and cause permanent damage to your vision. Anything that could affect our vision sounds alarming. To put it in perspective: it is much more hazardous to cross a street or drive a car than to have eye surgery.

Cora: Allergy Caused a Problem

Cora was a lovely woman in her forties. She had raised her family, embarked on a career, and solved, painfully, some marital problems. Her reward to herself was to have her upper lids done. They were heavy and saggy, especially compared to the rest of her face, which was youthful.

Cora had her surgery, which went well. After her surgery she developed swelling that was painless but much worse than most eyelid swelling. After trying various treatments, I realized that she was allergic to the ointment she was using to keep her eyes lubricated. We stopped the medication, and she had a perfect result. Cora confided in me that during the 3 days of severe swelling, if it weren't for her eye surgery, she'd have been in tears. "You have no idea how frustrating it is when you aren't even allowed to cry," she said, laughing, when it was over. Her eyelids were not permanently stretched by the swelling and her eyes looked bright and natural 2 weeks after her surgery. She was back to work 5 days after surgery, despite the swelling.

Rodney: No Longer a Grouch

Rodney was a successful middle-aged businessman. He didn't approve of cosmetic surgery—until his girlfriend, who was 5 years younger than he was, had a facelift. Then Rodney decided he had to have cosmetic surgery to keep up with her. His eyes were very tired looking. He worked long hours and had been a heavy drinker in the past. He was the strong, silent type and said little about his surgery until he was completely healed. At his last visit, he shook my hand and said, "Doctor, I felt stupid doing this in the first place. Now I feel stupid about feeling stupid—you don't know what a difference this makes. I don't look like a grouch anymore so I'm not acting like such a grouch. Explain that one!"

Effie: "Something Went Right at Last!"

Effie was in her midtwenties. Heavy upper lids ran in her family. In addition, she had lived a wild life as a teenager. "Drugs, drink—I did it all," she told me. "Can you erase it?" Effie had a lovely face, but her eyes made her look sad. She had upper lid surgery and had surgery on her nose at the same time. A week later I got an emergency call from her. "My eyelids are numb," she told me. "Tell me the worst." I explained that the numbness was normal—she had forgotten about it. Then she said, "Not only can I see my eyes for the first time in years, but it could be the first thing that ever went right in my life."

Sharon: An Early Psyche-Lift

Sharon was in her late forties when she decided to have her facelift, upper lids, lower lids, chin, and the tip of her nose all done. She was starting her life over as a single woman after a divorce. "My kids are all for it," she told me. "And I've been waiting for this for years."

Sharon had her surgery, and her son and daughter took turns nursing her afterwards. When she came to the office 5 days later to have some stitches out, she surveyed her face carefully in the mirror. "I can see what my face will be like," she said thoughtfully, "but it will take time. My eyes are perfect right now. That'll get me over the waiting period." (When you have a facelift and eye surgery at the same time, the fast healing and early visible good results from the eyelid surgery bolster your psyche while you wait for the longer facelift healing time.)

Tom: A Problem That Solved Itself

Tom was a pilot who had eyelid surgery during a stopover on one of his regular flights. He wanted to surprise his kids, who teased him about his eyes. Tom came into my office 2 weeks later in a state of shock—both his scars showed as a vermilion line above the natural crease. I wasn't sure exactly how this had happened: his surgeon either removed a fraction too much skin or muscle and/or made the incision a little too high. Regardless, I could tell Tom it would fade. It did. This disappointing result took care of itself. The scar was unnoticeable 2 months later without any treatment.

Jessie: Surgery Opened Her Eyes

Jessie was a teenager with heavy upper lids. They were typical of her family but she disliked them—largely because they reminded her of surgery she had had on her eyes as a child, which had frightened her. Jessie's mother thought that eye surgery could not be done until Jessie was at least 40. I explained that that was not the case. Jessie had her upper lid surgery done as an outpatient under local anesthesia. I removed a lot of excess fat in her upper lids. "I have never seen her so happy," said her mother afterwards. "She would never go to parties with her friends. Now she will—it seemed to open her up to people."

What Other Patients Say

- **Teacher, 26:** "My eyes were dry for a month, which worried me, but apart from that I had no problem. I look like 'me' again."
- **Female economist, 62:** "I had a facelift plus a brow lift. None of my friends can tell what happened to me. They all say it must have been my Caribbean vacation."
- **Manufacturer, 59:** "I had both upper and lower lid surgery. It opened my eyes—literally."
- **Real estate saleswoman, 45:** "I was sure I would go blind from this surgery. I'm just a pessimist. I didn't, of course. My eyes look bright again."
- **Female research scientist, 50:** "I had a facelift, a chin implant, and upper lid surgery. Frankly, I looked a wreck before the surgery. It all made a world of difference but the first thing everybody noticed was my eyes. They kept looking at me as though they'd never seen me before."
- **Social worker, 70:** "My eyes are sensitive. The stitches made my eyes tear until they came out. I wanted to rub my eyes, but I couldn't. I can't say surgery was fun. I didn't want a radical change but I wanted to look better. I needed a minor correction of my scar 6 months later. I'm pleased."

Cosmetic Lower Eyelid Surgery

What Surgeons Call It

The operation is known technically as a lower lid blepharoplasty.

What It Will Do

Cosmetic surgery of your lower lids should smooth out bulges, take away bags from under your eyes, and make the skin snugger. You'll look rested, and people will see your face instead of focusing on your unsightly lower lids.

What It Won't Do

This operation cannot remove wrinkles or "laugh lines," which are in the skin. Surgery can't remove this skin (or you would have no lower lid!). Nor can it pull the skin tight enough to flatten the wrinkles and lines, since pulling on the lower lid skin pulls the lid *down*, not the skin *up*. Surgery will correct the appearance of your *lower lids only*. Some people, especially those with allergies, have pockets of puffiness or bulging over the cheekbones, but so far there's no operation that can predictably improve this.

How Long It Will Last

Lower lid surgery tends to yield permanent or very long-lasting results. In time, the skin of the lower lid *may* become loose again or a bulge may reappear. If a small residual bulge remained, as does occur, it may in time become noticeable. Reoperation is generally not for ten years after successful surgery, if at all.

When to Have It

If it seems that you were born with bags and bulges under your eyes, there is no reason to delay surgery, even if you are a teenager. But if you always had smooth lower lids and are now noticing some changes with age—wait until the changes are marked enough to warrant surgery. A faint bulge that you can barely see after a late night is probably not enough to justify surgery yet.

Where to Have It

Lower lid surgery may be done in your surgeon's office operating room *or* an outpatient surgery center *or* a hospital's outpatient operating room. For this operation, an overnight hospital stay is rarely needed.

Conditions That Increase Your Risk

Note: All three of these factors are important because they may lead to irritation of the nerve of vision (the optic nerve) or put pressure on it. These conditions could affect your sight. If you have any **underlying eye disease**, your risk is higher because a surgical complication might worsen the eye disease. If you have any **bleeding tendency**, your risk is also slightly raised, because bleeding around the eye after surgery has been known to injure the nerve of vision, causing a temporary or even permanent change in vision. **High blood pressure** increases your risk, because you are somewhat more likely to bleed if your pressure is high. The high blood pressure may dislodge tiny blood clots so that you have renewed bleeding or more extensive bruising.

Usual Anesthesia

Local with sedation, given by your surgeon. Despite fairly heavy sedation, you may feel a pull, or sharp pain, when the excess fat is cut away, even when you are sedated and the fat is numbed with local anesthetic. This pain, if it occurs, is very brief.

How Long It Takes

Lower lid surgery tends to take 1 to 1½ hours. The most important factor is bleeding—if you have tiny blood vessels that don't bleed, surgery can proceed rapidly. However, *all* bleeding around the eye must be stopped. So your surgery could be prolonged, because you have large veins.

The Operation

(Figures 11-10 through 11-12)

Before

Lower lid surgery is usually done on an outpatient basis. You will arrive for your surgery about an hour in advance, having had nothing to eat or drink after midnight the night before. After you change into a hospital gown, you may be taken to a preoperative area where an IV will be placed in your arm so that you can be given a solution of saline and/or dextrose to keep you from getting dehydrated during surgery. The IV is also used to give you sedation. *Or,* you may be taken directly to the operating room, where the IV and sedation will be started immediately before surgery. Once you are on the operating table, a safety strap is placed across your hips, just like a seatbelt. The IV is placed in your arm (unless this was already done), and sticky pads are placed on your chest under your gown, so that your heart can be monitored. A blood pressure cuff is put around one upper arm to monitor your blood pressure during surgery. Finally, another sticky pad is placed on your hip or thigh. This is a grounding pad, so that surgical cautery can be safely used. (Surgical cautery consists of using an electrical instrument to seal off blood vessels and stop bleeding.)

You will probably be given a *small* dose of sedation first through the IV line to see how you react. Then your face is washed with surgical soap and sterile drapes are placed around your face and over your body. Shortly before the surgery, you will be given more sedation, until you are in a dreamlike or trancelike state. Local anesthetic is then injected with a tiny needle into the skin of your lower lids. Your eyes are covered and protected from the surgery by a special surgical contact lens, or by using a fine stitch to lift the lower lid up over the eye to cover it. You can *not* see the surgery.

During

Once your lids are numb, your surgeon will begin to operate. You may feel pulling, but no pain at this point. First, he cuts through the delicate lower lid skin. Next he lifts some of the skin off the underlying muscle. Then he separates the muscle fibers

Cosmetic Lower Eyelid Surgery

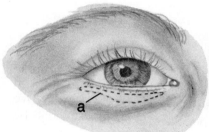

Figure 11-10.

The lower lid surgery removes only a small amount of skin. The incision is made just under the lashes. The dotted lines (a) show how much skin (at most) might be removed.

Figure 11-11.

The skin is lifted off. The "a" marks the muscle layer under the skin. The most important part of the surgery is removing the excess fat, which lies below the skin (b).

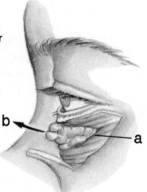

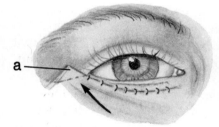

Figure 11-12.

The skin is pulled up and to the side so that the excess can be removed at the side of the eye (a) to avoid puckering of the incision under the eye.

to get to the fat deposits beneath the muscle. There are three areas of excess fat: an inner area, a middle area, and an outer area. *Most* of the excess is in the middle area. Each area of fat is gently freed, so that *only the excess* is removed, to avoid a sunken look around your eyes after surgery. You may be aware of a sharp stinging pain when the fat is cut, although extra local anesthetic and extra sedation are usually all you need to stay comfortable. Once the fat is removed, the excess muscle and the excess skin are trimmed also.

The sedation will gradually wear off, so after your surgeon has finished the operation on the first eye, you are usually given extra sedation to help you through the surgery on the other eye.

After

When the operation is over, cold packs are placed over your eyes to minimize bruising (see Tips). All the sticky pads are removed. You are taken by stretcher to the recovery room, where you may doze off for a while. You may need to urinate because of the extra fluid in your system from the IV. If so, the cold packs are removed, temporarily.

If your surgeon has recommended that you stay in hospital overnight, you will next be taken to your hospital room, but this is not common. Most of the time, once you are alert—about an hour after surgery—you can be taken home. At home, you go directly to bed to rest, and keep cold packs over your eyes.

The Process of Recovery

What to Do About Pain

Your lower lids will ache, starting an hour or so after surgery. Bending over may make them throb. Severe pain or intense throbbing is very rare, and you should call your doctor if this occurs. Possible reasons for such pain include a bandage that is too snug, a suture that has come out, or unexpected bleeding.

The Healing Process

Your lower lids will be swollen and sore for about 5 to 7 days. Bruising varies greatly, from minor (gone in 7 days) in one person to major (traces lasting up to 1 month) in another. Your eyes will be sensitive to light, wind, and dust for 2 to 4 weeks. The swelling of your lower lids may make your eyes irritated and teary for about 2 weeks. Because your eyes will be irritated easily, and to avoid pulling on the surgical incision, you will not be able to wear contact lenses for about 10 to 14 days.

Bandages

Bandaging is usually limited to tape or a strip of gauze over your stitches. Some surgeons will bandage your upper face with an elastic bandage and keep you in bed for the first 24 hours after surgery to rest your eyes. The trend is away from this, because it seems to be unnecessary.

Taking Care of Your Wound

You will want to avoid anything that irritates your eyes. You should not use eye makeup for 7 to 10 days. You may find eyedrops such as Natural Tears to be soothing if your eyes burn or itch or feel gritty. This usually improves once the stitches are removed (2 to 5 days after surgery). If your eyes tend to be dry, a lubricant such as Lacrilube should be used at night. This also helps if you wake up with "gummy" eyes, which mean that your natural eye secretions are thick because your eyes are dry. The lubricant will help counteract this temporary condition. If your lashes or your incisions build up crusts, which they may in the first week or so after surgery, you can clean them three or four times a day with water, eye makeup remover, or Lacrilube. Simply put a drop on a cotton swab and gently coat the crust. With each application, crusts will loosen and fewer, if any, will form. Cold packs on your eyes in the first 24 hours after surgery will help reduce bruising, but you may want to use cold packs for a week or two, in the evenings, for an hour or so. Your eyes will feel sore by the end of the day.

Stitches

The stitches are removed by your surgeon, or his nurse, on days 3 to 6 after your surgery.

Scars

The scar from this operation will be a fine line that lies under your lower lid lashes. It extends slightly beyond the lashes at the outer corner of your eye.

Tips

- You need to keep your eyes cold after surgery. You can use tea bags, plastic bags, or commercial eye packs.
- **Tea bags:** Before your operation, freeze wet tea bags. Tannin, a natural chemical in tea, helps combat swelling. The size of a tea bag is just right to fit over one eye. When you get home, place a frozen tea bag over each eye. When it melts, refreeze or

discard it, and apply another set. If tea bags feel *too* cold, put a gauze pad between your eyes and the tea bag.

- **Plastic bags:** Buy a box of the smallest Ziploc plastic bags. Like tea bags, these are the right size to lie comfortably over an eye. Half-fill the bags with water and freeze. After surgery, place a frozen Ziploc bag over each eye to keep the surgical area cold. When the ice melts, either discard the bag or re-freeze to use later. If the bag feels *too* cold, place a layer of gauze between your eyelid and the bag.
- **Commercial eye packs:** These are more expensive than the previous methods, but they don't involve any work for you. Buy at least two sets, one to use for your eyes and one to freeze for future use.
- You will want to conceal, as much as possible, the telltale signs of surgery. You can do this best by the following methods.
- Wear *lightly* tinted glasses to conceal your eyes without looking fake. You can do this even if you *don't* normally wear glasses. An added plus is that your eyes will be slightly light-sensitive after surgery, and lightly tinted glasses will make them more comfortable.
- You can cover the scars (they lie under your lower-lid lashes) with mascara. Your lashes are longer than they look, because the tips of eyelashes have little color. Thus when lashes are darkened with mascara, they will conceal the scar which lies beneath them. Although men *could* use this technique, most won't unless they have experience with stage makeup. (It is unappealing to most men.)
- You can camouflage the bruises on your cheeks with pancake makeup or concealer cream. (Virtually all makeup lines now make an opaque concealer cream or concealer stick.) Most men don't mind using this technique.

Back to Work

You will feel and look ready to work about 1 week after surgery. However, if you have bruised extensively or are very self-conscious about the surgery, you may decide to stay out of the public view for a few days longer—this applies to about 25 percent of patients. Even after 2 weeks, you may find that, although you are *much better than you were*, you can still feel stiffness and at times soreness in your lower lids.

Back to Parties

You can usually count on looking and feeling right for a party two weeks after your surgery. If you are *not* self-conscious and don't mind people commenting on your surgery, you *might* feel like a party as early as 1 week, but the late night (and alcohol) will leave you tired and make your eyes swell the next day. If you want to be *absolutely safe*, postpone parties for 3 weeks.

Back to Sex

Your stitches are removed early, so even a minor blow to your face could pull the fragile skin slightly apart. For this reason, sex should be postponed for 10 days at least.

Cosmetic Lower Eyelid Surgery: Recovery-at-a-Glance

This chart represents the *average* recovery times for this cosmetic operation.

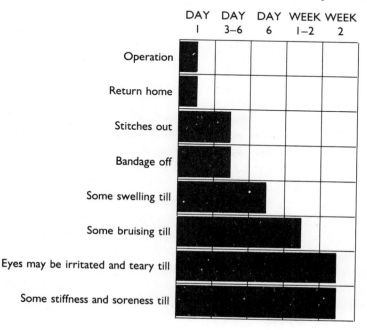

	DAY 1	DAY 3–6	DAY 6	WEEK 1–2	WEEK 2
Operation					
Return home					
Stitches out					
Bandage off					
Some swelling till					
Some bruising till					
Eyes may be irritated and teary till					
Some stiffness and soreness till					

Back to Sports

You can begin stretching exercises at the end of 1 week, but no bends or heavy lifting—it will make your eyes ache and swell. After 2 weeks, you can resume swimming, aerobics, and other sports—but not ball sports. (An exception is tennis—you can play a baseline game, but you should not play at net.) After 3 weeks, you can resume all sports, but start slowly and build up. You will not have your before-surgery endurance at first.

How Much It Costs

Your estimated cost for this operation is $1000 to $2000 for the *surgeon's fee* and $500 to $1,000 for the operating facilities. Remember, prices do vary, being higher in large cities, lower in rural areas, and rising every year.

Insurance Coverage

Insurance will not pay for, or reimburse you for, lower lid surgery. This is *strictly* cosmetic. The exception is the kind of executive plan that reimburses a person for *any* medical cost.

My Assessment of This Procedure

Eyelid surgery is a relatively easy operation to go through, and if your problem is visible lower lid bulges, you may get a *dramatic* improvement. For lower lids that are a little saggy and puffy, or that are thick from overactive muscle, the improvement *is* noticeable, but swelling may conceal it for a while, making the results less dramatic.

Your lower lids will feel stiff for several weeks until the swelling is gone. Also, the skin of the lower lids will be numb for weeks after surgery, but feeling returns as the swelling subsides. Major *and* minor complications are rare. You should remember that there will always be some slight asymmetry—one scar will heal a little sooner or look a bit better than the other one. This is normal.

Side Effects and Complications

Side Effects

There are a few side effects, minor and fairly predictable. Your scars may be slightly asymmetrical, and one may lie a millimeter lower than the other. A few lashes may have been cut during surgery, or may shed afterwards, but they will grow back. Once your stitches are removed, the tiny stitch holes may develop minuscule white cysts, called *milia*. These show as tiny white specks along the scar. Milia almost always disappear after 6 weeks. If they don't, your surgeon can remove them with a tiny needle.

Depending on how *you* heal, your scar may be pink or it may rapidly fade to dead-white. Sometimes a "perfect" white scar is more noticeable than a pale pink one. Either way, you can use mascara, concealer cream, or eyeliner to cover it up.

You will often have a temporary slight dryness of your eyes, along with a paradoxical teariness of your eyes. The cause is swelling from surgery which pulls your tear duct away from your lower lid, so that natural lubricating tears are not only diminished from the stress of surgery but also spill over the swollen lid instead of coating your eyes as they would normally do. You may have to use eyedrops for a week or two. Most often the problem is gone within 10 days. Surgery leaves your eyes temporarily prone to fatigue—reading and watching television, especially in the evenings, may make your eyes ache or feel gritty so that you need eyedrops. Your lids will be numb for a few weeks or even months. You will notice this when you put on eye makeup or concealer cream.

Minor Complications

Relatively common minor complications are cysts in the lower lid that must be removed by minor surgery. Your eyes may be so dry that eyedrops are needed three or four times a day for about a month, until natural tear production resumes at its normal rate. A variety of less common minor complications may be troubling but tend either to go away or to need minor touch-up surgery at a later time.

Marjory: Seeing Double for a While

Marjory was in her fifties and had large fat pockets in her lower lids. When I was removing the excess fat during surgery, I saw the muscle that pulls the eye down. It lies near the fat. Swelling in this muscle can cause it to malfunction. Afterwards, Marjory had swelling in the muscle: for 2 weeks, when she looked down, she saw double! The swelling in the muscle had put her eyes slightly out of synchrony. Two weeks after surgery her vision returned to normal.

Rodney: Scarring Caused a Bulge

Rodney, who was in his thirties, had had lower lid surgery done by another plastic surgeon. After his surgery, he noticed that one bulge remained. It bothered him. When I operated on him 6 months later, I found that some fat had scarred to the muscle so that it formed a visible bulge under the muscle. I trimmed the fat and Rodney's bulge disappeared. (Caution: In older people, around 60 or so, a bulge may persist after surgery not because of excess fat but because the muscles are weak. This is much harder to fix.)

Major Complications

Whenever you have eye surgery, there is a tiny chance that swelling or bleeding after surgery will put pressure on your nerves of vision, and temporarily or permanently diminish your eyesight. For this reason, cosmetic eyelid surgery is done with extreme care. Damaged vision is a rare, remote complication. A more likely (although extremely rare) complication occurred in Lee, who had cosmetic surgery done on her lower lids when she visited the Orient.

Lee: A Re-operation

Lee's plastic surgeon there removed too much skin from her lower lids. When Lee returned home and saw me, her lower lids were pulled down so that the lid lining was visible. Naturally she was distraught. I operated on Lee under sedation as an outpatient. I reopened her incisions, placed a small graft of skin, and rearranged the muscle. Although she wasn't happy to have had the complication, she healed well and looked normal with an adequate, although not fabulous, cosmetic result. Note: Lee's problem was from taking off too much skin. It shows why well-trained plastic surgeons tend to be cautious, rather than aggressive, in removing excess eyelid skin.

What Other Patients Say

- **College Student:** "These bags ran in my family and I hated them. I wondered why I had aged prematurely and I was thrilled to know it wasn't aging—it was the way I was made. I couldn't be happier with the way I look now."
- **Salesman, 48:** "No one ever commented on my eyes, but I felt that people assumed I had a drinking problem. I bruised after surgery—a lot—but it didn't hurt. I took some extra time off work, so people wouldn't ask me about surgery. Everyone thought I'd had a great vacation. All I can say is that sales are up!"
- **Executive secretary, 50:** "My eyes look better. Even though I was told it wouldn't remove the lines, I had hoped it would, in me. I could have a chemical peel but I don't want one. I'd have surgery again but I'd know more what to expect."
- **Housewife, 48:** "I remember all the surgery, even the pinch when she trimmed the fat, but I couldn't see it so it didn't bother me. My scar is red. I have to keep it covered with makeup."
- **Male lawyer, 37:** "I've been more nervous before a trial. It didn't bother me. It did what I wanted. No one noticed. I'm pleased."

Cosmetic Nose Surgery

What Surgeons Call It

Depending on what is done, the technical term for this operation is rhinoplasty or septorhinoplasty. It's a septorhinoplasty if the septum (partition) inside the nose also needs correction to improve breathing.

What It Will Do

A rhinoplasty will give you a smaller, narrower, more graceful nose and correct obvious problems like a hump. If your nose is *crooked*, the surgeon may or may not be able to straighten it, depending on what caused the crookedness.

If your nose is *straight, with no hump*, but the lower part of your nose looks broad, fat, or bulbous at the tip and the nostrils look too wide, you may not need the standard "nose job." Instead, you may need the "Tip Plasty" which is a more limited operation. This is cosmetic nose surgery limited to the tip of the nose. The operation—and your recovery—are much less involved than the usual cosmetic nose operation.

What It Won't Do

It won't give you the nose that you admire on someone else. And it won't necessarily make you look better in photographs or films, or improve your chances as a model.

How Long It Will Last

A rhinoplasty is permanent. If you injure your nose after rhinoplasty, even without breaking it, a humplike thickening may develop. Remember, a nose that's been operated on is *never* quite as strong as before. A little caution is all you need.

When to Have It

How soon? As soon as your nose is fully grown. For girls this is between 12 and 16. Boys grow later, so a boy's nose growth is usually not complete before 14 to 18. The "rhinoplasty rule of thumb" is "no cosmetic nose surgery before 16," but surgery can safely be done earlier if your nose growth is over. How late? After 40, nose surgery can be done but your nose tissues are thicker and harder to sculpt at surgery.

People who have been teased about their noses will usually be troubled by those memories until their nose has been reshaped. It makes sense to wait for the right time or until one has enough money. It doesn't make sense to wait for the negative impact of the teasing to fade. It rarely does.

Where to Have It

Rhinoplasty is usually done on an outpatient basis in a doctor's office operating room *or* an outpatient surgery center *or* a hospital's outpatient operating room. An overnight stay is unusual but not rare. It depends on your preference *and* your doctor's.

Conditions That Increase Your Risk

Surgery tends to be more difficult, with less predictable results, if you have broken your nose in the past. Operating on the outside *and* inside (septum) of your nose at the same time increases your risk of ending up with too small a nose, because when the outer bone and inner septum are *both* loosened, the nose can flatten.

Usual Anesthesia

A local with sedation, given to you by your surgeon or an anesthetist, is the most common. General anesthesia is unusual but not rare. It depends on your preference and extent of your surgery. It's more common when your cosmetic surgery is done at the same time as septal surgery.

How Long It Takes

Times are *approximate*. They vary from surgeon to surgeon and from operation to operation. Cosmetic nose surgery usually lasts *only* 1½ hours. Cosmetic nose surgery *plus* septal surgery may take 2½ hours.

The Operation

(Figures 11-13 through 11-15)

Cosmetic nose surgery is done from inside the nose, so there are no visible scars. The steps in cosmetic nose surgery are:

1. Bone is removed from the hump.
2. Cartilage is removed from the hump.
3. Cartilage and fat are removed from the tip.
4. (Optional) Cartilage *may* be removed from the end of the nose, where it meets the upper lip.
5. (Optional) Skin *may* be removed from nostrils at the crease where nostrils meet cheeks.
6. Bone is cut where nose meets cheek, and bones are bent in to narrow nose.

Before

Here's how cosmetic nose will feel to *you*. The experience will be much the same whether cosmetic surgery is done alone or combined with septal surgery. Assuming that you come to hospital on the day of your operation, you will change into a hospital gown and either be brought directly to the operating room, or to a preoperative area. You may be given sedation by an injection in your hip. An IV is begun through a needle in your arm so you can be given a solution of dextrose and/or saline to keep you from getting dehydrated during surgery. If you are not sedated, you may walk to the operating room. If you are sedated, you will be brought in on a stretcher. The room will seem cold. There will be bright lights. Once you are on the operating table, a safety strap is put across your lap. Sticky pads are put on your chest under your gown to monitor your heart. A blood pressure cuff is put on your arm. A sticky pad is put on your leg under your gown. This is a grounding pad to make surgical cautery safe to use on you. (Surgical cautery means using an electrical instrument to seal blood vessels and stop bleeding.)

If you are going to have general anesthesia, you will now be given pentothal or another intravenous drug to put you to sleep. You won't be conscious of what happens next.

If you are having local/sedation, you will be given some sedation now. Your face will be washed with surgical soap, and sterile drapes will be placed over your body and around your face. Then, after additional sedation, your nose will be numbed by local anesthetic injected around your nose and anesthetic-soaked swabs or packing in your nose. You may not remember this. If you do, you will remember snatches of what is done, perhaps a little discomfort, but nothing more.

During

If you are having surgery on your septum, this is usually done as the first step of your surgery. You may remember vibration or pulling. Once this is done, you are usually given additional sedation.

After this, your surgeon will begin to work on your nose (from the inside). This is what he does, but the sequence of steps varies from surgeon to surgeon. He will clean away the tiny hairs and then begin thinning the tip. You may feel pulling or slight pressure, but chances are that you will doze off.

Next, he will probably rasp down the bone that makes the hump. You may feel vibration. Then he carves away the excess cartilage on the hump. You may feel pulling. He may then narrow the nostrils. You may, at most, feel the tickle of a dangling suture on your cheek skin. If he shortens your nose at the upper lip, you may feel pressure.

So far you have probably dozed off and felt nothing. Now you may begin to be vaguely aware of what is being done. Your surgeon needs to chisel the side bones to narrow your nose. He may give you additional sedation before he works on the bones, because the chiseling of the bones creates vibration. It feels strange, not painful, but it isn't pleasant. Once the chiseling is done, your operation is largely over, except for stitches, removing the packing and putting on the bandage.

After

You leave the operating room on a stretcher. In the recovery room, the sedation tends to catch up with you, and you will probably fall asleep. When you wake up, your face will feel puffy and your nose may ache.

Cosmetic Nose Surgery

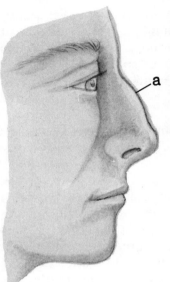
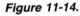

Figure 11-13.

Although the surgery makes the entire nose smaller, your most dramatic improvement will be in the profile, where the hump is removed (a). Notice that the chin is too small, compared to the nose. At times, a chin implant is done at the same time as cosmetic nose surgery.

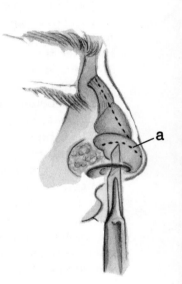

Figure 11-14.

Cosmetic nose surgery is done from *inside* the nose. Here the scalpel is trimming the excess tip cartilage (a). This step is also done in cosmetic surgery limited to the tip of the nose, which is described in the next section.

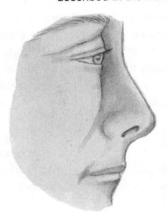

Figure 11-15.

The end result: Your profile will be straight or scooped, depending on what is best for you.

The Process of Recovery

What to Do About Pain

For the first 24 hours you'll feel throbbing and aching around your nose and eyes. Nausea and one to three bouts of vomiting may also occur, depending on how you react to the anesthesia.

The Healing Process

Immediately following surgery, you can breathe only through your mouth. Your nose is closed from swelling, surgical packing, or both. Your eyes will be puffy or even bruised for up to one week after surgery. Your nose will be swollen, noticeably for 1 to 2 weeks. From weeks 2 to 6 after surgery, your swelling is no longer noticeable to others, but you do not see daily improvement. You see your final result in about *one year*.

Your surgeon will usually see you once or twice the first week, to remove packing from your nose (day 2 or 3) and to remove the bandage from your nose (about day 6). You will usually see him again about 2 weeks after surgery and again about 6 weeks after surgery if all is well. If you have healed well, additional follow-ups are optional. There may be no need to be checked again if you are pleased with your result.

Bandages

I use plaster on top of the nose, a small pad under the nose and a little packing inside. Some doctors go to the other extreme, using a plaster bandage on the nose and forehead, wrapping the face with an elastic bandage, covering the eyes, and placing *deep* packing inside the nose. The trend is toward light, small bandages.

Taking Care of Your Wound

You may sneeze out your packing. Don't panic. Discard it; don't replace it. Call your doctor to notify him. Don't blow your nose for 2 to 4 weeks, because the pressure can make your nose start bleeding. (Vomiting can make your nose bleed also, but usually only during the first 5 days. The pressure is less great from vomiting because your mouth is open, which lessens pressure inside the nose.) If you sneeze, sneeze through your mouth, not your nose. Trying to hold in a sneeze only builds up pressure in your nose and can have a disconcerting result: Air may be forced out through the surgical areas into the deep layers of skin, resulting in a puffed-out nose with a Rice Krispy crackle from the air under the skin. (Crackling and puffiness are *temporary*.)

Mouth breathing will make your lips dry, so keep lips coated with lip balm or Vaseline. If your eyes become gummy from swelling, cleanse around your lashes gently with water, boric acid or an eye solution like Murine. Once your bandage is off, you can reduce stuffiness and crusting by holding a wet, warm washcloth over your nose and taking little breaths. This humidifies your nose. If your nose forms thick inner crusts, your surgeon may need to remove these in office, once they loosen. This procedure will make your eyes water, but it shouldn't hurt.

Stitches

Your surgeon may need to remove inside stitches if they don't dissolve. This shouldn't hurt. If your nostrils were narrowed at surgery, this area will have stitches which will need to be removed on days 4 to 6.

Scars

One surgical technique results in a small scar on each cheek at the side of the nose. A new technique cuts the nose skin off its supporting bone and leaves scars at the bottom of the nose. With this technique, the surgeon can see, as well as feel, what he does at surgery. *The standard nose surgery technique* leaves *no* outside scars, unless the nostrils are narrowed. Then there are scars outside in the crease around the nostrils.

Tips

- *Women:* Heavy eye makeup draws attention to the center of your face. For 3 weeks after surgery, avoid heavy eyeliner. Also avoid colored eye shadows (blue/purple/green/brown/pink) that will echo, and thus emphasize your bruising even when faint.
- Glasses draw attention *away* from your nose. You might wear lightly tinted glasses (even if you usually don't need glasses), starting about one week after surgery.

Cosmetic Nose Surgery: Recovery-at-a-Glance

This chart represents the *average* recovery times for this cosmetic operation.

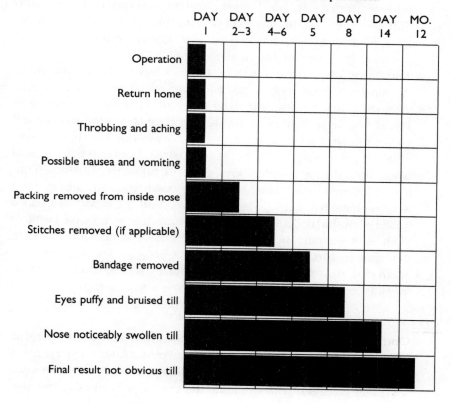

	DAY 1	DAY 2–3	DAY 4–6	DAY 5	DAY 8	DAY 14	MO. 12
Operation	■						
Return home	■						
Throbbing and aching	■						
Possible nausea and vomiting	■						
Packing removed from inside nose	■	■					
Stitches removed (if applicable)	■	■	■				
Bandage removed	■	■	■	■			
Eyes puffy and bruised till	■	■	■	■	■		
Nose noticeably swollen till	■	■	■	■	■	■	
Final result not obvious till	■	■	■	■	■	■	■

- You're likely to find glasses helpful in concealing telltale signs of surgery for another 2 weeks. A foam pad (as from the Dr. Scholl line) or even a tiny adhesive bandage where glasses rest on the nose will make heavy glasses comfortable.
- Makeup helps conceal the "fat" look your nose has when it is swollen. A *light* or white base or concealer cream along the top of your nose combined with a *darker* base or concealer cream on the side will emphasize the height of your nose, drawing attention away from the width so that your nose seems less fat. Men as well as women can use this makeup technique successfully.

- Crusts build up in your nose after surgery. To soften and loosen them, dip a cotton swab in water or Vaseline. Place the swab *gently* inside your nostril and let it rest next to the crust for a minute. Result: The hard crust absorbs moisture from the swab and becomes gelatinous. You can do this three times a day for as long as hard crusts form—a few days or a few weeks, depending on how you are healing.

- The lining of your nose will be dry, so sleep with a humidifier running all night. (The ultrasonic ones make less noise.)

- **Bleeding** after surgery is alarming and is most likely around day 6. If you get a nosebleed, it is probably from the lower third of your nose. Call your surgeon, but also *gently* pinch the lower third of your nose, including your nostrils, between your thumb and index finger, so that you feel firm pressure, but not pain. *Don't lie back* (the blood will trickle down your throat, making you nauseated). Sit up, lean forward, and let blood drip on a towel. Cough blood in your mouth onto a towel; don't swallow it. It isn't elegant, but avoids nausea from swallowed blood in an hour or two.

- **Bruising and swelling:** Keeping your eyes *cold* after nose surgery is soothing. It also helps to lessen swelling and bruising around your eyes and nose. These are the three easy ways to cool your eyes:

- Freeze wet tea bags before surgery. (Tannin, a natural chemical in the tea, combats swelling, an added plus.) After surgery, place a frozen tea bag over each eye. If they are too cold, put a layer of gauze between your eyes and the tea bags. When the tea bags melt, you can discard them or re-freeze them for later use.

- Or, again, before surgery, buy a box of the smallest Ziploc plastic bags. Fill them with water and put them in the freezer. After surgery, use one frozen bag per eye. Again, if this feels *too* cold, put gauze between your eyes and the plastic bag. You can re-freeze a bag when it melts.

- Or, buy commercial cold packs. The advantage of these is that they don't drip or get wet when they melt. The disadvantage is their feeling heavy on your eyes and nose.

- Your nose will be numb for weeks after surgery. As a result, your nose can drip when you aren't aware of it. To avoid embarrassment, carry tissues with you for several weeks.

Back to Work

Three-quarters of all rhinoplasty patients can return to work in one week. The rest will need 10 days to 2 weeks. Residual bruising and swelling will make your surgery noticeable, unless you use careful concealment. Your nose will look puffy to *you*. Makeup and glasses (see "Tips") help to hide this from others.

Back to Parties

Alcohol and late nights will make your nose ache, swell and redden, for 3 to 6 weeks. You will feel comfortable for an early dinner party at 2 weeks, a dance, late party, or ball at 3 to 4 weeks.

Back to Sports

Bending and heavy lifting will make your nose ache and swell for at least 2, and often 4 or even 6 weeks after surgery.

A blow to the top of your nose can cause a prolonged or permanent humplike swelling. Therefore if you can, avoid *all* sports for 6 weeks, and no *ball* sports for 6 *months*. But if you are an active person and don't feel you can make such a lifestyle change, your *minimum* restrictions are:

- Walking, hiking: 2 weeks after operation
- Most sports: 4 weeks
- Ball sports: 6 weeks
- Contact sports: 6 months. Ideally, you should postpone your cosmetic nose surgery until your football, contact karate, or ice hockey days are over.

Back to Sex

You should postpone sex for 10 to 14 days. Before then, the increased facial blood flow from sexual excitement may make your nose throb, swell, or even bleed if you have not fully healed. Sex at 10 days should be done cautiously. If your partner inadvertently bumps the top of your nose you can develop swelling that takes weeks, even months, to subside. After 3 weeks, you can resume sex without hesitation.

What It Costs

More or less routine cosmetic nose surgery only will probably cost you $2000 to $3000. Cosmetic nose plus septal surgery will cost about $2500 to $3500. These are surgeons' fees. Hospital costs are in addition. Complicated nose surgery to rebuild a shrunken, small nose costs up to $5000, rarely more.

In addition, anesthesia will cost you from $600 for sedation by the surgeon to $3000 if you need general anesthesia.

Insurance Coverage

Insurance will not pay for cosmetic nose surgery. If you have cosmetic nose surgery *plus* septal surgery, insurance pays for the cost of the septal surgery. This will usually end up being about half of your total cost.

Note: Although you do have a somewhat higher risk of a poor result when cosmetic nose surgery is done with septal surgery, it is *nevertheless very common to do these two operations simultaneously.* You may need the septal surgery to straighten your nose; also you benefit financially, because your insurance pays half.

My Assessment of This Operation

This is a very common operation. You will probably find it easy to have. Most cosmetic surgeons find nose surgery challenging but artistically satisfying, with a (relatively) low complication rate. The most dramatic change will be in your profile. The revolution from a hump to a nice profile helps to keep you happy while you wait for the swelling to go down.

If your profile change is subtle, your first weeks or months of recovery may be frustrating. But don't despair—the waiting will be worth it. Most people find recovery from nose surgery to be surprisingly easy. In fact, in some circles, having a "nose job" is considered a status symbol!

Side Effects and Complications

Side Effects

Your side effects may include prolonged swelling, a temporary loss of or decrease in your sense of smell, trouble breathing or a *feeling* that your breathing is blocked, and throbbing of your nose when you bend over to wash your hair, lift groceries, or do exercises.

Phyllis: Some Whiteheads Developed

Phyllis, a young woman of 25, wanted to keep her nose swelling to a minimum. I showed her how to tape her nose every night. This kept the swelling down, but the tape brought out a cluster of milia (whiteheads). For Phyllis this was worse than the swelling, so she stopped the taping. The milia went away. The swelling returned but gradually subsided of its own accord.

Doug: Allergies Were a Problem

Doug happened to have his cosmetic nose surgery during the pollen season. Unfortunately, he was allergic to pollen. His allergy was not a bad one, but the surgical swelling along with his allergies, caused him to have trouble breathing for 2 weeks. It took a month for his sense of smell to return.

Complications

Possible complications include bleeding, infection, a flat nose, and such rarities as the bone chisel cutting the lacrimal duct at the corner of the eye. Also, your sense of smell comes from tiny nerves in the back of the nose, and in the septum, so extensive septal surgery can damage these nerves in rare cases. A change in your sense of smell may occur without nerve damage if your new nose shape changes the air flow so that the air you breathe in through your nose doesn't reach these tiny nerves.

The most common complications *soon after* surgery are bleeding and infection. The most common *late* problem is dissatisfaction with your nose. About 10 percent of people after nose surgery need, or want, something more done. This may seem a lot, but it's to be expected. Here's why: A cautious surgeon will tend to leave your nose a shade too big. Removing a little more later on is easier and safer than trying to "put something back."

A more aggressive surgeon will tend to remove too much. Your nose will look perfect—until the swelling is all gone. Then you will need more complicated surgery to enlarge it. Most operations turn out fine—10 percent is not much when you consider that this surgery is the most complicated cosmetic operation of all!

Minor Complications

Angel: A Minor Bleeding Problem
I did cosmetic nose surgery on a young woman named Angel. When I saw her in my office five days later, everything was fine, but three hours later her mother rushed her back. Her nose had started to bleed. I examined her nose, cauterized one internal incision, and put in a little packing. The packing fell out on its own in three days. She did fine after that.

It takes 5 days for enzymes in your nose tissues to dissolve the blood clots in your nose that stopped the bleeding at surgery. That's why you are more likely to have bleeding after nose surgery around the fifth day than at any other time.

Ethel: Further Surgery *Desired*
I did cosmetic nose surgery on Ethel, a woman of 30 who wanted to keep some of the ethnic character of her nose. It was a beautifully chiseled nose but long, with a high hump. One year after surgery, she decided it was almost, but not quite, what she had hoped. Under local anesthesia, I shortened her nose a fraction and smoothed the hump with a fine rasp. The result was perfect for her.

Sam: Further Surgery *Required*
I was in a grocery store and was stopped by a friend to check out the nose of his friend, Sam, who had had cosmetic nose surgery. They both agreed that the new nose, which had been done six months before, had been totally messed up. It looked "weird" and crooked. But in fact the nose itself was not crooked and the result overall was good. However, one piece of cartilage on the lower left side had become dislocated from the bone. By shifting slightly, it made the whole nose look crooked. To correct this "catastrophe," all that was

needed was a small graft of bone or cartilage slipped in under the skin. Sam told me his surgeon's name. I knew that this surgeon was good, and that he would re-operate on a dissatisfied patient up to one year later, without charge. Sam hadn't gone back to the surgeon because he thought the surgeon had proved himself to be incompetent. Not so. If you are dissatisfied with your surgery, you should go back to your surgeon first before going elsewhere.

Major Complications

Stephanie: Major Bleeding

Stephanie called me at 7:00 A.M. I had operated on her nose five days earlier. Stephanie said she had been bleeding for four hours and it looked like a lot, but she hadn't liked to look too closely. She felt awful. I examined her in the hospital emergency room and found a small artery bleeding briskly in one of the surgical incisions. I cauterized the artery and the bleeding stopped. However, Stephanie had lost more than a unit of blood, which made her feel faint and sick. She spent one night in hospital—a little scared but fine.

The risk of bleeding can be lessened if you follow suggestions in the Tips section.

Grant: A Major Infection

I did cosmetic nose and septal surgery on Grant, a boy of 16. Grant had sinus infections, and I gave him antibiotics during surgery. About a week later, his mother called me at midnight, to say that Grant had terrible pain in both cheeks. He had a severe sinus infection, stirred up by the surgery, despite the antibiotics. I prescribed more antibiotics, which his mother got at an all-night drugstore. Within 6 hours Grant felt better. Within a week he was fine.

Infection is rare after any nose surgery. It is more likely if you have had trouble with nose or sinus infections in the past.

Steve: Re-operation for Dissatisfaction

Steve, who was 19, had cosmetic nose surgery. He thought he had sworn off contact karate for life. But 2 weeks after surgery a friend wanted to show him a twisting kick to the face. The kick inadvertently landed on Steve's new nose. Of course Steve's nose swelled up and bled a bit at the time. However, as the swelling subsided it became apparent that Steve's nose was now—too small. The kick had pushed the bones out of place. Fortunately he could still breathe. He needed corrective surgery with a cartilage graft to rebuild the top of his nose.

What Other Patients Say

- **High school boy, 17:** "This was great. I don't remember the surgery. My hump was gone, and I could see that right away. A breeze."
- **Housewife, 26:** "I was told about the swelling but it didn't make an impact on me until after the operation. I worried for the first three weeks, and then I decided I'd have to live with it forever. It was really true what the doctor said, though. It took a year for all the swelling to go away, but I was pleased after six weeks."
- **Computer salesman, 30:** "I guess I like my nose. It didn't have a big hump, and it took time to see the change. I almost wish it was smaller, but everyone else says it's great."
- **Mother of three, 40:** "It was the easiest thing I've done in years. It looks super. Now the rest of my family is getting rid of our family nose!"

Cosmetic Nose Tip Surgery

What Surgeons Call It

The technical term for this operation is tip plasty (molding of the tip) or an alar cartilage reduction with alar wedge resection.

What It Will Do

Cosmetic nose tip surgery makes the tip of your nose more delicate and better shaped. The *tip* should be thinner and less bulbous. Remember, though, that swelling will obscure your result for as long as a year. The surgery also aims to make your nostrils less wide. This result is not obscured by swelling, so you see the improvement sooner. Remember that your profile will *not* be changed.

What It Won't Do

This operation cannot give you someone else's nose. It can improve the size and shape of your *own* nose. This operation will not give you a *dramatic* change, because the operation is limited and the results take time to appear. If you are hoping for a psychological boost from your surgery, you need to remember that you'll likely be seeing the improvement slowly, over months.

How Long It Will Last

The results of a nose tip operation are permanent. The excess skin in your nostrils and the excess fat and cartilage in your nose tip are gone. However, if you have this surgery in your teens or twenties, you *may* notice that by age 40 the tip of your nose has thickened slightly, since cartilage thickens in time. But even if this occurs, you're unlikely to consider it marked enough to make another operation worthwhile.

When to Have It

You can have this operation any time after your nose stops growing. This means from about age 15 to 70!

Where to Have It

Nose tip surgery is usually done on an outpatient basis in a doctor's office operating room *or* an outpatient surgery center operating room *or* a hospital's outpatient operating room.

Factors That Increase Your Risk

If the tip of your nose reddens easily in cold or in the sun, this operation may make the reddening worse. Also, if you are cold sensitive, the surgery tends to make your nose tip especially cold sensitive for the first winter after surgery. Allergies also may be temporarily worsened by surgery on the tip of the nose.

Usual Anesthesia

A nose tip operation is done with local anesthesia with sedation, given by your surgeon. You may need only sedation by mouth, but intravenous sedation may be used.

How Long It Takes

The "tip plasty" operation will take 1 hour, sometimes less.

The Operation
(Figures 11-16 through 11-19)

Before

You arrive on the day of your surgery, having eaten nothing since midnight of the night before. You will change out of street clothes and into a hospital gown. You may go to a preoperative room, where an IV will be placed in your arm so that you can be given a solution of dextrose and/or saline to keep you from being dehydrated during surgery. Alternatively, this may be done in the operating room. Once you are on the operating table, a safety strap is put across your hips. Then sticky pads are placed on your chest to monitor your heart. A blood pressure cuff is placed on your arm to measure your blood pressure. Finally, a sticky pad is placed on your leg under your gown to serve as a ground so that surgical cautery can be used, safely. (Surgical cautery means using an electrical instrument to seal off blood vessels and stop bleeding.) Your face is washed with surgical soap, and sterile paper or cloth drapes are put around your face and over your body.

You may now be given more sedation. If you are having only sedation by mouth, you have been given the pills before coming into the operating room. It would be beginning to take effect by this time. Your nose will be numbed by tiny needle injections. The inside is numbed with liquid anesthetic on gauze packing or cotton swabs. Your eyes will be covered to protect them from the bright surgical lights. If your sedation is light, you will re-member the surgery, but time will seem to go quickly. If you are heavily sedated, you may remember nothing at all.

During

Your surgeon will probably begin by trimming the inside nostril hairs. Then he will cut inside the nose, near the tip. He will remove excess fat under the skin, as well as the cartilage where it is broad and thick. He may need to free all the tip cartilage and re-shape it and/or place a small cartilage graft at the tip, to give it a finer point. He may need to narrow your nostrils as well. Like most cosmetic surgeons, I usually make this my last step. The inside as well as the outside nostril incisions are usually stitched—then the packing is removed from your nose and you can breathe through your nose again. Tape is placed across the tip of the nose to minimize the swelling. A gauze pad is taped under your nose to absorb any dripping. You are often wide awake by now.

If in addition to the nose tip operation you have a graft placed to make your nose taller, it can be done at the same time. If a silicone graft is used, a tunnel is made from the tip of the nose along the top. The long, narrow silicone graft is inserted. This kind of graft is easy to place but is often rejected—the incision simply won't heal until the silicone is removed. Other grafts are made from bone or cartilage. A sliver of bone taken just below your elbow may be used. Or, the cartilage may come from the septum that divides the inside of your nose. The graft is placed in a tunnel, just like a silicone graft. Because they are not pre-shaped, cartilage and bone grafts take time to trim and shape. But your body does not object to them—once they are in place, your tissues will accept them.

After

Apart from recovering from the sedation, having your stitches and tape removed and waiting for your swelling to subside—this is all.

Cosmetic Nose Tip Surgery

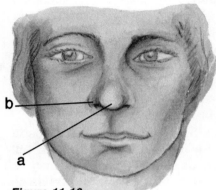

Figure 11-16.

The tip of the nose (a) is broad from excess cartilage and fat. The nostrils (b) are also too broad for the face.

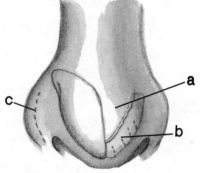

Figure 11-17.

The tip cartilage on this side (a) has now been trimmed. The rim of the cartilage has been scored beneath (b) to change its shape and give it more curve. The dotted line (c) shows where the nostril skin will be cut to narrow the nostril.

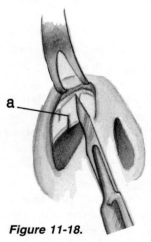

Figure 11-18.

The work on the tip cartilage is done from inside (a) by holding up the nostril. The cartilage may be reshaped by cuts on either side of the inner surface. If the cartilage is already well shaped, no such cuts may be needed.

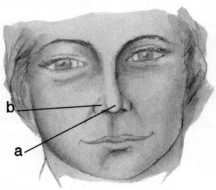

Figure 11-19.

The tip (a) now is smaller and better shaped, and the nostrils (b) are narrower, too.

The Process of Recovery

What to Do About Pain

You should have no pain after a nose tip operation. The tip of your nose will ache a few hours after surgery while the anesthesia wears off. After that you may have occasional throbbing, which will be worse when you bend your head over. But you should have no pain.

The Healing Process

The surgery makes the tip of your nose puffy. No one else will notice this once the bandage is off—about 5 days after surgery. However, the swelling will be noticeable to you, because it will look as though there's little or no improvement compared with before the surgery. You *may* see a big improvement after 6 weeks, but it takes a *year* for most people to see the difference.

You need to see your surgeon several times in the 2 weeks after surgery. Crusts may form in the tip of your nose, and you need to be checked to be sure you are healing without infection.

Bandages

You will have tape on the tip of your nose. This will be removed in your surgeon's office about 5 days after surgery. You may have a little packing inside each nostril—your surgeon may re-move this or instruct you to remove it. It usually is removed by the second day after surgery. If your nostrils have been nar-rowed, you will have a small gauze and tape bandage around each nostril.

Taking Care of Your Wound

You may find that crusts form inside your nostrils or that the inside of your nose feels dry. This is best treated by soaking a cotton swab in water or Vaseline and letting it rest on the crust for a minute three or four times a day. The crust will absorb the water or ointment and become soft, loosening from the inside of your nose.

Some crusts may also form on the outside where your nos-trils are narrowed. These are usually best treated by dabbing gently at them with a cotton swab soaked in a mixture of half peroxide/half water. This will loosen the crust so that it can separate by itself.

Stitches

The stitches inside your nose are usually absorbable. However, they often don't absorb completely, so your surgeon may remove them 1 to 2 weeks after your surgery. The outside stitches where your nostrils are narrowed will be removed within 5 days to avoid permanent stitch marks on your skin.

Scars

The scars inside your nose are not visible. However, there will be a scar at the base of each nostril where it meets the cheek. This lies in a natural crease line and should be unnoticeable—and in time virtually invisible. It may take 6 weeks to 6 months in some people to soften and fade.

Tips

- Makeup helps conceal the "fat" look your nose has when it is swollen. A *light* or white base or concealer cream along the top of your nose combined with a *darker* base or concealer cream on the side will emphasize the height of your nose, drawing attention away from the width so that your nose seems less fat. Men as well as women can use this makeup technique successfully.
- Crusts build up in your nose after surgery. To soften and loosen them, dip a cotton swab in water or Vaseline. Place the swab *gently* inside your nostril and let it rest next to the crust for a minute. Result: The hard crust absorbs moisture from the swab and becomes gelatinous. You can do this three times a day for as long as hard crusts form—a few days or a few weeks, depending on how you are healing.
- The lining of your nose will be dry, so sleep with a humidifier running all night. (The ultrasonic ones make less noise.)
- Bleeding after surgery is alarming and is most likely around day 6. If you get a nosebleed, it is probably from the lower third of your nose. Call your surgeon, but also *gently* pinch the lower third of your nose, including your nostrils, between your thumb and index finger, so that you feel firm pressure, but not pain.

Nose Tip Surgery: Recovery-at-a-Glance

This chart represents the *average* recovery times for this cosmetic operation.

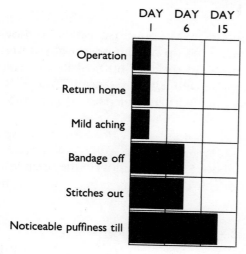

	DAY 1	DAY 6	DAY 15
Operation	■		
Return home	■		
Mild aching	■		
Bandage off	■■		
Stitches out	■■		
Noticeable puffiness till	■■■		

Don't lie back (the blood will trickle down your throat, making you nauseated). Sit up, lean forward, and let blood drip on a towel. Cough blood in your mouth onto a towel; don't swallow it. It isn't elegant, but avoids nausea from swallowed blood in an hour or two.

Back to Work

If the bandage on the tip of your nose does not bother you, and if you do desk work, you can return to work once the sedative effect wears off—about 2 days after surgery. However, most people don't want to be seen with such a bandage, so plan to return to work on days 6 or 7.

Back to Parties

You can go to a party at the end of a week after surgery but that would be too soon to cover the nostril incisions with heavy makeup. Also, alcohol may make your face flush and make the surgical area feel hot. Dancing—other than slow dancing—will make the surgical area swell and probably ache. Besides, your nose will tend to hurt at the end of the day, for several weeks. Unless it is an early-evening dinner party, it is best to put parties off for 2 weeks.

Back to Sex

Sexual excitement will tend to make your nose swell and ache. Also, a bump or mild blow to the tip of your nose will not only make it hurt, but may pull apart the healing nostrils, causing them to bleed and leaving you with a widened scar. To be safe, postpone sex for 10 days after surgery at least and preferably for a full 2 weeks.

What It Will Cost

Your surgeon's fee will be about $1000. The cost of the operating room will be around $500 to $700.

Insurance Coverage

Nose tip surgery is purely cosmetic. Insurance will *not* pay.

My Assessment of This Procedure

About 15 percent of people who "hate" their nose only need a tip plasty. If the upper half of your nose is fine and you have no bump on top of your nose, the tip plasty could be what you need. This is a surprisingly easy operation to go through. Some blacks who have wide flared nostrils find that narrowing the tip is their cosmetic solution. But blacks and Orientals who have low noses and want a "Caucasian" look usually need more than just a tip plasty. They also need the nose made higher. This is done with grafts of bone, cartilage, or (sometimes) silicone.

Side Effects and Complications

Your biggest obstacle is waiting—for a year—until your final swelling is gone and you can see your new tip shape. If the skin on your nose is thick, you may be disappointed even then, because the thick skin may still make the tip look thick.

Your nose tip will be numb for months because the nerves to the tip of your nose are bruised and cut during surgery. You may notice that your breathing seems different. Because your nostrils have a different shape, air enters your nose in a new flow-pattern. Bleeding and/or infection are extremely rare. The tip of the nose has an excellent blood supply but no major arteries or veins. The blood flow washes away any bacteria, minimizing the risk of infection.

Clara: An Easy Operation

Clara was in her thirties. She had a nicely shaped nose, but the tip was broad and the cartilage thick. Although her face was pretty, the round thick tip of her nose drew attention to itself, away from her prettiness. Clara had a tip plasty on a Thursday. She had her bandage removed in my office on Monday morning, and she went to work after that. Clara was thrilled. Although it took months for the final swelling to go down, she could see—and feel—the new softness and shape in the tip of her nose. Best of all, she found that the recovery from her surgery was easy and it left no telltale signs.

What Other Patients Say

- **Executive secretary, 40:** "My nose always bothered me. The tip looked so masculine. I could feel the result right away—the tip of my nose felt soft. I would say for me the swelling was all gone by 6 months. This was easier than grocery shopping!"
- **Telephone repairman, 27:** "My fat nose was all in the family. I didn't see the difference after surgery and I was pretty down about that. Frankly, I had forgotten about it until my next birthday. I was getting ready to go out and I realized that my nose wasn't shaped the way it used to be."
- **Teenage girl, 17:** "My mom was more terrified of my surgery than I was. I wanted it done. All I remember was going into the operating room. I could kind of see the change within a few weeks, so I didn't mind waiting for the rest to appear. My only problem was that for weeks the tip of my nose felt like pins and needles when you touched it. It bothered my boyfriend because it made me jump when he kissed me."

Brow Lift

What Surgeons Call It

This procedure is technically known as a brow lift.

What It Will Do

A cosmetic brow lift aims to smooth out forehead lines and furrows and to prevent their return, to raise the eyebrows and upper lids, and to soften or flatten deep frown lines between your eyes.

What It Won't Do

This operation won't remove all forehead lines. It won't make your forehead completely smooth or expressionless. It can't lift your forehead without also lifting your brows and upper lids.

How Long It Will Last

Brow lifts are done differently now than ten years ago. Today we cut out muscle as well as skin. This makes the effect of the surgery last 5 to 10 years, or longer.

When to Have It

Although there are no age restrictions, it's uncommon for anyone under 40 to *need* this operation. Most men and women having a brow lift will be between 45 and 60. Sometimes, deep cross lines in the forehead, low brows, and a low hairline occur in young people. *Age* is not the problem; their appearance is usually inherited. Thus the surgery *may* be done for patients in their twenties or thirties.

Where to Have It

A brow lift is usually done on an outpatient basis in a doctor's office operating room *or* a surgery center operating room *or* a hospital operating room.

Conditions That Increase Your Risk

Scars may become visible in a man or woman whose hairline recedes. A scalp infection or condition such as rosacea may increase the chance of infection after surgery, although infection is rare. If you have had cosmetic upper lid surgery in the past, a brow lift may pull your upper lids so tight that you cannot close your eyes properly. Your surgeon should evaluate this possibility carefully before surgery. People with a high hairline may need to have the scar placed at the junction of hair and scalp. This carries the risk of a visible scar.

Usual Anesthesia

Brow lifts are usually done under local anesthesia with sedation, even if they are being done along with other cosmetic facial operations.

How Long It Takes

Your brow lift surgery will take between 1½ and 2 hours to do. When it is done with a facelift, the upper part of the facelift incision becomes the lower part of the brow lift operation. This means that the combined operating time may be slightly less.

The Operation
(Figures 11-20 through 11-23)

Before

You will arrive for your surgery about one hour before it is scheduled, having had nothing to eat or drink since midnight the night before. You will change into a hospital gown and be taken to a preoperative area or directly to the operating room. An IV will be placed in your arm so that you can be given a solution of dextrose and/or saline to keep you from becoming dehydrated during the operation. You may be given a preoperative dose of sedation by mouth or through the IV. Unless your hair is very short, it will be tied up in rubber bands in front of and behind the surgical area to keep it out of the way. Long hair directly over the strip of scalp that will be removed will also be cut before surgery. (Your head will not have to be shaved.)

You may be given a dose of antibiotics through your IV, but infection is rare and many surgeons will not do this. Your surgeon will mark the incision line with purple surgical ink. If you are having other surgery—for instance a facelift and/or a chin lift—he will mark all the incision lines at the same time.

Once you are on the operating table, sticky pads are put on your chest to monitor your heart. A sticky pad is also put on your hip under your gown. This is a grounding pad that makes the surgical cautery safe to use. (Surgical cautery means using electrical heat to seal off bleeding blood vessels.)

You may already have been given a small dose of sedative, but now in the operating room you will be given a larger dose, which makes you very drowsy or puts you completely to sleep. Your scalp will be washed with surgical soap. Sterile drapes will be placed over your body and around your face and scalp.

During

Your surgeon will inject local anesthetic above your eyebrows, right across your brow. He will also inject local anesthetic along the incision line. Next, he will make the incision across your scalp, along the marked line. The incision is usually a long curved one that goes just above one ear, over the top of the head a few inches behind the hairline, and down to the other ear. A variation of the incision is the "gull-wing," which curves back, bringing it nearer the front hairline at the top of the head. This helps hide the scar if your hair is thin on the sides. (For a third variation, see Scars.) The scalp tends to bleed profusely. He will stop the bleeding with cautery or with stitches or clips across the scalp that pinch the skin.

He will then lift up the scalp and forehead, including the forehead muscle, which is called the frontalis. This is the muscle that creases your forehead. He will remove several strips of frontalis muscle right across the forehead. The forehead is peeled right down to the eyebrows. In between the eyebrows is a vertical muscle, called the corrugator muscle, which makes the frown lines. The surgeon will cut out all or part of this muscle, depending on the depth of your frown lines. Finally he will pull your brow up and back and cut off the excess scalp skin. He will stitch the scalp closed with either a series of 50 or more single stitches or metal staples, or with one long continuous suture, or a combination of both.

If you had much bleeding, he may put in a small drain under the scalp on one side of your head to permit blood and fluid to drain onto your bandage instead of collecting beneath the skin.

Brow Lift

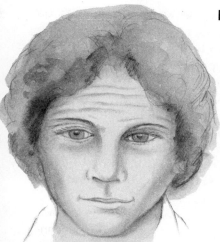

Figure 11-20.

In this procedure, the deep forehead creases and the low eyebrows will be lifted.

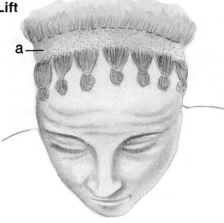

Figure 11-21.

Before the brow lift incision is made in the scalp, the hair is trimmed where it will be cut off (a). Hair is pulled into rubber bands to keep it out of the way of the surgery.

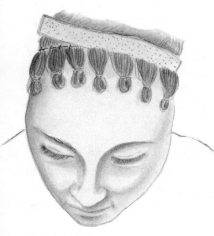

Figure 11-22.

The excess skin is being cut off. The deep work on the muscle has already been done.

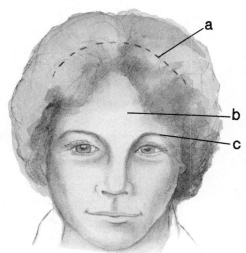

Figure 11-23.

The scar lies behind the front hairline (a) and extends down to the tops of the ears. The brow is pulled up (b), and the deep creases are smoothed. The eyebrows are higher (c), and the upper eyelids are pulled tighter, too.

Your surgeon will now proceed to the other operations you are having.

If this is the only procedure to be done, he will now wash your face and hair to prevent soap and bloody drainage from irritating your scalp. He will remove the bands from your hair, place gauze padding across the incision, and wrap your head with a stretch or elastic bandage.

If you are having your upper lids done as well as your brow lift, your surgeon will almost always do your brow lift *first*. He then will check your eyelids. If the brow lift stretched out the excess eyelid skin, he may decide not to do your eyelids after all.

After

After the operation you go to the recovery room for about an hour or two. From there you are taken home to go to bed and rest.

The Process of Recovery

What to Do About Pain

You may have quite a severe headache for a day or two. The pain comes from the surgery and from throbbing in blood vessels in the scalp. Not everyone has such a headache. Sometimes long-acting local anesthesia is injected at surgery to prevent a headache, especially if you are headache prone. However, it may not be possible to do this if you are having other operations because the dosage of local anesthetic needed for all your operations may make the long-acting anesthetic unsafe to use.

The Healing Process

Bruising may be quite extensive. It will sink down your face over the first 10 days, making your eyes and then your cheeks alarmingly discolored. (Bruising always moves downward due to gravity.) Tinted glasses will help conceal the bruising around your eyes.

You will need to return to your surgeon on day 3 or 4 to have your bandage changed or removed. You will return a second time between 7 and 10 days to have your sutures removed, between 4 and 6 weeks after that for a final check.

Bandages

Your entire head and brow will be wrapped with a bandage: either a white gauze, an Ace wrap, or an elastic cloth. Your hair is tucked under the bandage. If it is long, it will come out as a ponytail at the back of your bandage. This avoids a bulky wad of hair putting painful pressure on your scalp.

Taking Care of Your Wound

You will probably be allowed to shower and brush out your hair the day your bandage is removed or the day after. I let my patients use shampoo about day 5 but only at the back of the head. (There are stitches at the front.) You can gently brush or comb your hair and blow-dry it with cool air. You can wrap your head in a scarf if the weather is cold or the sun very hot. It is best to avoid sun exposure on any surgical wound for at least 6 weeks.

Stitches

Stitches may be removed all at once or in two stages, depending on what kind of stitch is used and how you are healing. Often the brow lift incision is closed with metal staples, which don't tangle in the hair like thread sutures. Sometimes one long thread suture is used, or many separate ones. If your scalp is irritated by the staples or stitches, your surgeon may remove half of them early at day 4 and leave the rest in for another 7 days. All your stitches/staples will be out by 10 to 12 days after the operation.

Scars

Besides the two kinds of surgical incisions mentioned in The Operation, there is another one which may be your only option if you already have a high brow. That is to make the incision where the hair *meets* the brow. This will, however, leave a visible, thin white scar which can be covered by either combing your hair over it, or by wearing bangs.

Almost always, the hair surrounding the scar will thin temporarily (6 to 18 months) because of the stress of the surgery, but there will still be enough hair to hide the scar. Bald patches can occur if you suffer a complication such as bleeding or infection, or if your scar widens (scars don't grow hair, and all scars are bald).

Tips

- If your hair is *very* light, white, or thin, your scar may show. You may want to consider tinting your hair a slightly darker shade.
- If your hair is thin and straight, a permanent will help conceal the scar by making your hair curly so that it clusters over the scar instead of separating and allowing the scar to show through.
- Bangs won't help conceal the scar because it is not *at* your brow (in most cases) but several inches *behind* your hairline.

Back to Work

You can go back to work between days 8 and 11 if the brow lift was your only operation. Your limiting factors will be fatigue and bruising. Your face swells after this surgery, but the obvious swelling around your eyes should be gone by a week. Your face will be more swollen in the morning, less so as the day goes on.

Back to Parties

If you will only feel comfortable when *all* the bruising is gone, you should allow 3 to 4 weeks before going to parties. However, if you are willing to hide the bruising with makeup, you can go to an early, short dinner party as early as day 11. You will find it tiring, though. A late party or cocktail party where you stand for a long time at the end of the day will tire you and make your wound throb if you try it before 3 weeks are up.

Back to Sports

You can do a few limbering-up exercises (knee bends, arm swings) at the end of a week. At the end of two weeks you can take long walks, do short jogs, swim a few laps. After 3 weeks, you may resume all sports, but you won't be up to speed for another week or two. Contact ball sports such as soccer should be avoided for 4 to 6 weeks. A blow to your head can cause the healing scar to rupture, leaving you with a wide, thin, sunken scar.

Back to Sex

It is best to avoid sex for about 10 days. You are unlikely to hurt the surgery, but you will be tired, and the stimulation may bring on a severe headache.

Brow Lift: Recovery-at-a-Glance

This chart represents the *average* recovery times for this cosmetic operation.

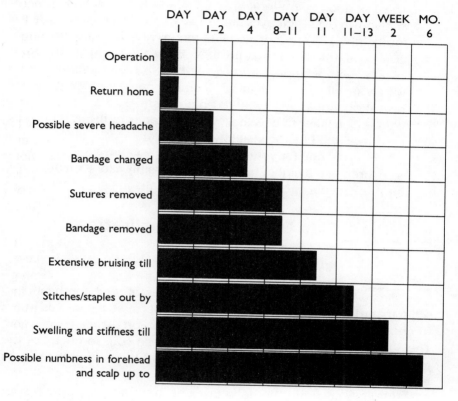

	DAY 1	DAY 1–2	DAY 4	DAY 8–11	DAY 11	DAY 11–13	WEEK 2	MO. 6
Operation								
Return home								
Possible severe headache								
Bandage changed								
Sutures removed								
Bandage removed								
Extensive bruising till								
Stitches/staples out by								
Swelling and stiffness till								
Possible numbness in forehead and scalp up to								

How Much It Costs

Your surgeon's fee will range from about $1500 to $2500. The hospital fee (anesthesia, operating room) will range from $800 to $1500 if the surgery is done on an outpatient basis with local/sedation.

Insurance Coverage

Insurance will *not* pay for this operation unless you can *prove* that your upper lid skin is blocking your vision and that the brow lift is the best way to correct this. Ask your surgeon if this might apply to you. If not, don't waste your time.

My Assessment of This Procedure

This is a good operation for men and women whose brows have sunk down over their eyes and those with furrowed and wrinkled foreheads. The surgery also lifts the eyelids and in some cases is a substitute for upper-lid lifts. Brow lifts tend to be more popular with women, and at least half the time they are done with a facelift or other facial cosmetic surgery. Men have the operation, but for men with receding hairlines, or those in whom baldness is likely to develop, the advantages of the surgery may be outweighed by the visibility of the scar.

In exchange for your improvement, you have a less expressive forehead, a higher hairline, and possibly a look of unnatural surprise if your brows are raised too high.

Side Effects and Complications

Side Effects

Side effects of a brow lift include numbness of your forehead and scalp that may last for 6 months or longer, because the nerves in the forehead are stretched by the surgery, and won't work for a while. The stretched nerves may work imperfectly, so your forehead or the front of your scalp may feel prickly or itchy at times until the nerves heal.

Although stitching the deep layer of the scalp helps keep your scar narrow, some scars will stretch. They may end up a quarter to half an inch wide. If your hair is thick, the wide scar may not be noticeable, but it may require a change in your hairstyle to conceal.

Your forehead will feel—and be—slightly swollen and stiff for weeks after surgery. As in all surgery, the vestiges of swelling persist for 6 to 12 months. You will look fine, but you may notice that with fatigue, or early in the morning, your upper face looks slightly puffy for several weeks or months.

Minor Complications

The surgical trauma of having your scalp lifted may cause hair follicles to go into a resting state. Resting hair follicles may take 6 months to grow again. It may be 18 months before you get back your presurgical thickness. Thus, if your hair seems thinner after surgery, it is *not* your imagination—but neither is it a catastrophe. It will grow back. (Some women have the same thinning occur after childbirth. If this happened to you, you may be more likely to have the thinning from surgery, too.)

Major Complications

Serious complications from the brow lift include poor healing from stretching the scalp too tightly, bleeding, infection, and nerve damage. **Infection** is very rare—the scalp's wonderful blood supply fights off infection efficiently. The most common complication, understandably, is **bleeding**. This may only be extensive bruising, or a small blood clot that forms under your skin and must be drained by removing a stitch. In rare cases, severe bleeding may require a transfusion or a trip back to the operating room to drain a hematoma (large blood clot). Such bleeding is upsetting at the time, but it should not affect your final result.

Poor healing may result from pulling the scalp too tight, or it may result if you have unexpected swelling after surgery. In this case, the swelling is what pulls the scalp too tight. In either case, one or more areas of your incision will not heal but will gape open about half an inch. These will heal slowly in two weeks or so but these slow-healing areas will leave bald patches because they heal with your scar. If this happens, you may be distressed, and it may require much attention to your hair to conceal. However, after 6 to 12 months, it may be possible to cut out these wide bald scars and shift the hair around the area to give you a narrow unnoticeable scar.

Nerve injury can occur, either to the nerves of feeling in the forehead or to the nerve to the forehead muscle. If feeling does not return over a year or so, your nerve may have been injured when the muscle strips were cut. Although theoretically it would be possible to try to repair the nerve by surgery under the microscope, the problem rarely seems worth the effort. The forehead is not very sensitive, and you may readily adapt to patches of numbness. On the other hand, if the nerve to the muscle is injured you might not be able to raise your forehead or wrinkle your brow on one side. Thus your forehead expression is asymmetrical. If the nerve is weak, it may improve in time. If the nerve is not working at all you might need surgery to fix the cut nerve, or to *cut the normal nerve* to make your forehead expression symmetrical.

Here are some examples of patients who had this operation, with and without complications.

Ida: A Troublesome Scar

Ida was in her late forties when she decided to have her entire face "re-done." She had a brow lift, along with a facelift, upper and lower lid surgery, a chemical peel, and a chin enlargement. This was a lot of surgery, and she had a great deal of swelling in her face and eyelids, as expected. She healed well, except that a one-inch length of her brow incision did not heal and pulled apart when the stitches were removed. Ida was distraught. The area healed on its own, but it took several weeks. After it healed, Ida had a wide patch of scar that could be seen through her light blond hair. She concealed the scar with a hairpiece. After a year she had minor surgery to cut out the scar. Although the scar was not visible any longer, she had become fond of the hairpiece and did not give it up.

Susan: A New Phase of Life

Susan had a brow lift because at 40, her always furrowed brow seemed to her worse—and more unsightly—than ever. Also, after an unfortunate marriage, she didn't want to carry her worry lines with her into her life. Susan had a brow lift under local anesthesia. She went back to work after a week—still bruised but not bothered by it. For the first time in her life, she had a smooth forehead. She couldn't believe the difference to her expression. She felt she looked content for the first time.

Beverly: Not "Mad" Anymore

Beverly had a habit of frowning, and deep frown lines ran in her family. Also, she felt her brows were sagging, a sign of aging that bothered her. She was 50 and happily married. She had a brow lift, despite her family's bewilderment as to why she wanted it done. The surgery lifted her brows and converted her deep frown grooves into smoother, although still present, lines. She healed but complained for months that the numbness made it hard to use her curling iron. She felt it was worthwhile when her youngest son told her that he liked her not looking "mad" at him anymore.

What Other Patients Say

- **Real estate executive, 63:** "I can see the difference but I had so much done to my face it's hard to tell what changed the most. I like looking calm for a change."
- **Tennis pro, 47:** "I've squinted and scowled in the sunlight so much all my life, that this was a must. I couldn't believe the difference for me."
- **Office manager, 41:** "I guess I'm satisfied. I wanted all my lines and wrinkles gone. It didn't do that."
- **Financial planner, 52:** "I bled like a stuck pig during my surgery. Afterwards, I looked like I got mugged after a Friday night bash. But when I healed it looked good."

Cosmetic Chin Surgery

What Surgeons Call It

Depending on what is done, this procedure is generally called an augmentation mentoplasty.

What It Will Do

Cosmetic chin surgery aims to give you a stronger, firmer chin, with a better *profile*. If you have an unusually *long* chin, surgery may change the way you look face-on. However, 90 percent of patients will see their improvement largely in profile or oblique views of their face.

What It Won't Do

It *won't* improve alignment of the teeth or correct a bone problem in the *jaw*; it changes only the *chin* (i.e., that part of the lower jaw that sticks out in front). Jaw problems and tooth problems are corrected by orthodontia or by bone reconstruction of the whole jaw or sometimes the whole *face*. These are *complex reconstructive problems*.

How Long It Will Last

The improvement is permanent.

When to Have It

About a half of cosmetic chin surgery is done alone; usually this surgery is combined with another cosmetic operation such as a "nose job" or a facelift. You can have chin surgery once your chin growth is *mostly* over—about 16 for girls and 18 for boys. But your chin will grow a bit more until you are in your early twenties. So, if you are a *teenager*, and are having a chin implant placed to enlarge your chin, choose a small to medium-sized implant. A large one might be too large in five or ten years and you might want the implant replaced with a smaller one later on.

Bone surgery to reshape the chin can be done at the same age.

Where to Have It

This operation is usually done on an outpatient basis in an office operating room *or* an outpatient surgery center *or* a hospital operating room. If bone surgery is done, an overnight stay may be necessary.

Conditions That Increase Your Risk

Any condition that makes you prone to infections in your mouth or on your chin will increase your risk of complication. The *most common* factors are severe facial acne *or* being a heavy smoker (important only if the surgery is done via the mouth). *If* you are a smoker *and* your surgery is via your mouth *and* you continue to smoke in the week after surgery, you are much more likely to have an infection. An infection will make your body reject a chin implant. If your chin bone is reshaped, infection in the bone can make it shrink.

Usual Anesthesia

When an implant is used, the surgery is usually done with local anesthesia and sedation given to you by your surgeon. If the chin bone is being reshaped, local anesthesia with sedation or general anesthesia will be used. Either way, you can go home the same day.

How Long It Takes

The operating time will be *about 1 hour*. When the bone is re-shaped, it tends to be a bit longer.

The Operation
(Figures 11-24 and 11-25)

Chin Implant: Before

You will arrive for your surgery about an hour before it is scheduled. You will have had nothing to eat or drink since midnight the night before. You will change into a hospital gown and will then go either to a preoperative area or directly to the operating room. An IV will be placed in your arm so that you can be given a solution of dextrose and/or saline to prevent your becoming dehydrated during surgery. You may also be given preoperative sedation through the IV. (If you are a very stoical person, you may need only sedation by mouth. In this case, you would be given sedative pills before your surgery, but you may not need any IV, and may not need a heart monitor.) Once you are on the operating table, a safety strap is put across your lap. Sticky pads are placed on your chest so that your heart can be monitored during surgery. Also, a sticky pad will be placed on your hip under your gown if cautery will be used. This is a grounding pad, which makes the cautery safe for you. (Surgical cautery uses electrical heat to seal off bleeding blood vessels.)

Next, your face is washed with surgical soap, and sterile drapes are placed over your body and around your face. If you are having intravenous sedation, you will be given a small dose of sedation to test your reaction. Then you will be sedated until you doze. Then your surgeon will inject local anesthetic into the nerves and tissues in your chin and mouth. Your eyes will be covered to protect them from the bright surgical lights.

Chin Implant: During

Your surgeon will make an incision in the skin under the chin or inside your lower lip just above your chin. He will gently lift the tissues off the bone to make a space large enough for a chin implant to fit—1½ to 2 inches wide. Next, he will use implant "sizers" to test the right size for you. He will have a general idea, but sizers are often used to be sure that the implant chosen is the right size. Your implant may be solid silicone or a "gel" implant. Gel implants are solid outside but have a core of gel-silicone, so that they are soft and can move with your facial expression. (However, since the gel can leak out if it is hit hard or punctured with a needle, your surgeon will choose the implant for your individual lifestyle and needs; for example, a solid implant if you play soccer, and a gel if you have thin tissues and a hard implant might show through the skin.) Your surgeon will next place the actual implant in the space he has made. Then he sews in the implant and sews up the muscle and skin (or the lining of the mouth, if he does your surgery through the inner lower lip).

The surgical soap is washed off your face. Tape is strapped over your chin. You are now awake. You are taken to the recovery room, and within an hour or two you will be released to go home—to bed.

Chin Implant: After

In the recovery room, an ice bag may be placed over your chin. You may want to do this at home, for comfort and to help decrease the swelling.

Chin Reshaping: Before

If you are having surgery to reshape the bone of your chin: The preliminary steps are the same as above, except that you *always need an IV, and you may have general anesthesia.*

Chin Reshaping: During

Once you are asleep, your surgeon makes an incision about 3 to 4 inches long through the inside of your lower lip. This avoids a long outside scar. The surgeon lifts the tissues off the bone and lifts the chin bone up and out. He will use an electrical saw to cut off that part of the chin bone that is poorly placed. Then he drills holes in the bone to wire the chin bone into a better position. He may use a small metal plate instead of wires to hold it there.

This may *sound* simple, but the bone cuts have to be made exactly right. At the end the bone may not look perfectly positioned and new drill holes may need to be made. If this happens, your surgery will take extra time to do. You can still end up with a great result.

Once the bone is in place, the muscle and mouth tissue are sewn up. Your bandage—usually an extensive elastic wrap around your chin and head—is put on. You may be awake if you had sedation.

Chin Reshaping: After

If you had general anesthesia you will wake up feeling *cold*. (General anesthesia dilates blood vessels in your skin, so you lose body heat during surgery.) You can go home, but it will be at least 2 hours before you feel strong enough. If the general anesthetic made you very dizzy or nauseated, you may stay in the hospital overnight.

Cosmetic Chin Surgery

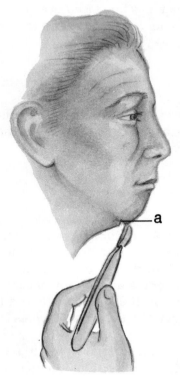
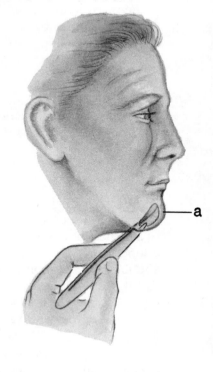

Figure 11-24.

An implant is being placed to strengthen a weak chin. The incision can be done as here, under the chin (a), or the implant can be put in place through an incision in the mouth.

Figure 11-25.

The implant is now put in place. Note the new fullness of the chin (a). Bone surgery can create the same effect by reshaping chin bone.

The Process of Recovery

What to Do About Pain

Chin implant surgery causes *virtually no pain* afterwards. Pain after surgery is worse in body areas that *move*. Your chin does not move a great deal, and it moves less after surgery when you eat soft or liquid food. However, your chin will tend to ache on and off. After *any* operation, the aching is more noticeable the first two days after surgery. After that, aching occurs only when you are tired.

If your chin bone has been reshaped, you may hurt for a day or you *may* only ache. This operation is more extensive than a chin implant. Your chin will be more bruised and swollen.

The Healing Process

Your chin will be numb for *at least* 2 weeks, and often as long as 6. Some numbness may last up to 6 months, although it should be slowly subsiding. You may be bruised, but bruising works its way downward from the pull of gravity. You are likely to find that your bruising is under your chin or in your upper neck.

Your chin will be *visibly* swollen for about 2 weeks. After that, although it will still be swollen (remember that surgical swelling persists for months), the swelling will be noticeable to *you and your surgeon* but not others.

Bandages

The bandage after a chin implant is often only tape strapping across your chin, to keep down swelling and to support your chin when you talk and eat.

When the bone is repositioned, you need more support and will probably have an elastic wrap around your head and chin. Bandages are removed by day 6 after surgery. Tape tends to loosen, especially in men, whose beard literally lifts the tape off as it grows.

Taking Care of Your Wound

Men can shave and women can apply makeup as soon as the bandage comes off, but everything has to be done more gently than usual. Besides feeling numb, your skin will be sensitive. Shaving is done gingerly at first; making up is best limited to brushing on powder or patting a little concealer cream on the bruises.

Because your chin is stiff, brushing and flossing your teeth will be more difficult than usual—your mouth won't open as fully as it usually does, especially if your surgery was done through an incision in your inner lower lip. About half of chin implants and almost all chin bone reshaping are done this way.

If you have such an incision, you will be given detailed instructions for caring for it. These almost always consist of:

Chin Enlargement: Recovery-at-a-Glance

This chart represents the *average* recovery times for this cosmetic operation.

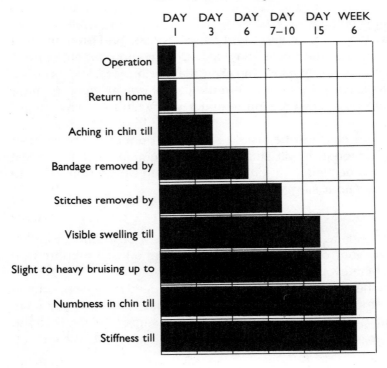

	DAY 1	DAY 3	DAY 6	DAY 7–10	DAY 15	WEEK 6
Operation						
Return home						
Aching in chin till						
Bandage removed by						
Stitches removed by						
Visible swelling till						
Slight to heavy bruising up to						
Numbness in chin till						
Stiffness till						

- Gentle or no flossing for a week
- Gentle brushing, often with a *child's* toothbrush
- Rinsing your mouth three or four times a day with salt water, salt and peroxide in water, or an antibiotic mouth wash
- Liquid food for the first day. Soft food for the next 5 days: soup, ice cream, milkshakes, puddings, possibly ground meat, but nothing that requires chewing or is highly salted or spiced.

These are all *commonsense* precautions. Most people follow a soft diet on their own. You won't feel like "testing" your surgery with anything that might hurt or irritate your mouth.

Stitches

Mouth stitches usually dissolve by themselves, but sometimes "dissolving" stitches don't dissolve. If this happens, your surgeon will remove them after about a week to 10 days. Skin stitches are used if your surgery was done through an incision *under* your chin. These are removed by day 6. Sometimes a surgeon will use a "buried" skin stitch—this is fine nylon running entirely under your skin except at either end of the incision. It is less irritating than standard skin stitches and stays in about 10 days.

Scars

If your surgery is done through your inner lower lip, you have *no* visible scars. If your surgery is done through an incision under your chin, you will have a short scar *under* your chin (about 1½ to 2 inches). These will usually heal with a flat scar. About 20 percent of people will heal with a lumpy red scar in this area— it will flatten, but may take up to a year to do so. This is annoying because you *feel* it, but being under your chin, it won't show.

Tips

- Men will want to buy an electric shaver because the skin may be numb for weeks after surgery and will tend to be easily nicked.
- If you need dental work, wait about a month between the chin surgery and the dental work. Otherwise your mouth may become unduly sore.
- If you have severe acne, have your dermatologist treat this before surgery. Besides reducing your infection risk, it will also help your skin tolerate the bandages.

Back to Work

After a **chin implant** you can usually go back to work on day 6—as soon as the bandage is off. I have had patients go back to work on day 3 when they had little sedation and had the kind of job where they could "hide" from public view. If you had *general* anesthesia, you will need at least a full week off, and often *two*.

Back to Parties

Because the surgery makes your chin stiff, even if not sore, it won't feel comfortable to talk at first. Crunchy party food is out for at least a week. Unless you must make an appearance, wait 2 weeks for a party—and probably 3 weeks if your bone was reshaped.

Back to Sports

You should do no sports for a week. Otherwise your chin will ache and swell. *Ball* sports are *out* for 2 weeks—a blow on your chin with a tennis ball or baseball can cause bleeding, swelling, and thick internal scarring. In general, wait 3 weeks for any sport other than swimming, jogging, or hiking. Wait 6 weeks for a contact sport.

Back to Sex

You should avoid sex for a full week. For the second week, avoid facial contact—an inadvertent bump or blow can open up your healing incisions or cause pain and swelling in your chin.

How Much It Costs

Cost will vary from a minimum of $1500 for a chin implant, to $3000 or more for chin bone reshaping. These are the surgeon's fees. Anesthesia will range from $500 for local anesthesia to $2000 or more for general anesthesia. Cost *may* be a factor in deciding what operation and/or anesthesia you choose—discuss your options with your surgeon.

Insurance Coverage

Insurance *may* pay, if you can prove that your chin is malformed from a birth defect or an injury. This is not common. Ask your surgeon. If he thinks yours is an unusual case, discuss payment with your insurance company *before* the surgery. *Remember*: In these cases, your insurance is unlikely to pay, *unless they agree to do so before surgery, and commit themselves in writing as to exactly how much they will pay.* They may, for instance, pay the hospital fee but not the surgeon's fee.

My Assessment of These Procedures

The **chin implant** is easy for you during and after surgery. The recovery is short, and there is little if any pain. It is an excellent operation to improve a small chin.

Chin **bone surgery** is somewhat more extensive. Swelling, bruising, and discomfort are all more pronounced. It is an excellent operation to reshape your chin, but it is done only if the simpler implant operation will not correct the cosmetic problem.

Note: Oral surgeons, who are dentists, not medical doctors, operate on the jaw. Chin reshaping is a cosmetic operation which is done by some oral surgeons. If your plastic surgeon doesn't do chin bone reshaping, he may refer you to another plastic surgeon or to an oral surgeon for this operation.

Side Effects and Complications

Side Effects

The most common side effects of chin surgery are numbness and swelling. The numbness is from chin nerves being bruised or stretched during surgery. Swelling of your chin is inevitable after surgery. Until it goes down after six months or so, it may make you wonder if your surgeon didn't make you too strong-chinned. The swelling is not obvious, but it may trouble you.

Complications

If you had a **chin implant,** the most likely thing to actually go wrong is for the implant to shift out of position. This is not dangerous, and it is not usual. Correcting it requires *redoing* the operation—taking out the implant, enlarging the pocket, and/or putting in a different implant. The most common cause of an implant shifting is its pocket being a little too big or too small. Next most troublesome is infection. This is rare, but an infection around an implant will cause your body to reject the implant. It can be replaced in about 6 months.

If your chin bone is **reshaped,** your most common complication will tend to be injury to a nerve. Here your chin, and even your lower front teeth, are numb for months or even a year. This is less likely to happen after a chin implant, because the surgeon does not have to stretch the chin tissues—and hence the nerves—as much as he does when cutting the bone. In rare cases, a nerve will not recover. You may have to live with it—or may choose to have another operation to try to repair the nerves if they have been torn, not just stretched. In such cases, a torn nerve can be sewn back together. Over the months, feeling *may* return. A nerve can be so damaged, however, that it won't work, even after it has been sewn back together. Grim? Not really. You may think that having a chin that looks right for you is well worth the risk *and* the (rare) complication.

Andy: An Implant That "Popped"

Andy was 28 when he had his big nose made smaller and his small chin made bigger with a chin implant. He thought his chin looked lopsided when his surgeon took off the tape. Andy moved to a new job and consulted me about his lopsided chin. The swelling had gone down, and the lopsidedness was even more noticeable. No one had commented, but Andy could feel the implant lying crooked. He could even see it, and it bothered him. He decided to have the surgery redone, for peace of mind. At surgery, I found that the pocket was a little too small for his implant, which had popped out of place. I enlarged the pocket and replaced the implant. Andy was pleased but felt put out at having to go through another healing period.

Cindy: One Step at a Time

Cindy had a small chin and her nose was too large. She was terrified of surgery and decided to have her chin done first (unlike most people) because it was less complicated than nose surgery and besides, if she didn't like the result, she could always have me remove the implant.

It took me about 45 minutes to do Cindy's surgery. I removed the tape from her chin on the fifth day. She returned to work straight from my office. Her chin looked puffy but she was not bruised and had no pain. At two weeks, with most of the swelling gone, she was pleased. At six weeks the last trace of stiffness faded and her new chin felt like "part of me." A year later—buoyed by the success of her chin surgery—she decided to have her nose operated on too. Note: Usually nose surgery is done before, or at the same time as, chin enlargement. This makes it easier for your surgeon to enlarge your chin in proportion to your new small nose.

Joan: A "Witchy" Chin

Joan was 21 when she decided she hated her chin enough to have it "fixed." She was lovely, but in profile her chin curved up slightly, giving her an ungraceful point. She decided to have cosmetic nose surgery and to have her chin reshaped. At the same operation, I operated on Joan's nose, and then, working with a maxillofacial surgeon, reshaped the bone of her chin.

It took Joan longer to recover from the bone surgery than from the nose surgery. Her chin was still slightly sore after 2 weeks and her neck was bruised. She covered this with a scarf and returned to work. Six weeks after surgery, with most of the swelling and all of the bruising gone, she could see her new profile and was pleased.

What Other Patients Say

- **Airline stewardess, 31:** "I was afraid that my chin would end up too big. No one ever noticed that I'd had it done, and once the swelling was gone I felt comfortable with how things turned out. It didn't hurt at all. I got called for work the fourth day after surgery. I took the bandage off myself and headed in to work, after I called the doctor to tell her what I had to do. It turned out fine."

- **Male account executive, 24:** "I hated the thought of the hospital and had my surgery done with almost no sedation. I can take a lot of pain, but it didn't hurt. I could feel the pulling. I felt groggy for about an hour and then I went home. I wanted to go to work. I didn't think the bandage was that bad. But the doctor said I had to go home and rest. My chin was numb *for weeks but* I look good!"

- **Veterinarian (female), 33:** "I had revision of my chin *bone*. It hurt afterwards. I was sick to my stomach twice. I went home the same day, though. After I got over all that part of the surgery, it was great, but my chin sometimes aches when the weather is cold."

- **Male high school senior, 18:** "I had a weird chin. It hung down. I wanted to be asleep for the surgery. I was. If I press really hard I can feel the metal where the chin was wired. I don't get comments about my face anymore."

Cheek Implant

What Surgeons Call It

The technical name for this procedure is cheek implant or malar implant.

What It Will Do

Cheek implant surgery aims to create a higher cheek line, giving your midface more definition.

What It Won't Do

If your facial bones are naturally rather flat, this operation will not radically alter the bone structure of your face. It will, however, give it more shape. The operation is often helpful to actors, actresses, and models who need the cheek prominence to give them facial projection on film or in a photograph.

How Long It Will Last

The surgery result is permanent because the implant is a permanent one.

When to Have It

You can have a cheek implant whenever you decide that your cheekbones need more fullness. Age tends to flatten the tissues over the cheekbone, so many men and women have the surgery at the same time as a facelift. Younger people are most likely to have cheek implants done without other surgery. For them, cheek flatness is from a family tendency to flat cheekbones.

Where to Have It

This operation is done on an outpatient basis in a doctor's office operating room *or* an outpatient surgery center *or* a hospital outpatient operating room.

Conditions That Increase Your Risk

The cheek implants are tolerated well by your body unless an infection occurs. So you and your surgeon need to be alert for anything that might increase your risk of an infection. Smoking is most important. It delays wound healing, especially in the mouth—and this operation is done through an incision inside your upper lip. *Stop smoking* if at all possible—or accept the possibility that your smoking could totally undo the result of your operation. If you have an infection in your mouth, your surgery should be postponed until the infection is controlled. If you have a dental infection, it too should be treated.

Usual Anesthesia

Cheek implants are usually done under local anesthesia with sedation. The operation is limited to a fairly small area, so a few patients will tolerate local anesthesia and only sedative pills, without the heavier intravenous sedation.

How Long It Takes

This operation will take about one hour to do.

The Operation
(Figures 11-26 through 11-28)

Before

You will arrive for your operation about an hour before it is scheduled, having had nothing to eat or drink since midnight the night before. You will change into a hospital gown and will be taken either to a preoperative area or directly to the operating room. Your surgeon will mark on your cheeks where he wants the implant to lie. An IV will probably be started in your arm, and you will be given a solution of dextrose and/or saline to prevent dehydration during surgery. You'll also receive a dose of antibiotics, although no one is sure that giving them preoperatively is necessary or effective in preventing infection. (If you are having only sedation by mouth, and no IV, you will probably be given antibiotics by mouth.)

Once you are on the operating table, sticky pads will be placed on your chest to monitor your heart. (Again, these may not be used if you are having minimal sedation.) A sticky pad will be placed on your leg, under your gown as a grounding pad, which makes surgical cautery safe to use. (Surgical cautery uses an electrical heat device that seals off bleeding blood vessels.) Sometimes it is not needed for this operation.

You will then be given intravenous sedation which will make you drowsy. Your face will be washed with surgical soap, and sterile drapes will be placed around your face and over your body. Your surgeon next will inject local anesthetic into your cheek to numb the nerves in the cheek. He will also lift up your lip and inject local anesthetic inside your upper lip. Your eyes will be covered with moist gauze to protect them from the surgical lights overhead.

During

If you are having a facelift as well, your surgeon may put the implants in place through the facelift incisions. If not, your surgeon will lift up your upper lip and make an incision in the groove inside your upper lip where your lip and gums meet. He will then lift the tissue of your cheek up from the bone beneath, being careful not to cut the nerve of feeling in your midcheek that goes to your upper lip. When he has done this on one side, he will proceed directly to the other side. He will then inspect the implants, probably already knowing the size he expects to use, and will select an implant size conforming to the space over your bones. Then, holding the implant with an instrument, he will push it in over your cheekbone. If the space seems too small, he may enlarge the space over your cheek, or he may choose a smaller implant.

Once the two implants are in position, your surgeon will stitch up the incisions. Your mouth is wiped with water and the soap is washed off your face. Your face is dried and tape strips are placed over your cheeks to support the implant.

After

You will be wheeled to the recovery room, where you may spend an hour or so. You should then be able to go home to rest, and probably to sleep. You will be more comfortable if you keep your head up on a few extra pillows and if you keep a cold pack over your cheeks for the rest of the day.

Cheek Implant

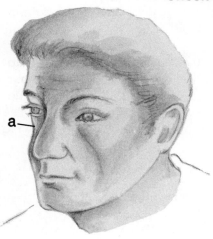

Figure 11-26.

Cheek implant surgery will correct the flatness in the cheek (a)—best seen in an oblique, not a full-face view.

Figure 11-27.

An instrument holds up the lip while the implant is inserted via the groove between the teeth and upper lip (a). If you put your tongue in that groove, you can feel how close it lies to the cheek prominence.

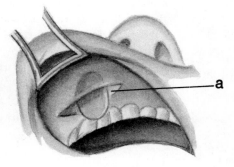

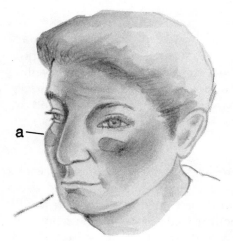

Figure 11-28.

The implants are in place on top of the cheek prominence (a).

The Process of Recovery

What to Do About Pain

You should not have pain after this operation, but your cheeks will feel stiff and unnatural. You will not talk naturally both as a result of the anesthesia numbing facial nerves and from swelling. You will be unable to smile comfortably for several days. The swelling may affect your jaw joint, so that yawning and chewing feel temporarily uncomfortable.

The Healing Process

The stiffness in your face subsides rapidly after the first 5 days and is gone within 7 to 14 days, although you may feel aware that you aren't back to normal for another month. You will be able to drink right after surgery, but you will not be able to eat solid food for several days, as it may irritate the incision inside your upper lip. After a day or two, you may develop some faint yellow or bluish bruising on your lower cheek, which should fade in 7 to 10 days.

Although your cheeks are swollen for about 2 weeks, this is often a symmetrical puffiness that attracts little attention.

Bandages

Usually you will have tape strips placed across your cheeks. This not only helps keep the swelling down and the implant in place but also reminds you not to move your face too much. The more your face rests, the faster the wound can heal and the swelling subside. These strips will be removed five days after the surgery. Your head and face are not wrapped, unless you have had additional surgery that requires such bandaging.

Taking Care of Your Wound

You will be asked not to brush your upper teeth until the incisions are healed—about day 6. You can use a gentle Water Pik. Use a child's toothbrush so that you don't have to open your mouth wide to brush your back teeth, but don't brush the front near the incision. You will also be asked to avoid strong mouth rinses, but you should swish out your mouth several times a day with slightly salty water.

After about day 6, you can brush regularly. After 10 days, you should be able to return to regular dental care such as floss and gum picks.

Stitches

Your stitches are inside your mouth, between your upper lip and teeth. The stitches will usually dissolve, but not always. After about a week to 10 days, if the stitches have *not* dissolved, your surgeon will remove them.

Scars

You will have no *visible* scars. There will be a scar inside your upper lip. It may feel hard and swollen for several weeks or longer.

Tips

- Since this operation will make your cheeks more prominent, you may want to stop using blush-on for a while to avoid drawing attention to the change in your face.
- The surgery will make your cheeks and upper face feel stiff and swollen for several weeks. So don't schedule dental surgery or dental care for the first 6 weeks after surgery. (Extensive dental work *might* stir up a late infection around the new implants.)

Back to Work

Because there are so few telltale signs from this surgery, you can usually return to work by day 6.

Back to Parties

Although you can start going to parties at the same time as you go back to work, you will find that your cheeks ache by the end of the day. Also, alcohol may increase the blood flow around your surgery, making your cheeks burn or even flush slightly. It may be better to postpone late night social events for another week.

Back to Sports

You can resume stretching exercises by days 6 to 8, but bending over will make your cheeks swell and ache. Avoid any heavy lifting or vigorous workouts such as aerobics or Nautilus for 2 weeks. As for ball or contact sports—a blow to your cheek can

Cheek Implant: Recovery-at-a-Glance

This chart represents the *average* recovery times for this cosmetic operation.

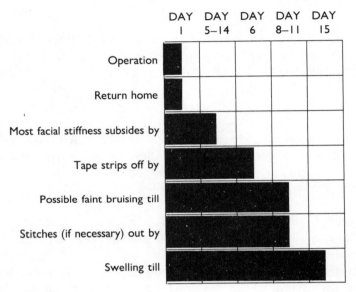

	DAY 1	DAY 5–14	DAY 6	DAY 8–11	DAY 15
Operation					
Return home					
Most facial stiffness subsides by					
Tape strips off by					
Possible faint bruising till					
Stitches (if necessary) out by					
Swelling till					

cause bleeding around your implant at this stage. If, for instance, you must play tennis, avoid the net and play a baseline game. Don't resume soccer, football, basketball, etc., for 6 weeks after surgery.

Back to Sex

Your mouth won't feel comfortable for passionate kissing for about 2 weeks. Sexual arousal will make the surgical area ache or swell during the first week, and an unexpected bump to your cheek could lead to bleeding around the implant. Avoid sex for 10 days.

How Much It Costs

Your surgeon's fee will range from $1000 to $2000. The cost of the implants will be between $250 and $400. The operating room cost will range from about $500 to $1000. So your total cost could run as high as $3400. Usually it's somewhere between two and three thousand dollars.

Insurance Coverage

Insurance will *not* pay for this operation unless you can prove that you have an injury or birth defect that has caused a bone defect in your cheek.

My Assessment of This Procedure

A cheek implant is fairly straightforward for you to have. You should not have a difficult recovery, and complications are uncommon. It is often done in conjunction with other facial cosmetic operations to enhance the result, but if it's done alone, you are likely to have a subtle rather than a dramatic change in your face.

Side Effects and Complications

Side Effects

The side effects of this operation include temporary numbness of your upper lip or the side of your nose. This is because the surgery may stretch nerves in your cheek. The numbness feels as though your anesthesia has not worn off. It poses a problem when you try to kiss (you can't feel with the numb part of your lip) or when you shave in that area or try to put on lipstick. The numbness will often begin to fade within 2 weeks. Feeling usually has returned by 6 weeks, but occasional patches of numbness may persist for many more months. Rarely, numbness is permanent.

Your scar inside your upper lip is rarely a problem but if, for instance, you sing or play a clarinet you may find that for a while the swelling and the scar make you uncomfortable when you try to perform.

Complications

Infection is rare. Once an infection begins, it seems reasonable to treat it with antibiotics, but invariably the implant must be removed because the antibiotics can't reach a high enough concentration around it to kill the germs. Signs of an infection would be pain, fever, redness in your cheeks, and swelling out of proportion to the surgery—that is, not puffiness but balloonlike swelling in your face. Infection occurs less than 1 percent of the time.

Under normal circumstances, most people find this operation easier to recover from than they had expected.

Mary: Her Career Took Off

Mary was a model in her late teens. Wanting to become as photogenic as possible, she had cheek implant surgery with sedation as an outpatient. She felt groggy and a little nauseated from the sedation, but felt better by that evening. Her cheeks were puffy but not tender 3 days later. She said the swelling was similar to what she had when an upper wisdom tooth was removed. I removed the tape after 3 days, because it was irritating her cheek skin. On the fifth day Mary went out on a "shoot" and no one noticed what she had had done. (These were not close-up photographs of her face.) She didn't know if she got more jobs because of her surgery, but she thought so. Her lack of cheek definition had been pointed out after a video analysis by a modeling consultant—and certainly her career took off after her surgery.

Jerome: No Longer a "Nebbish"

Jerome was dissatisfied with his facial appearance after a serious illness. Time did not seem to correct it. He felt all the strength in his face had been drained. Jerome decided to have chin and cheek implants. (He had had a cosmetic nose operation as a teenager.) He had the surgery with sedation as an outpatient and found that it left him tired for several weeks. He had arranged a week off from work but stayed out a week and a half. He was delighted with the result and found that besides not feeling so "nebbish-y" any longer, his boss gave him more challenging assignments, with the comment that Jerome looked as though he'd finally recovered from his illness.

Harriet: Having It All Done

Harriet decided to have her face "rejuvenated" and had a facelift, eyelid surgery, neck suction, and cheek implants. She opted for general anesthesia, because she did not want to be awake, and money was no object for her. She couldn't tell at first what the implants had done for her, because her face was swollen from all of her surgery. In fact, it took 3 months, and with most of the swelling gone, she realized that she had "cheekbones" that she had never had before.

What Other Patients Say

- **Part-time runway model, 22:** "I model for fun, not because I have to. I've always liked a strong face, and with my cheek line higher, I feel my face stands out on the runway in a way it didn't before."
- **Art teacher, 37:** "I knew I had to stop smoking, and I did a few days before surgery, but I smoked three packs in the first 2 days after. I got an infection 5 days later, and both implants had to be removed. That was done in the office. I'm waiting until I stop smoking until I try again."
- **Legal secretary, 43:** "I bruised a lot, but I have a thin face and I bruise easily. I was numb for weeks. My cheeks were so flat I had nowhere to put my blush on. Now I do, so I'm pleased."
- **Director of nonprofit institute, 59:** "I had my face redone. It took forever to recover, but I had a lot of surgery. I never noticed the implant part. That healed without a hitch. I look fine."

Correction of Prominent Ears

What Surgeons Call It

The technical name for this procedure is otoplasty, meaning shaping of the ear.

What It Will Do

An otoplasty corrects prominent ears so that they lie flat (but not squashed) against your head.

What It Won't Do

This operation does not change the size or shape of your ear, although that can be done at the same time. Some ear shapes are difficult or impossible to correct. Fortunately, an odd ear shape is *much* less noticeable when the ear is flat against your scalp. Also, surgery will not make your ears perfectly symmetrical. No person has two identical ears. You will notice slight differences between your ears, if you look closely, both before *and* after surgery.

How Long It Will Last

Permanently, once it is fully healed. However, the commonest complication of this surgery is relapse, in which the ear, which is completely composed of cartilage, fails to hold its new shape. It may stick out again, although not as much as before. This happens during the first 6 weeks, when your body is "gluing" your ear in its new place with scar tissue.

When to Have It

You can have this done as early as age 5, because your ears have reached 90 percent of adult size by then. Generally, surgery is done when a child is young, to avoid unnecessary teasing, which causes its own adjustment problems.

Where to Have It

This operation is usually done on an outpatient basis in a doctor's office operating room *or* a surgery center *or* a hospital operating room.

Conditions That Increase Your Risk

These are few. However, if you have had a previous severe ear injury, such as a burn or an extensive laceration, you have an increased risk of infection or slow healing because your ear is damaged. Surgery should still be possible.

Usual Anesthesia

Adults and teenagers usually prefer local anesthesia with sedation, given by the surgeon. Once your ear is numb, the surgery may be boring, but not painful. General anesthesia is necessary for young children because they cannot hold still. The sedation may excite children instead of calming them, and the needle injections, which they don't understand, are frightening. There are rare exceptions in which sedation is used in a calm, grownup child of 10 or 11.

How Long It Takes

Surgery takes between 1½ to 2½ hours. The cartilage in children and teenagers tends to be softer and easier to work with. Surgery can extend to 3 hours—even more—if the cartilage proves difficult to mold into the right shape.

The Operation
(Figures 11-29 through 11-30)

Before

You will arrive for surgery about an hour before it is scheduled, having had nothing to eat or drink since midnight the night before. You will change into a hospital gown and will usually be taken to a preoperative area to have an IV placed in your arm so that you can be given a solution of dextrose and/or saline to prevent dehydration during surgery. (If your sedation is going to be light, this may not be done.)

You are then taken to the operating room and are helped onto the operating table. A safety strap is placed across your hips and sticky pads are placed on your chest to monitor your heart. Another sticky pad is placed on your hip under your gown if surgical cautery will be used. This is a grounding pad that makes the cautery safe to use. (Surgical cautery uses an electrical heat device to seal off bleeding blood vessels.)

At this point, if you are having general anesthesia, you will be given medicine through your IV to put you to sleep. If you are having sedation instead, you will first be given a small dose to give the surgeon an idea of how much more you'll need (you'll feel slightly drowsy). Next, a little pack is put in each ear to keep liquids from dripping in, and your face and ears are washed with surgical soap. Sterile drapes are put around your face and over your body, and you are given more sedation.

During

Once you are dozing, your surgeon will inject anesthetic around (not into) your ears, numbing the nerves. He will use one of three basic methods of reshaping your ear or a combination.

- Simply putting in stitches to hold it in its new position
- Tunneling under the skin in front of the ear to scrape down the cartilage with a rasp (which is like a fine file) to weaken it, and then putting the stitches in to hold it back
- Cutting the ear cartilage at the back to weaken it and then putting in the stitches to hold it in place

Often, all three steps are done: the cartilage is thinned in front, cut in the back, and sutured in place.

First, your surgeon makes the incision in the crease behind your ear. You may feel pulling or scraping as he lifts the skin off the cartilage. If he rasps the front of the ear, you may feel a pull on the lower end of your ear and then a rocking feeling as the delicate rasp is slipped from the back to the front of your ear under the skin. You may not be aware at all when the cartilage is cut at the back. Cartilage is soft and your ear will be numb so you will probably feel nothing at this step.

The stitches are crucial because they fold your ear into its new shape. During this time you think that nothing is happening, except you may feel the skin of your face tickled as the dangling end of the stitching material (suture) touches your skin where it is not numb. When the stitches are tied, you may feel a pulling, and a squeaky sound as the suture rubs across itself. By the time the first ear is finished, you may be awake and bored. You will probably be given more sedation before the other ear is done.

Correction of Prominent Ears

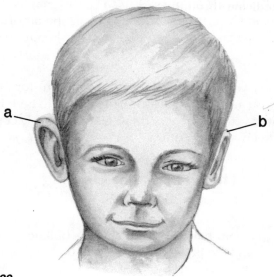

Figure 11-29.

Side (a) shows a typical prominent ear sticking out from the side of the head. Side (b) shows the corrected ear—it should lie naturally against the head, not "plastered" against the scalp.

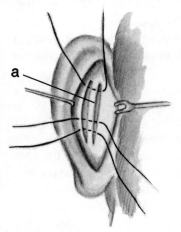

Figure 11-30A.

The cartilage (a) has been cut—one of several techniques of correcting the ear cartilage. Stitches are in place and will be tied, folding the cartilage into its new position, so that the ear does not stick out.

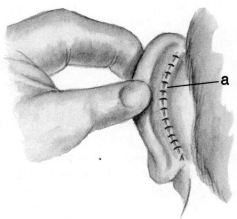

Figure 11-30B.

The scar lies on the back of the ear, hidden in the natural crease (a).

After *both* ears are set back, your surgeon will check that they match as much as possible. If not, he may have to redo some stitches. Once the operation is over, the surgical soap is washed off your face and then the bandage is put on.

After

After surgery, you will be in the recovery room for an hour or two. When you are ready, you go home to rest in bed. Keep your head elevated with two or more soft pillows. This is comfortable and helps keep swelling down.

The Process of Healing

What to Do About Pain

You should have *no* pain, unless a stitch is pulling on your bandage, or the bandage is too tight. This can be relieved by cutting your bandage (as *directed by your surgeon—don't do it otherwise*) or having your surgeon or his nurse apply a new bandage. Your ears will throb the day of surgery while the local anesthetic wears off, and they may throb or ache a little, especially in the evenings, for a day or so. You're very unlikely to need more than one or two pills of a narcotic painkiller such as Demerol (many people take none) but you will need some acetaminophen, a nonaspirin pain reliever that is sold in all drugstores without prescription.

The Healing Process

Your recovery will be from the anesthesia: 2 to 5 days of grogginess, if you were sedated, and 10 days to 2 weeks of great fatigue, if you had general anesthesia. You may also be nauseated or sick for a day after general anesthesia. Children recover very quickly from general anesthesia, and for a child of 6, the recovery period will be only a few days of fatigue—less than a weary parent hopes for an active child. Anesthesia makes children cranky, too.

Bandages

Your head is wrapped for 2 to 5 days in a bulky bandage covering your scalp and ears and sometimes going around your chin.

Once the bandage is removed, you will wear a headband or a light bandage such as an Ace bandage wrapped around your head and over your ears for a week or so. What happens after that depends on your surgeon. I ask my patients, especially the children, to wear a headband as much as possible for up to 6 weeks—this avoids bending the ear the wrong way by sleeping on it and having some "friend" think it is "funny" to tweak your newly operated ears.

Taking Care of Your Wound

You will need *no* special care. Your stitches lie behind your ears. Once the bandage is off, you can bathe normally. Pat behind your ear gently to dry.

Stitches

Your stitches are behind your ear. These are removed in 5 to 7 days, unless they are "subcuticular pull-out stitches." These run below the surface of the skin and can stay in for 2 weeks without inflaming your skin.

Scars

You will have a long (2 to 3 inch) scar in the crease behind your ear. Since your ear now lies close to your scalp, the scar doesn't show.

Tips

- You will need several headbands to support your "new" ears while they heal. Also, the headbands keep them warm—your ears will be super-sensitive to the cold for about a year after your surgery.
- Earrings *can* be worn once your bandages are off, but be sure they are *light and small* so that they don't drag or pull on your tender new ears.

Back to Work

You can go back to work on day 5 after surgery—when your bandage is taken off. Even if your bandage is removed sooner, it is unlikely that you will have recovered adequately from your sedation to go to work earlier. If you had *general* anesthesia you should give yourself 7 to 10 days.

Back to Sports

Your ears will throb when you exercise during the first two weeks, so postpone any vigorous exercise. You can take long walks and do stretching exercises at 7 days. You can swim by the tenth day, but it is best not to swim for 2 or 3 weeks if you have had swimmer's ear (otitis from swimming pool bacteria). If you *did* get an infection, it could spread to your wound and ruin your result.

You can jog, hike, and do Nautilus after 2 weeks. *Please, no* contact sports for 6 weeks and no noncontact ball sports (basketball, tennis) for 3 weeks. A blow to your ear could cause bleeding around the cartilage and leave you with a misshapen "boxer's ear."

Back to Sex

One week, but wear your headband!

How Much It Costs

Your surgeon's fee will range from $2000 to $3000. The hospital fee could range from as low as $800 for local/sedation to $3000 for general anesthesia.

Insurance Coverage

Insurance is *much* more likely to pay for this operation when it is done on a child, because this cosmetic problem comes under the heading of "congenital anomaly"—something wrong, present at birth. For teenagers, you may need to argue to get the surgery covered. For adults, insurance payment is less likely. If the insurance company says "yes," get written approval including the *dollar amount* they will pay, before the surgery. You may need a report from your doctor and even photographs to give to your insurance company for review by their plastic surgery consultant. This takes time. You should plan on *at least* a month of calling your insurance company and getting and sending the necessary reports, for which there may be an additional charge. It is worth the effort and the cost of the report. Regardless of what your insurance company decides, you will still pay your surgeon in advance for the surgery and collect afterwards from insurance.

Correction of Prominent Ears: Recovery-at-a-Glance

This chart represents the *average* recovery times for this cosmetic operation.

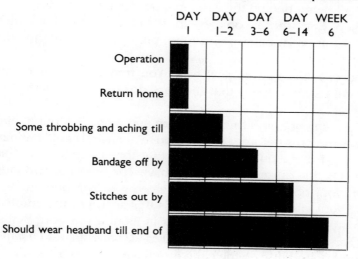

	DAY 1	DAY 1–2	DAY 3–6	DAY 6–14	WEEK 6
Operation					
Return home					
Some throbbing and aching till					
Bandage off by					
Stitches out by					
Should wear headband till end of					

My Assessment of This Procedure

This is a good operation. Apart from the nuisance of wearing a headband, most people are surprised by how little recovery is involved.

Side Effects and Complications

Side Effects

One of the most common side effects is the sensitivity of your ears to cold weather. This is worst the first year after surgery, so you should plan on wearing a hat, scarf, or earmuffs, even if you never have before, for that first year at least. The ear itself will tend to change color in warm and hot weather for the first year. It may be numb for weeks after surgery, and the numbness may return in cold weather. Your skin may be puffy over the front of your ear for months.

Minor Complications

Although the scar can become lumpy, this is rare since it's the cartilage, *not* the skin, that is holding the ear in position. Besides, the scar is hidden, being behind the ear. Most people find that their ears hurt or are sore when they lie on them for the first several weeks after surgery. Two soft down pillows or a foam pillow with a "cut-out" for your ear will help.

Also, no one has symmetrical ears. You may notice when you study your ears after surgery that the ears do not match perfectly. This is *normal*.

Your ears may not hold the new shape and may stick out again, though not as much as before. This is called relapse and could happen during healing from a pull on your ear that tore the stitches. This would *hurt*. Or, the surgery might not have changed the cartilage enough. Or, your body might not have healed with a strong enough scar to hold your ear in its new place. It is this scar, not the surgical stitches, that permanently holds your ear in its new position. Statistically, the ears relapse in one of every *10* or *20* patients, and usually require another operation on the ear 6 months after surgery. At times the ear does not relapse but the new ears look so asymmetrical or artificial that the surgery must be redone, usually 6 months later.

Major Complications

The *worst* complication would be a serious infection of the ear cartilage, leaving you with a misshapen or thick ear—not a happy exchange for one that stuck out. This can be so severe that you end up in the hospital on intravenous antibiotics. It may even require emergency surgery to drain the infection and/or remove infected tissue, plus later surgery to repair the ear. Such infections are extremely rare.

Joseph: Some Upsetting Bleeding

Joseph was 14 when he had ear surgery. He went home the same day. He called me the next morning. Blood had soaked through his bandage. He came to my office with his father. I took off the bandage, which was soaked with blood from behind his left ear. I found one of my stitches stuck to the bandage in such a way that the skin was pulled apart. The bleeding was from the skin behind the ear. I injected local anesthetic to numb the skin and put in one stitch. The bleeding stopped. I rebandaged Joseph's ear. This complication had no effect on his final healing. It upset him dreadfully—he thought he was dying when he saw his blood-soaked bandage.

Pietro: An Optional Re-Do

Pietro had me operate on his ears while he was visiting this country one summer. He wanted his ears set back to a specific point, a little further out from his head than usual. I did his surgery. In my effort to get his ears just where he wanted them, one turned out perfectly and the other, over a few weeks, relapsed, sticking out more than he or I thought looked good. In addition, after seeing his ears where he had thought he wanted them before surgery, he decided that he preferred them flat against his head. I re-operated 6 weeks after his first surgery. This was an early re-operation but he was leaving the country soon. I did not charge him, but many surgeons would, since redoing his ears involved to a great extent his change of mind. He did have to pay for the operating room. I made both ears flat against his head. Pietro was pleased and there was no further relapse.

Noreen: One Ear or Both?

Noreen had very protruding ears, one much worse than the other. She was 18. At first, Noreen only wanted me to correct the ear that looked worse. I explained to her that correcting one ear to match the other can be almost impossible. The operated ear tends to look better than the other instead of matching it. Noreen agreed to let me operate on both ears. She had her surgery as an outpatient with local anesthesia and sedation. She went home the same day. Once her bandage came off and she saw her ears, she said "Oh yes. You were right to do both."

Anna: A Major Reshaping

Anna was in her thirties and had hated her ears for years. They not only stuck out, but one was so thick that it actually hurt her to sleep on that side. She wanted her ears corrected so that they looked and felt better. I told her that I could make them look better but I didn't know if I could get rid of her discomfort when she lay on the one thick ear. On her way into the operating room, Anna told me that she "knew" I would have to take out a lot of cartilage. Usually in ear surgery, we reshape the cartilage but we don't cut it out. However, Anna was right. I shaped the thick ear cartilage and put in the stitches *but there was too much cartilage. I had to cut out about 15 percent of her ear cartilage! Anna was delighted. Her ears looked great and felt better, but the more extensive surgery made her ear hurt for 2 weeks where the cartilage had been cut out.*

What Other Patients Say

- **Boy, 7:** "I can't see them anymore!"
- **Administrator, 28:** "I can't see the scar. My ears looked pink and puffy for months."
- **Girl, 15:** "I guess I'll go swimming this summer. My ears don't poke through my hair anymore!"
- **Male accountant, 40:** "I never noticed, before surgery, but my left ear is bigger than the right. For some reason that bothered me for weeks after surgery."
- **College freshman, 18:** "The surgery was easier than I thought it would be, but the bandage was awful. I wanted my ears totally flat against my head. My surgeon didn't do that the first time. I asked him to re-operate, and he did."
- **Boy, 6:** "I don't get called 'Dumbo' anymore."

A Note About Children

When ear surgery is done on little children, before they have been teased or made self-conscious about their ears, their parents are usually happy with the result of the surgery. The child is usually accepting but is a bit baffled about it all.

Once a child has been teased, he or she may *ask* to have surgery or may go along with it—being delighted with the result.

However, some children say that they *don't* want surgery. Their request should be heeded. A child who is not (yet) bothered by having protruding ears, is going to be bothered a lot by having surgery that they don't want and that has some risks. I have had teenagers as well as children brought in to my office to have cosmetic ear surgery when they like their ears, but their parents don't. *Remember:* The person who *wears* the ears, should make the surgical decision—always.

The Chemical Peel

What Surgeons Call It

Some surgeons call this procedure a chemical face peel; others call it chemabrasion.

What It Will Do

This treatment aims to smooth out your skin by chemically removing the outer skin layers and the fine wrinkles.

What It Won't Do

A chemical peel will not tighten or plump out your skin, nor will it remove deep grooves or folds. It will not necessarily erase all the lines, although it should erase many and soften and flatten others.

How Long It Will Last

The wrinkles removed by a peel usually don't come back, but new lines may gradually show up over many years. Some people seem to have a permanent result from the peel, with few new lines forming as long as 10 or even 20 years afterwards. Your results will depend on your skin, sun exposure (sun makes the skin line again) and whether or not you smoke. (Smoking contributes to loss of elasticity in the skin.)

When to Have It

A chemical peel can be done at any age, but people in their forties and fifties are likely to heal somewhat faster and to have less pain than people in their seventies. Some women form fine lines around the lips at an early age—before other signs of aging in their face. For them a chemical peel around the mouth could be done in the thirties. (A variation of the chemical peel can be done for *very* early lip lines. The peel is painted, but not taped, right along the red lip line. This is a light peel, but may smooth out tiny lipstick-bleeding lines that are a nuisance but not bad enough for extensive treatment.)

A chemical peel around the mouth can be combined with a facelift or other facial cosmetic surgery, but a full-face peel is usually done alone. There tends to be considerable swelling of the face and eyes. For this reason, the facelift would be done first and a full-face chemical peel about 6 weeks later.

Where to Have It

A chemical peel is often done on an outpatient basis in a doctor's office operating or treatment room *or* in an outpatient surgery center. A hospital operating room, a treatment room, or the hospital room itself may be used if you're staying overnight.

Conditions That Increase Your Risk

Orientals and sallow-skinned people, especially those whose skin discolors easily, *should not* have this done. They may develop permanent blotchy skin color. Underlying heart disease may make this treatment unsafe for you. Phenol, the common chemical used to peel your face, is absorbed into the bloodstream during treatment and may irritate the heart temporarily. This would not be a problem for a person with a normal heart, but might be unsafe if you have arrhythmias or another serious heart problem. Your surgeon should discuss it with your heart doctor, if there is any question.

Usual Anesthesia

You are given sedation to make the burning from the chemical used in the peel tolerable. However, your skin is *not* injected with local anesthetic in most cases. The application of the chemical is done slowly to make it less uncomfortable for you.

How Long It Takes

A full-face peel will take about an hour to apply. Smaller areas will take 15 to 30 minutes.

The Procedure

(Figures 11-31 through 11-33)

Before

You will arrive for your procedure about an hour before it's scheduled. You will change into a hospital gown in your room if you are staying overnight, or in a preoperative area if you are an outpatient. An IV will be placed in your arm, through which you are given a solution of dextrose and/or saline to prevent dehydration during the procedure. Next, you are taken to the treatment or operating room. Sticky pads will be placed on your chest, and attached to a heart monitor. You will next be given a small dose of sedation in order to judge how large a dosage you require. (You will feel slightly drowsy.)

Your face is washed with a surgical soap, and then the skin is wiped with ether to remove all oils. Oil on your skin would interfere with placement of the adhesive tape later on.

During

The chemical peel solution is applied to your face with cotton swabs. It is swabbed down each wrinkle and an inch or two below the jawline if the lower face is being peeled. Those areas are then taped, first with short, narrow strips and then with an outer layer of wider (1 inch) longer strips. No tape at the lips may be used, if you also are having a facelift. The "peel" takes place underneath the tape—your skin is not peeled off like a facial masque.

After

After the treatment, you are taken to a recovery area. You are given lots of fluid either by mouth or by IV, and are encouraged *not* to talk. By the end of the day after a full-face peel, your eyes may be swollen shut. Once you have recovered from the sedation, you are generally sent to your hospital room (if you are staying overnight after a full-face peel) or home, if you had a small area done.

Chemical Peel

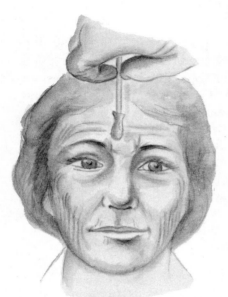

Figure 11-31.

The surgeon uses a cotton swab to place chemical on the skin, being sure to put it into the crevice of each wrinkle.

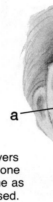

a

Figure 11-32.

The face is bandaged with two layers of adhesive tape (a). If a peel is done around the mouth at the same time as a facelift, there may be no tape used.

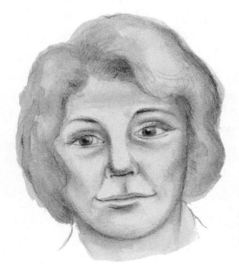

Figure 11-33.

After the peel the skin is *smoother* but not tightened; tightening would require a face-neck lift.

The Process of Recovery

What to Do About Pain

Your peeled skin will ache, burn, or hurt for about 2 days. This is enough to require narcotic pain medication and sedation. You will be in bed or in a chair for those first 2 days, although you'll be able to walk around a bit. Many people find it much easier to recover in the hospital unless they have a friend or family member who is going to be able to care for them intensively for those first two days. Around your mouth the peel will not only ache, but motion may irritate the peeled area, so you'll need to avoid talking and eating except for a small amount of liquid.

The Healing Process

You will need to see your doctor on the third day to have the tape bandage removed. You will see him again 3 to 5 days after that, and again 3 to 5 days after *that*, unless you are so healed that the next visit can wait a week or so.

Your face swells dramatically after a full-face peel. Even with your skin healed at a week, you will look puffy. After you heal (about 7 days) your peeled skin will be *red*. You should use *no* makeup on the peeled skin for 2 weeks after the peel. Your peeled skin will take at least 6 weeks to fade. It may be months before you can go without makeup in public.

Bandages

Your bandage will be two layers of adhesive tape strips over the peeled areas. This tape is pulled off after 2 days. This hurts, and further medication is required before it is done.

Taking Care of Your Wound

You don't have to do anything for your wound for the first 2 days because the peeled area is covered with two layers of adhesive tape. (Your sedation will require someone to help you in daily activities.)

On day 3, when the tape is removed, your surgeon will usually cover the peeled skin with a thymol iodide powder to dry the weeping areas and help fight infection. Your skin will be moist at first and then dries to a brown crust. You will *not* want to be seen in public. You may be given a powder to apply to your skin at home. On day 4, you will be instructed to put a lubricating ointment, such as A&D, on your skin to soften it. You can begin to gently soak your skin with plain water, and apply more ointment to crusted areas. (You can't use soap for *weeks*. It will dry and irritate your peeled skin.)

You must avoid suntanning and intentional sun exposure for the first 3 to 6 *months* after your chemical peel. Sunblocks are drying and irritating to most skins to some degree. You may not be able to use a sunblock for 4 to 6 weeks after the peel. After that you must remember to use a sunblock on the peeled skin whenever you are out in the sun. If you live in a northern climate, you only need to be concerned about this in the spring and summer. For those in the South, a *daily* application of sunblock in the morning would make sense.

The peel permanently removes your normal tanning ability, which means you can *very* easily get a severe sunburn. Also, you are almost certainly at a higher risk for developing sun-stimulated skin cancers, if you expose your peeled skin, without sunblock protection, to the sun.

Men can have chemical peels, but women have thinner skin and tend to be the ones with the extensive fine lines that the chemical peel treats best. A man who has this treatment would be able to use an electric razor, gently, about 5 to 7 days after the chemical peel, avoiding areas that haven't healed. Astringents such as after-shave or cologne are kept off the peeled skin for 4 to 6 weeks.

Stitches

This is not an operation—there is no cutting of your skin. The treatment is done by the chemical. Thus, you have no stitches and no incision in your skin.

Scars

The chemical peel does not cut your skin, and thus scars are not an inevitable part of your surgery. However, the phenol in the peel is a caustic chemical. It is possible for it to burn one area more deeply than another, leaving a small scar. This is likely to appear as a slow-healing area that leaves a shiny pink lump instead of being smooth like the skin around it. A few small scars such as this, although uncommon, may need no treatment. In 6 months, when the swelling in the scar is gone, it may be a flat, smooth spot in your skin that is only noticeable on close inspection. *Severe* scarring can result from this treatment, although it is rare. It is extraordinarily unlikely to occur when your peel is done by a conscientious cosmetic surgeon. (In some states, non-physicians have done peels, and as would be expected, problems arise when this is done by those without medical expertise.)

Tips

- This treatment will bleach your skin and will leave you without your normal suntanning ability. Besides, you shouldn't sunbathe at all for 3 to 6 months after a peel.
- If you are a sun worshiper, this procedure may not be for you.
- If only part of your face is being peeled (for example, around the lips) there may be a noticeable contrast between peeled and unpeeled skin if you have many freckles.
- I want to stress again that people with dark skin, especially Orientals, will have such prolonged or permanent blotchy skin color from a chemical peel that this procedure is *not* advisable for them.

Back to Work

You can go back to work about 2 weeks after your chemical peel. You could go back earlier, but your red and swollen skin will probably make this unacceptable for you. Back to work is when you can cover the redness with makeup. The makeup should be nonallergenic and lightly applied (to cover the redness more than to make you look your absolute best, at this point). Men will have a problem concealing the redness unless they are willing to experiment with a concealer cream or a makeup line such as Clinique, which has makeup products for men.

Back to Parties

Your social activities will depend on how fast your redness fades and how comfortable you are with your makeup. If you work all day with makeup on, then go out that night with makeup on two weeks after a peel, you're likely to find that your skin is dry, irritated and red the next day. Also, if your skin tends to flush when you drink alcohol, the alcohol you drink at a party two weeks after a peel may make your skin temporarily redder, or may make it feel hot or burning. For most people, 3 to 4 weeks is the earliest you'll be happy at a party. For a few people, who are reluctant to appear until they feel "just right," it may be 6 weeks.

Back to Sports

You will need to avoid all sports in the sun for the first 6 weeks after a chemical peel. You can begin to do stretching and limbering up exercises once your skin is healed, but exercise will make your peeled skin temporarily red, and perspiration will make it burn or itch. Avoid vigorous exercise for 2 weeks after the peel, and then limit your exercise for another week, until you know what your skin will tolerate.

Exercise outdoors in a cold wind can be irritating to your skin, leaving it dry, chapped, and even crusted in areas. Avoid skiing and other outdoor snow sports for 4 to 6 weeks. (Besides, the reflected sunlight can burn your skin, especially on a clear day at high altitude.)

Back to Sex

You can resume sex once your skin is healed. However, your fatigue from your sedation and from the healing of your skin may make sex unenjoyable. Preferably, give yourself 10 to 14 days.

How Much It Costs

Your cost depends on the extent of the peel and whether you have it done as an outpatient. A chemical peel around the mouth, done in a doctor's office as an outpatient, may cost less than $1000. On the other hand, a full-face peel done in the hospital with a two-day stay may involve a surgeon's fee of $1500 to $2500 or more, and a hospital fee of $1500—or more if the treatment is done in the operating room.

Chemical Peel: Recovery-at-a-Glance

This chart represents the *average* recovery times for this cosmetic operation.

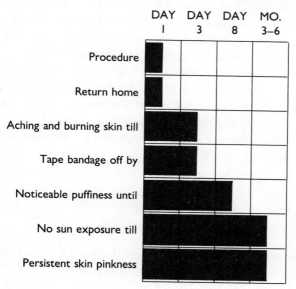

	DAY 1	DAY 3	DAY 8	MO. 3–6
Procedure	■			
Return home	■			
Aching and burning skin till	■■			
Tape bandage off by	■■			
Noticeable puffiness until	■■■			
No sun exposure till	■■■■			
Persistent skin pinkness	■■■■			

Insurance Coverage

Insurance will *not* pay for this treatment. A rare exception may be made if the chemical peel is done to remove superficial cancerous or precancerous skin growths on your face. (These may result from years of overexposing your face to the sun.) You can *try* inquiring if your insurance company would consider reimbursing you for the treatment, but it's unlikely that they will. If they say that they might, *remember to have in writing the dollar amount that they will reimburse you, before your peel.* If you don't get a commitment in writing in advance, they are likely to decide afterwards that the appropriate reimbursement is much less than they suggested it would be.

My Assessment of This Procedure

The chemical peel is able to change the skin in a way in which no other procedure can. Therefore, it is extremely useful. However, it hurts, the recovery is tedious, and the redness in your skin may last for months. The peel can scar the skin, and the chemical phenol can cause heart arrhythmia during a peel.

Chemical peel is *not* recommended for the skin on other parts of the body. The excellent blood flow and thinness of facial skin make it possible for the face to heal without scars after a peel. This is not true on the hands and arms, where the skin reacts to the peel by forming scars. These can be disfiguring and may require surgery to correct.

Side Effects and Complications

Side Effects

The chemical peel will always alter your skin color because it removes the outer layers of your skin. A person with extensive freckling who has a partial face peel may find that the peeled area looks fine but the contrast of no freckles with surrounding freckled skin is unattractive or unnatural and requires permanent makeup camouflage.

The pores of your skin are enlarged by the peel. The skin will burn easily in the sun and will always require sun protection. It *won't* tan. If only one part of your face has been peeled, and you forget your sunblock, suntanning will give you a piebald look—part tan, part not. Also, the peel may stimulate moles to darken, temporarily or permanently. These are all side effects, not complications. They are caused by the technique itself. You need to be sure that the wrinkles that you don't like are worth the exchange.

Minor Complications

Milia (whiteheads) and skin discoloration may occur if you go out in the sun after a peel, or if your skin is dark. People of Hispanic, Native American, Indian, and Mediterranean extraction tend to be at a higher risk for this. Oriental women seem to develop such predictable, permanent blotchiness that the technique is not recommended for them.

Blotchy dark skin patches after a peel can be treated by repeeling the darkened skin, and after that, by avoiding the sun assiduously or protecting your skin with a high-number skin block.

Scars may develop from a chemical peel, especially around the mouth and jawline where the skin tends to move under the tape. People who tend to heal with thick scars may be at a higher risk for scarring after a peel. Overall, perhaps 5 to 10 percent of patients after a chemical peel have a small area of scar that will eventually fade.

Major Complications: A Warning

Chemical peel should not be taken lightly on the grounds that it is not an operation. The chemical phenol is potentially dangerous and can cause such problems as convulsions if it reaches a toxic level in your body. A doctor who wants to do your full face peel in 10 minutes and send you home is risking not only your result, but your health. Too cavalier an attitude toward this treatment suggests that you might seriously consider a second opinion.

Cheryl: A Minor Problem With Freckles

Cheryl was in her fifties when she had a chemical peel around her mouth. She was not a smoker and had a fair, slightly freckled skin. She loved the result and thought her recovery was easy. However, the skin color around her lips was bleached, compared with the slightly freckled skin on her cheeks. This did not improve with time and would not be expected to. However, she was so pleased with her appearance that the contrast in color between lip and cheek did not bother her.

Vera: Some Minor Scarring

Vera was in her sixties when she had her chemical peel. She had an area of scarring at her jawline. This developed under the tape and may have occurred because she talked constantly after her peel, but also because she had extreme swelling. This long scar was obvious but flattened and faded by the end of a year. Vera was not happy with the scar but felt in balance that her appearance was much better with the scar than with the facial wrinkles.

What Other Patients Say

- **Retired land broker, 41:** "I hurt afterwards, but the result was worth it. I would have liked all my lines to be gone forever. I got little ones coming back in a few years. Also I had a few small scars."
- **Model, 50:** "I never go out in the sun, and I was told I had a perfect skin for this. I looked fearsome for a week and like a lobster for two months but after that it looked nice."
- **Housewife and avid gardener, 67:** "I knew I'd forget to wear my sunblock and I did, of course. And of course I got a mark on my face that looked like a coffee stain. I had that done and it wasn't as bad as the first time because it was a small area. My lines are definitely not all gone, but they are much better."

Dermabrasion and Dermaplaning

What Surgeons Call It

The technical names for these procedures are the same as the common ones: dermabrasion and dermaplaning.

What It Will Do

These treatments will give you a smoother skin, often with few or no telltale signs to show where the treatment was done. **Dermabrasion** "sandpapers" the skin surrounding scars, which are thinner than normal skin, so that the scars blend in better. **Dermaplaning** actually shaves off sheets of scarred skin to a measured distance, just like taking skin for a graft.

What It Won't Do

Neither technique will *remove* scars, correct deep, pitted scars —these go right through the skin into the deep tissues.

How Long It Will Last

Permanently. However, the dermabrasion/planing causes swelling that takes up to months to fully absorb. Ironically, as the swelling subsides, scars that the procedure could not reach may become more noticeable. Such changes will not be dramatic, but if you watch your skin closely, you will see them.

When to Have It

Anytime after the cause of the skin scarring, for example, acne, is under control. It can be done during an active acne flare-up, but the risk of infection is slightly higher.

Where to Have It

Dermabrasion is done on an outpatient basis in a doctor's office operating room *or* an outpatient surgery center *or* a hospital operating room. **Dermaplaning** may require an overnight hospital stay. If so, it will be done in a hospital operating room or a doctor's operating clinic with overnight facilities.

Conditions That Increase Your Risk

If you have a tendency to get **fever blisters** (cold sores), they may flare up after facial dermabrasion. Black skin, Oriental skin, and dark "Mediterranean" skin may become blotchy after dermabrasion/planing, and thus it is usually *not* recommended for these skin types. Dark black skin may heal with a smooth color, unlike Oriental, or a lighter shade of black skin. Having had **previous chemical peel or dermabrasion** increases the risk of scarring. Having had **radiation** of the skin (even if done years ago for acne—once popular but risky) increases your risk of infection and of poor healing. Finally, having had a **bad skin burn**—one that left scarring, not a "normal" sunburn—increases the risk of infection and scarring.

Usual Anesthesia

For **dermabrasion**, skin is numbed with local anesthetic via needle injections, combined with sedation, *or* numbed with a freezing spray such as Freon. Extensive **dermaplaning** requires general anesthesia (see The Procedure).

How Long It Takes

About one hour or less, for **dermabrasion** of part or all of the face. **Dermaplaning** is a three-step procedure and can take 2 hours, or more.

The Procedure
(Figures 11-35 and 11-36)

Dermabrasion: Before

You will arrive for your procedure about an hour before it is scheduled. You will change into a hospital gown and probably go directly to the operating room. If you are having heavier sedation than just a pill, an IV will be placed in your arm so you can receive the sedation and a salt or sugar solution that will prevent dehydration during surgery. Sticky pads will be placed on your chest to monitor your heart.

Your surgeon will then mark the area to be dermabraded, and will numb your skin with an anesthetic spray, by injection, or both. Spraying the skin makes it stiff so that it's difficult for your surgeon to tell if he has dermabraded deeply enough. On the other hand, if only an injection is used, you may need heavy sedation, unless only a small area is being dermabraded.

Dermaplaning: Before

This procedure usually requires general anesthesia. You will come to the operating room about an hour before your surgery, having had nothing to eat or drink since midnight the night before. You will change into a hospital gown, and an IV will be started in your arm. Once you are on the operating table, sticky pads will be placed on your chest under your gown and another sticky pad may be placed under your gown on a hip if surgical cautery is to be used. (Cautery means using an electrical device to seal bleeding blood vessels.) Then you will be given intravenous anesthetic and you will go to sleep for the surgery.

Dermabrasion: During

Once your skin is numb, the dermabrader is turned on. The dermabrasion instrument is a small, round metal brush or file. It is attached to a metal handle that is attached to an electrical cord or to a tube of compressed air. If you are being treated near your eyes, they will be protected by a shield. Each area is worked on several times. You will feel pulling, stretching, and vibration. Your head will be turned from side to side as different areas are dermabraded. Once the anesthetic wears off, your skin will burn.

Dermaplaning: During

Once you are asleep, the surgeon will make two outlines in purple ink for each area to be treated: the central scarred area and the surrounding area which must blend with it. Chemical peel solution is next put on the whole area to be treated (see Chemical Peel). The peel is not deep but is done to blend surrounding skin color with the planed skin. A gauze pack is put in your mouth to stretch the cheek skin and then scarred strips of skin are cut off by the dermatome, a skin-graft cutting instrument that looks like an electric shaver. If cysts beneath the skin are uncovered, they are cut or scraped out. Finally, dermabrasion is used to complete the treatment in selected areas such as at the base of the nose (where the dermatome can't cut a skin strip easily).

Dermabrasion and Dermaplaning

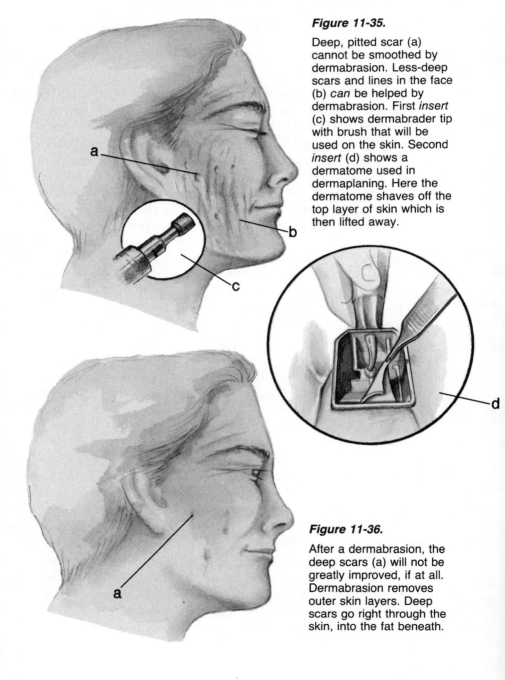

Figure 11-35.

Deep, pitted scar (a) cannot be smoothed by dermabrasion. Less-deep scars and lines in the face (b) *can* be helped by dermabrasion. First *insert* (c) shows dermabrader tip with brush that will be used on the skin. Second *insert* (d) shows a dermatome used in dermaplaning. Here the dermatome shaves off the top layer of skin which is then lifted away.

Figure 11-36.

After a dermabrasion, the deep scars (a) will not be greatly improved, if at all. Dermabrasion removes outer skin layers. Deep scars go right through the skin, into the fat beneath.

Dermabrasion/planing: After

A bulky wet bandage is put on your face (see Bandages).

After the surgery, you will go to the recovery room—where you will wake up. Depending on how extensive your dermaplaning was, you may be sent home or you may stay in the hospital a day or two while you recover.

The Process of Recovery

What to Do About Pain

Your skin will tingle and burn as the anesthesia wears off. After dermaplaning, your face may ache or throb. The skin will have a burned feeling, like a raw sunburn. Pain medication is usually needed. This may be acetaminophen, a mild pain reliever available over the counter, or a narcotic prescription such as Demerol. Your face will feel swollen, and eating and talking will be difficult. If you try to force your mouth open, it will hurt.

The Healing Process

It will be at least 5 to 10 days before you can go out in public, and even then your skin will be pink. The deeper the dermabrasion, the longer the healing time.

Bandages/Wound Care

If you stay in the hospital, the nurses take care of your bandages. If you go home, your surgeon will give you specific instructions. For a small dermabrasion, I may ask my patient to take the outer gauze off the day after surgery, leaving one layer of fine gauze. Then they're asked to soak the gauze three or four times a day and, leaving it in place, to blow-dry the area thoroughly. This process softens the crusts that form and keeps the gauze dry, so that infection cannot set in.

For larger areas of dermabrasion/planing, I put on a wet bandage at surgery and remove all the layers of gauze the next day. Antibiotic ointment is put on over the treated skin, which is blow-dried with low heat four times a day. Needless to say, you will look unsightly until you are healed: 7 to 14 days.

For 6 weeks your skin will be thin and pink and may blister or crack easily: sun, wind, heat, and cold are avoided as much as possible. Makeup is possible in 2 to 3 weeks. A non-allergenic brand is preferable, because your healing skin may hurt or develop a rash from your usual cosmetic brand.

Scars

There should be no scars. Too deep a dermabrasion will cause thick red scars in the deepest areas. These areas may be lumpy at first and fade with time or with the use of steroid cream. A particularly bad scar *may* need to be removed surgically, but this is *rare*. (The risk is higher if your skin has been previously treated with a chemical peel, radiation, or dermabrasion.) A sunscreen or sunblock to protect your skin from the sun is *mandatory*; use a *#15 or higher* for 6 months. You can gradually decrease the strength of the sunscreen, depending on the natural color in your skin, but you should never go without.

Tips

- The dermabrasion (or dermaplaning) is usually easier than your recovery—be sure your surgeon gives you detailed instructions on what to do.
- Resign yourself: your dermabraded/planed skin will be noticeably pink for 2 to 6 weeks.
- Doing the procedure in the spring or fall avoids the extreme heat and cold that will make your healing skin chapped and raw (if cold) or sore and inflamed (if hot).

Back to Work

One week—but only if you can hide out in your own office. Your face will be pink to red, with patches of crusts. Also it will feel swollen and tight. Most people need 2 weeks—your skin will be pink, and the color may be quite blotchy. A few small crusts may persist. Light makeup is possible but your skin will be dry and itchy.

By the third to fourth week, your skin will not feel dry or stiff during the day (although it may, transiently, when you wake up in the morning). You will be able to wear makeup. Your skin will look pink, but you may be able to go in public without makeup.

Back to Parties

You can plan on a party in 3 weeks—with makeup. If you *won't* wear makeup, 4 weeks is the earliest. Even at this time, you *may* feel your skin flush or burn after drinking alcohol.

Back to Sports

You can walk, jog, and do exercises at 2 weeks—but you will want an immediate shower. The sweat will make your skin burn otherwise. If you swim (indoors, to avoid sun and wind) keep your face out of the water (no Australian crawl) for 4 weeks because the chlorine will dry your skin and new crusts may appear temporarily. Wash your face under a cool shower and put cream on your skin afterwards.

Limit your sports to a half hour at a time for the first month. Sweat and body heat will irritate your healing skin, just as if it had been burned. No ball sports for 4 to 6 weeks, unless you are *very* careful, because being hit on the dermabraded skin area with a tennis ball or basketball would be painful and might leave a scar.

Dermabrasion/Dermaplaning: Recovery-at-a-Glance

This chart represents the *average* recovery times for this cosmetic operation.

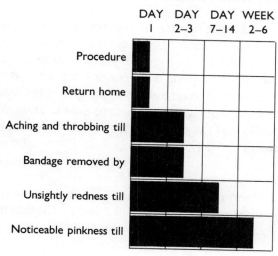

	DAY 1	DAY 2–3	DAY 7–14	WEEK 2–6
Procedure	■			
Return home	■			
Aching and throbbing till	■	■		
Bandage removed by	■	■		
Unsightly redness till	■	■	■	
Noticeable pinkness till	■	■	■	■

Back to Sex

Seven to ten days, once your face is healed.

What It Costs

Cost depends on the extent of the dermabrasion/planing. It may be $1500 to $2500 for a full-face dermabrasion, plus $500 for the operating room. For dermaplaning, the cost will be about $2500 to $3500 and about $2000 for the operating room and general anesthesia.

Insurance Coverage

Insurors will *usually* pay if dermabrasion/planing is done to remove extensive scars—for example, acne scars, precancerous keratoses from too much sun, or scars from an accident. Insurance will *not* pay for dermabrasion to remove wrinkles. *Remember:* If there is any doubt about what your insurance will pay, submit your surgeon's proposed surgery and his fees to your insurance company *in writing, before your surgery.* Ask them to tell you *in writing* if they will pay for the surgery, and if so, *how much they will pay.* When payment is uncertain, insurance will tend *not* to pay if you ask them afterwards.

My Assessment of These Procedures

Dermabrasion is most often used to treat extensive acne *scars.* It's not usually used today to treat active acne because new skin-treatment medicines make it less necessary. Dermabrasion can be done several times if the surgeon does not dermabrade deeply the first time. Surgeons tend to go lightly, since giving too deep a treatment would leave you with new, worse scars. Thus you might be able to have, and might need, two or three dermabrasions. **Dermaplaning** usually goes deep and cannot be repeated.

Besides treating scars, dermabrasion is used to smooth wrinkles on the face and around the mouth. However, collagen injections and chemical peel are also used for this. Collagen is probably best if you have only a few wrinkles that don't seem worth the cost and risks of a chemical peel or dermabrasion. As for chemical peel versus dermabrasion—it tends to be a matter of the surgeon's preference, since both techniques remove the outer skin, one chemically and the other mechanically. Chemical peel seems to be increasingly chosen because it does not require a machine or an operating room.

Side Effects and Complications

If you are a pale to medium-skinned Caucasian, your skin will be pink and blotchy—with some brown and some light areas—for 6 weeks. If you are black, you will find your skin startlingly light. However, discoloration will usually fade in 6 weeks, and your black skin color returns. If you are Oriental, your blotchy skin discoloration may last a year or longer, and for this reason dermabrasion is usually *not* advised for you—or for Causasians with dark "Mediterranean" skin, the kind that tends to blotchy skin color.

Unless you wear your sunblock regularly for 6 months, your skin will burn badly, or it may develop permanent light and dark patches.

Dermabrasion may make normal skin pores larger—permanently or for up to 6 months while swelling subsides. Tiny white specks (milia) may appear in the skin. These will often absorb by 6 weeks after surgery, but your surgeon may have to remove them. Some patients will get a "crop" of milia over their faces. The treatment is daily swabbing of your skin with alcohol, brushing it with a complexion brush, and cleansing it with an astringent product such as Therapads. A severe case may take months before the milia are gone.

Peg: Some Long-Term Results
Peg came to see me for a facelift, 25 years after a dermabrasion for acne. She was fair-skinned. However, the dermabrasion had permanently lightened her face, with faint brown freckles all over. She had been pleased with her dermabrasion result, but surprised that the discoloration did not completely fade. This may not happen today, since we have sunblocks to prevent discoloration from the sun after dermabrasion. The condition of her face had no effect at all on her facelift, which didn't change her freckles but tightened her face.

Sophy: Ignoring Criteria Led to Disappointment

Olive-skinned Sophy had her cheeks dermabraded for acne the summer she graduated from high school. She worked in the hospital as a volunteer and consulted me for a second opinion after she healed. She had developed extensive milia over both cheeks 2 weeks after her dermabrasion. These showed up as white dots highlighted by the surrounding dark color of her skin. Milia occur, but rarely to this degree. Sophy's surgeon did not know what to do—he had never seen severe milia before. Sophy needed months of treatment, during which she scrubbed her face daily, went without makeup to avoid more milia, and went weekly to the office to have milia snipped out. In addition, it was summer. She found the sunblocks made her skin sting, so she sometimes didn't use them. Although her acne scars were better, her olive skin was blotchy, from her skin type plus the sun. Once the milia were gone she had to use makeup to conceal her blotchy skin color. She was not pleased. Note: Skin color is the most important criterion for dermabrasion; next is whether you can stay out of the sun.

Arnold: Erasing Acne Scars

Arnold was in his late twenties when he saw me for dermabrasion. He had had mild acne but the scars bothered him terribly. I dermabraded his skin once so that his skin wasn't so rough and the scars were not so deep. Arnold also had some pitted scars which I cut out and stitched at the same operation. He was pleased with his improvement and didn't want more treatment.

Angie: Telltale Lip Wrinkles

Angie was in her early fifties and wanted a facelift. She decided at the same time to have dermabrasion around her mouth, where her lipstick "bled" into the wrinkles. I did the facelift and the dermabrasion. Angie actually found the facelift recovery easier. The dermabrasion made her lips sore, she had to drink with a straw and her dermabraded skin was pink for weeks. After she healed she was content; her lipstick stayed in place.

What Other Patients Say

- **Teenage boy:** "I thought I'd never have this done. It seemed like a lot to go through—and it was. I was sore. I had a slight infection. But once it healed it made a big difference, so I didn't care."

- **Female executive, 41:** "My acne left me an absolute disaster. When I took off my makeup, most doctors' mouths dropped when they saw the horrendous scars. Dermabrasion didn't do any magic miracle for me—I know nothing can—but I only need half the makeup now because my skin is smoother, the color is better, and I feel okay."

- **Politician, 39:** "This was worse than running for reelection, which was why I had it done in the first place. It's not perfect but my skin looked smoother, and that plus some collagen made me look better on camera."

- **Model, 25:** "I want normal skin. I hate my face. I've had two dermabrasions and collagen and I admit I'm better but I wanted my skin *perfect* again and it's not."

Eyeliner and Other Surgical Tattooing

What Surgeons Call It

The technical term for this procedure is surgical skin pigmentation. *Important Note:* This is not a tattoo done in a tattoo parlor. It is a sterile surgical procedure that places sterile nonallergenic pigment under the skin. The surgical equipment is licensed only for medical use.

What It Will Do

The surgical tattooing process can be used to:

- Darken the upper and lower rims of your eyes so that you do not need to apply eyeliner every day.
- Fill in thinning eyebrows (which are *very* difficult to reconstruct surgically) so that the eyebrow looks as normal as possible.
- Reconstruct the areola around the nipple after breast surgery to create the look of the areola without the need for surgical reconstruction with grafts.
- When the technique is used for areas of skin color loss, for instance after a burn, the goal is to shade in skin color, so that the damaged skin blends in with the surrounding normal skin and matches it as closely as possible.

I will be primarily discussing eyeliner tattooing in this section, because that procedure is the most commonly performed one.

What It Won't Do

This technique cannot perform miracles. For instance, it will enhance your eyes, but if you normally wear heavy eye makeup, it will not make your eyes look completely "made up." If you have the technique done to fill in eyebrows that were lost from overplucking, it will *sketch in* your brow, but someone looking closely will see that the color is in your skin and not from real eyebrow hair.

How Long It Will Last
Permanently.

When to Have It
You can have eyeliner tattooing at any age from 15 to 80! However, I recommend that teenagers wait until their twenties before having this done, because teenagers' faces change so much that what looks good at 15 may look wrong at 25—and this procedure is permanent.

Where to Have It
The operation is done on an outpatient basis in a doctor's office operating room (usually) *or* an outpatient surgery center *or* a hospital operating room.

Conditions That Increase Your Risk
You may be *allergic* to the pigment used in this procedure, although this occurs less than 1 percent of the time. To be on the safe side, your doctor will usually test you about a week before your "tattooing." The test scratches a little pigment into an area that won't show (I use the scalp). If redness, swelling, or a rash develops around the test area, you are allergic, and your tattooing would *not* proceed.

If you are allergic to eye makeup, but wear it anyway, because you feel you can't go without it, *you will have to discontinue wearing it* at least 2 weeks before the tattooing procedure is done. Nonallergenic makeup should be used for 2 weeks prior to the tattooing. *Any* infection you have *must* be cleared up before tattoo surgery.

Usual Anesthesia
The procedure *can* be done with only local anesthetic, but I prefer to give my patients sedation by mouth, as well, for their own comfort.

How Long It Takes
Depending on the equipment used, the procedure can take 30 to 60 minutes for the eyeliner and about 60 minutes for other areas of the body.

The Procedure

(Figures 11-37 and 11-38)

Before

You will arrive for your eyeliner tattooing about an hour before it is scheduled. You will already have discussed with your surgeon the desired shade and shape of your tattoo. (For more information on your options, see Tips.) If the procedure is in the morning, you will probably have been instructed to have nothing to eat or drink after midnight the night before. If it is done later in the day, you will probably be allowed a liquid breakfast, since you will only be lightly sedated. If you and your surgeon have decided on *no* sedation, then you will have been permitted to eat. However, since surgery makes most people nervous, it is advisable to eat *lightly*.

After you change into a hospital gown, you are taken to the operating room. If you are having local anesthesia, and you have not already been given sedation in the pre-op area, you are given it now, making you feel relaxed and drowsy. Sticky pads *may* be placed on your chest to monitor your heart. (This is not necessary unless you are going to be *heavily* sedated.) Once you are on the operating table, a safety strap is placed across your hips.

During

The nurse may have tested the tattooing instrument (about the size of a pen) before you came in the room. If not, you may hear or see her click on the machine, which makes a whirring noise, but not as loud as dental equipment. You will also hear a tap—when the tiny, almost microscopic needle is attached to the handle.

Next, you will be given anesthetic drops into each eye to keep your eyes from blinking. Then, using a *tiny* needle, your surgeon will give you three or four injections of local anesthetic, starting at the corner of each eye. An ice compress will be kept over one eye, to prevent swelling or bruising from the injection, while the *other* eye is numbed. You may doze on and off during the procedure, depending on how much sedation you are given. This is what is done:

First, your eyes are cleansed with ointment. Next, a flat metal eyelid clamp is gently applied to the first eye to hold your lower

Eyeliner Tattooing

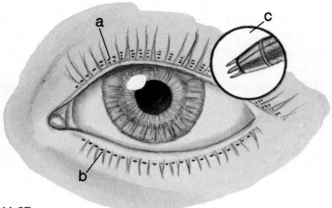

Figure 11-37.

Eyeliner tattooing on the upper lid (a) is done with three tiny lines of dots. For the lower lid (b), the eyeliner tattooing is put in between the lashes, in one line. A close-up of the tattooing instrument (c) shows the three fine points that permit microdots of pigment to be placed in the skin.

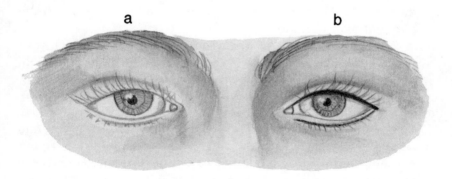

Figure 11-38.

Before eyeliner tattooing (a), eyes lack definition. After eyeliner tattooing (b), eyes are outlined, making eyes look bigger, lashes thicker.

eyelid up over your eye. This protects your eye. You can't see the surgery.

When the lower lids are being colored, the needle vibrates along the lashes, putting tiny dots of color *in between* your eyelashes, not below them. This makes your lash line look dark without looking unnatural. Once this lower lid is done, your surgeon will usually remove the little clamp and do the upper lid next. When the clamp is placed on your upper lid, the lid is pulled *down*. Again, this covers your eye. To create the desired effect for your upper lids, more pigment is needed. Thus *three* tiny lines of pigment are made just above your lashes. At the *inner corner* of your eye, the three lines converge into one line. This avoids a broad, heavy look at the inner upper lid. The pigment will *not* extend beyond the corner of your eyes. Some women do wear their eyeliner far beyond their eyes, depending on current fashion. The pigment is permanent, so it is done to suit your looks, permanently.

When one side is finished, your surgeon will put gauze dipped in ice water over this eye and do the other one. Your *treated* eye may burn.

If you are having the procedure somewhere other than your eyes, the technique is the same: The area is numbed and the pigment placed in the skin.

If the pigment goes in the wrong place during surgery, your surgeon will scrape it out. It is much more difficult to scrape out pigment once your skin has sealed over it (in about 3 days).

After

You will be awake but groggy after this procedure, if you had sedation. If you had no sedation, you will be awake but your eyes may burn quite a bit. Either way, your surgeon will probably have you rest in a recovery area for an hour or so, keeping ice over your eyes, until letting you go home.

The Process of Recovery

What to Do About Pain

Your eyelids (or whatever area is treated) will burn after the surgery. However, you should not have *pain* after this procedure.

The Process of Healing

Your eyes may tear for a day or two after surgery. This will *not* wash out the pigment, as it would mascara or other eye makeup. Your lids, or whatever area was treated, will be *slightly swollen* for about 5 days. The treated area will also be slightly pink, but bruising is *rare* because the pigment goes into the skin, not into deep tissues.

If your eyes were treated, you will *not* be able to wear eye makeup for *1 week*. It may irritate the treated areas and cause an infection.

Bandages

If your eyes are treated, none. But if the pigment is placed on the nipple or other clothes-covered body areas, you would wear a gauze pad over the area to prevent clothes from rubbing against it.

Taking Care of Your Wound

After your operation you go home and keep ice compresses over your eyes. Ways of doing this are also described in the sections on Upper Lid or Lower Lid surgery. However, after pigmentation, you won't be heavily sedated, you'll want to be able to move around more than after upper or lower lid surgery. Your eyes won't be hurting. I think your best two choices are:

- **Icy-cold gauze pads.** Prepare these by putting ice lumps in a bowl half-filled with tap water. Dip in a gauze pad, wring it out, and place over your eye. When it is no longer cold, dip it in again. If you need to get up or your eyes feel too cold, just put the gauze in the ice water until you need it next.
- **A commercial cold pack** for the eyes.

You will need to apply antibiotic eye ointment to your eyelids (or whatever area was treated) for 5 days. Your doctor may give you a sample or a prescription. This ointment prevents crusts from forming around the pigment and keeps down infection.

Stitches/Scars

This procedure requires no stitches and leaves no scars.

Eyeliner Tattooing: Recovery-at-a-Glance

This chart represents the *average* recovery times for this cosmetic operation.

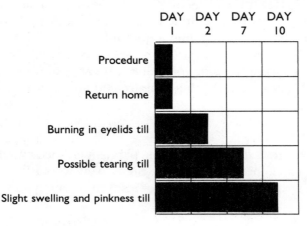

	DAY 1	DAY 2	DAY 7	DAY 10
Procedure	■			
Return home	■			
Burning in eyelids till	■■			
Possible tearing till	■■■			
Slight swelling and pinkness till	■■■■			

Tips

- A range of colors from cream to dark brown is available. *Mahogany* was originally recommended as a "universal brown" for the eyes and is still the commonest eye pigment color used.
- You can also specify whether you want the underlining to be *just* on your lower or upper lids, as well as whether or not you want the line to go from the outer corner all the way to the inner corner.

Make sure you discuss these options with your surgeon.

Back to Work

Three to seven days. If you *must* wear makeup to work, you will have to wait the full 7 days.

Back to Parties

One week. If you have too much activity earlier than a week, you probably won't *hurt* yourself, but your eyes will get puffy, pink and sore. Remember: After surgery, fatigue makes pain or soreness noticeably worse.

Back to Sports/Sex

One week, for the same reasons noted above for parties.

What It Costs

This will be from $1000 to $2000 for both the surgeon's fee *and* use of the operating room, for eyeliner. Other areas may cost more or less, depending on what is done.

Insurance Coverage

Insurance will *not* pay for any cosmetic pigmentation. Eyeliner, eyebrows, and enhancement of hair transplants are all *out* for insurance. However, if the treatment is for a scarred area, or for nipple reconstruction after a mastectomy, contact your insurance company *before* you have the pigmentation. Ask them to make a decision on your case *in writing*. If they agree to pay for the procedure, have them commit themselves in writing as to exactly how much they will pay before you have it done.

My Assessment of This Procedure

Surgeons have been trying to develop a medically acceptable technique of tattooing for years. This relatively new technique, which has been used for about 4 years, seems to be the answer. It is becoming increasingly widely used. The technique is *delicate* and requires special training. But it is an excellent solution to problems for which previously there was no treatment except makeup or complicated surgery.

Side Effects and Complications

There are four main problems with eyeliner tattoos. The most common is that the tattooing may leave a little skip area that must be retattooed. This can be done at any time after surgery, but it's usually a good idea to wait 6 weeks because the pigment lightens as you heal over it. It looks more natural, and skip areas become much less obvious. You may decide you don't want it touched up.

Second, the tattoo may be put into the wrong place. For instance, if it goes too deep, it may reach the muscle and form a small fan-shaped stain. This is scraped out during surgery if it is noticed then. If not, you'll need a minor re-operation to scrape and trim out the pigment.

Third, your surgeon may put the pigment *in the wrong place*. In the early days of eyeliner tattooing, some surgeons put the lower-lid pigment *under* the lashes. When the lower lid skin stretched even a little, the pigment showed up as a dark line and did not blend with the lashes. (You can't smudge in the color, as you do with eyeliner.) Treatment: cutting out the pigmented skin!

Finally, any treatment around your eyelashes can damage the lashes, causing them to fall out—possibly permanently.

Although all of these complications are uncommon, you should remember that they do happen.

What Other Patients Say

- **Girl, 14:** "I lost part of my eyebrows after an infection. I looked like a freak, and when they first tried surgery to make me new brows they looked even worse, ugly and thick. I had them take those out. I wouldn't have had tattooing done except makeup wouldn't stick on my skin, so my eyebrows wore off by the end of school. This was a snap. It looks good so I can forget about my eyebrows. It didn't hurt. You couldn't see I had anything done."
- **Doctor (female), 40:** "My eyes burned like crazy. I wasn't prepared for that, but it looks great. I don't have time for eye makeup and I don't look good enough to go without."
- **Administrative assistant, 29:** "I wanted to be able to go without makeup. It didn't do that for me. Also I need a second treatment because the first wasn't dark enough. It's okay."

Hair Transplant Surgery

What Surgeons Call It

Depending on what is done, this procedure may be called hair punch grafts, hair strip grafts, hair-bearing flaps, or scalp reduction.

A Word About Hair "Restoration"

Graft vs. Flap. To understand hair transplants you need to know the difference between a graft and a flap. A **transplant** means that the hair is moved from one place to another. If this is done by means of a **graft**, a portion of skin with hair follicles is cut entirely out of the scalp and put into a new part of the scalp where the *bald* skin has been cut out and discarded. It is like moving a piece of sod from one part of a lawn to another. A "punch" graft simply means one that is circular; a strip graft is long, not round. If the transplant is done with a **flap**, a piece of scalp with hair is cut, but left attached to the scalp on one side. The flap is swiveled into a new position where the *bald* skin has been cut out and discarded. The flap keeps its own blood supply. The graft has no blood supply of its own and will die unless new blood vessels grow into it quickly to keep it alive. **Scalp reduction** means that the scalp is made smaller by cutting out bald skin on top of the scalp and discarding it. This pulls scalp with hair up over the sides and top of the scalp.

Hair Weaving. Hair transplant surgery should *not* be confused with hair weaving, which either weaves hair—real or synthetic—into your own hair to make it look thicker or implants synthetic hair into your scalp. The first is an accepted technique, but implanting synthetic hair into your scalp *does not work*. In time—sometimes months—your body rejects the synthetic hair, and may leave your scalp scarred or temporarily infected. If a surgeon suggests synthetic hair surgery for your scalp, get a second opinion. The only accepted implant material—as of now—for correcting baldness is *your own scalp*.

Hair Growth Drugs. Minoxidil was developed as a blood-pressure drug and then was found, more or less by accident, to make hair grow. In time, drugs may be able to prevent baldness, but Minoxidil is not the final word. When you start to go bald, your hair follicles are resting but still alive. After a few years, those hair follicles will die. Minoxidil will work *only on hair follicles that are still alive*. It cannot bring dead follicles back to life. Also, the hair growth from Minoxidil tends to be short and curly, which may not be right for you. Finally, Minoxidil is absorbed into your body when you put it on your scalp as a lotion. It has side effects related to its effect on blood pressure, including dizziness and impotence. (This stops when you stop the drug.) Still, for those men whose hair is *beginning* to thin, this drug could be worth trying.

What It Will Do

The goal is to decrease the bald areas on your scalp and to conceal the remaining baldness so that your hair appears as normal as possible.

What It Won't Do

Hair transplant surgery won't change the nature of your hair. If your hair follicles are placed far apart, surgery cannot produce a thick growth of hair. Also, none of this surgery will give you *more* hair, since your hair is simply being moved from one place on your head to another. Finally, the surgery will neither stop you from going bald nor *prevent* you from going bald. It can only redistribute your hair during and/or after the time that you lose it.

Your scalp is genetically coded to go bald—or not—in certain places. For instance, if your family hair pattern is to thin at the temples and on top, then hairs taken from the back and sides aren't "coded" to go bald and will continue to grow hair, regardless of where they are put. Thus, hair grafts and flaps will grow new hair, unless the site from which they *came* begins to go bald. Then the transplanted hair will stop growing also.

When to Have It

If your hair is thinning, you should first consult a dermatologist to find out if there is a reason—other than genetic—for you to be losing hair. Although genetics will be the most common answer, a hormone imbalance, recent illness, skin disorder, or even a vitamin overdose can cause hair to thin. Besides, even if you are genetically coded to go bald in spots, good care of your scalp may slow down the problem. Once you have lost hair at the temples, or elsewhere, you should consult your dermatologist (if he does hair transplant surgery) or a cosmetic plastic surgeon—or both—to decide what surgery is best for you.

You can have hair transplant surgery at any age. Although it is uncommon for teenagers to need it, some teenagers will notice that their hair is already thinning. Hair transplant surgery is common in men from their twenties to their sixties. Who won't have a problem? People of Irish descent tend not to go bald. When we find out why, we may be able to prevent hair thinning on other people.

Where to Have It

This procedure may be done in a doctor's office or an outpatient operating room. Both plastic surgeons and dermatologists do such surgery. However, dermatologists usually do only grafts and not hair flaps and scalp reductions, which are larger operations.

Conditions That Increase Your Risk

- An infection or disorder of your scalp skin must be treated before hair grafting or it will interfere with the healing of your grafts. Such disorders include psoriasis, eczema, seborrhea (dandruff), and acne in and around the scalp.

- An underlying illness, such as diabetes or lowered immune resistance, increases your risk of infection, poor healing, and poor growth of the grafted hair.

- As mentioned under Tips, wearing a hairpiece over the grafts will cause the new hairs to fracture at the shaft.

Usual Anesthesia

Grafts are done with local anesthesia, usually with sedation. Flaps and scalp reductions are done either with local sedation or with general anesthesia.

How Long It Takes

Duration will vary with what is done. A session of 30 to 50 hair grafts may be done in 1 to 2 hours. A complicated scalp flap may take several hours or more. A scalp reduction (in which bald skin is cut out and discarded) will take between 1 and 2 hours to do.

The Operations
(Figures 11-39 through 11-41)

Before

You will come to the operating room about an hour before your surgery, perhaps less if you are having only hair punch grafts. You will change into a hospital gown. (For hair grafts, you may keep on your street clothes, but only change out of your coat and shirt.) An IV is placed in your arm. (Again, this may not be needed for hair punch grafts.) You are given some sedation and you go to the operating room, where your surgeon will trim hair only from the scalp on which he will operate. Sticky pads will be placed on your chest if you are having heavy sedation or general anesthesia. A sticky pad may be placed on your leg as a ground to make the surgical cautery safe to use. (Surgical cautery uses an electrical instrument to seal off bleeding vessels.) It is not often needed for grafts, but is used for flaps and scalp reductions. Next, you will be put to sleep if you are having general anesthesia. If not, you will now be given the sedation.

During

Your scalp is then washed with surgical soap, and sterile drapes are placed over your body and around your face. You will have one or more of the following procedures done.

If **punch grafts** are being done, your surgeon injects local anesthetic into the scalp where he will take the grafts, and where he will put them. He will use a small instrument—like a tiny cookie cutter on a handle—to cut out the bald skin, leaving spaces in between to allow blood flow to the living grafts. Next he will cut out hair grafts—slightly *larger* than the holes in the bald scalp, so that they will fit snugly. He will trim off excess fat from the grafts. The donor areas may not be sewn up depending on your surgeon's preference. The grafts are gently fitted into their holes and arranged so that the hair will grow in the right direction. At the end, your scalp is cleansed. (The scalp will bleed—this is a messy procedure.) Tape may be put over the grafts, then a layer of gauze, and your head is wrapped in a bandage.

Strip grafts are most often used for the front hairline. They may be rectangular, or intricately zigzagged to avoid an unnaturally straight hairline.

Your surgeon will inject local anesthetic into the hair at the back of your head and into the area of your front hairline. Next he will cut out the bald skin in front, splitting the tough fibrous layer under the scalp so that the graft will fit. At the back of the head he will cut out the strip graft with its hair. This donor site is sutured closed. The strip graft is delicately handled—if it is bruised, it may not survive. It is gently sewn in place at your front hairline with fine sutures, usually under magnification. Your scalp is then cleansed. Gauze is placed over the graft, and your head is wrapped in a bandage.

To do a **scalp reduction**, your surgeon will move your scalp about to decide how loose it is and how much bald skin he can take out. Then he will mark the area to be cut out and inject it with local anesthetic. He will cut out and discard the bald skin. Next he will snip the deep fibrous tissue in the scalp to make it stretch. He will lift the scalp in all directions to loosen it even more and then sew the incision closed. Your head is cleansed and gauze is placed over the sutures. Your head is wrapped in a bandage.

To do a **scalp flap**, your surgeon will mark the bald skin where he wants to put the flap and the hairy scalp that he will use for the flap. He will inject both areas with local anesthetic. He will cut out and discard the bald skin. Next he will cut the flap—usually a long broad (2-inch) strip, tapering to a point at the end. The flap is then cut away from your scalp—until it is attached only on one side. It can then be swiveled into the open area where the bald skin was cut out. It is sewn in place. The place where the flap was taken is called the donor site. It is also sutured closed. Your scalp is then washed. A layer of gauze is placed over all the stitches and your head is bandaged.

Hair Transplants

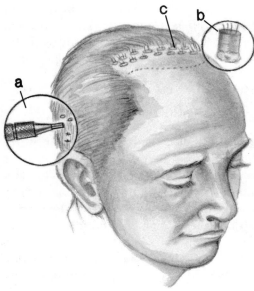

Figure 11-39.

A close-up (a) shows the hair-punch instrument taking punch grafts from the back of the head. These areas may be stitched, as shown, or not. A close-up of a punch graft (b) shows the skin and fatty layer, which carries the deepest hair follicles. With the punch grafts in place (c), notice that the grafts cannot be put next to each other. At a second session, the gaps can be filled in with more grafts.

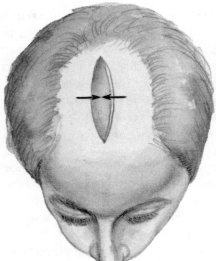

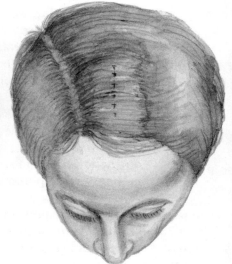

Figure 11-40.

For a scalp reduction, the central bald scalp skin is cut out so the surgeon can make the bald area smaller by pulling the hair closer together.

Figure 11-41.

Hair can be grown to cover the remaining bald area. Or, hair grafts may be placed in it.

After

Once the surgery is done, you go to the recovery room. (Or, if you only had hair grafts with minimal sedation, you may be able to go directly home.) At home you keep your head up as much as possible, to minimize the swelling.

The Process of Recovery

What to Do for Pain

Your scalp will ache and throb where the surgery was done. You may need narcotic painkillers by prescription or only over-the-counter acetaminophen (Tylenol).

The Healing Process

You will be sore for at least a day. For some people, the discomfort lasts several days. If you have had a scalp flap or scalp reduction you'll also feel tired, because of the heavy sedation or general anesthetic that was needed.

You will need to see your surgeon after about 5 days, if you had **hair grafts**. If you had a **scalp flap** or **scalp reduction** you will probably need about three visits in the first 2 to 3 weeks to check your healing, change the bandages, and remove stitches.

Bandages

If you had 30 or more hair grafts you will have a bandage wrapped about your head for 2 to 5 days. (If only a few grafts were done, you might need only a light tape bandage.) If you had a large scalp flap or a scalp reduction—your head will be bandaged for at least 5 days.

Taking Care of Your Wound

You can rinse but not vigorously wash your hair for 10 days. If you do, the grafts may become dislodged, bleed, and fail to grow new hair. You will be allowed to brush or comb your hair where your surgery wasn't done. Also you can use a gentle blow dryer—on a cool setting—to dry your hair.

Stitches

Punch grafts are not usually stitched in place. They are so delicate that a stitch, unless it's a fragile one put in under magnification, may damage the graft. Scalp flaps, scalp reductions and strip grafts will be stitched. These stitches are left in for 5 to 10 days and removed by your surgeon or his nurse.

Scars

There will be scars at the *donor* site (where the hairy scalp is taken *from*) and there will be scars at the *recipient* site (where the hairy scalp is *put in*). All the *donor* site scars will be hidden by your remaining hair. However, the scars may be up to a half-inch thick and pink. The **flap** may leave a long, wide (2 inch) scar, and if that is vertical at the back of the scalp, your remaining hair may tend to fall aside, revealing the scar.

The **scalp reduction** may leave a broad pink scar across the top of the scalp. This is visible if you bend over. However, a scalp reduction is usually only a first step in treating baldness and other steps will place grafts to cover the scar.

The scars in the *recipient* areas (i.e., where you were bald) will be faint, and concealed once the new hair grows—in about 3 months.

Tips

- Your result will depend to some extent on your own hair texture and thickness. If your hair is fine and thin, hair grafting may be disappointing because your hair grafts will contain only a few hairs. The new growth of hair may be sparse, regardless of what the surgeon can do.
- If it is not clear that your hair is thick enough to graft, your surgeon can do test grafts, putting about five small hair grafts in a bald patch and waiting 5 months to see how they grow.
- If your hair is thin all over, as often happens with women who suffer hair loss, then grafting will not succeed—the surgical result can only be as good as the scalp hair that you have.
- Hair graft procedures are not usually done all at once but in stages over a year and a half or longer.
- You will have to wear a bandage after each procedure. You might experiment with hats and scarves to conceal your bandage at those times.

- It will take about 3 months for your new hair to grow in, each time.
- You will have to wait at least 3 to 4 months between further grafting to an area of scalp.
- If you wear a hairpiece, you must decide to get rid of it if you want hair grafting. If you wear the hairpiece over the hair grafts while you wait for them to grow, the hairpiece itself will cause breaking of each new hair shaft at its base, and hair cannot grow.

Back to Work

Most people will be too self-conscious to go to work with a head bandage. If you are not, you could go back to work after about 2 days, if you had only light sedation. If you had heavy sedation or general anesthesia, you will need about 5 days to recover.

Back to Sports

Exercise will stimulate blood flow in the scalp and your grafts may be hit. Either event can cause bleeding or dislodge a flap or graft. This could lead to wide scars or cause the hair to grow out improperly, or not at all.

After 1 week, you may be able to swim—without a swim cap—or jog, but both should be done at half-speed and for a short time. Noncontact ball sports should be avoided for 2 to 3 weeks. Any contact sport—ice hockey, football, soccer—is out for 3 to 4 weeks, longer if you play a rough game.

Back to Parties

You can go to parties once your bandage is off and your stitches are out: days 6 to 11, depending on what procedure(s) you had done. Actually you *can* go to a party even with stitches in if they don't show. (Stitches are short and dark, and may look exactly like hair.)

Back to Sex

You should wait 10 days or more. Sexual activity will greatly increase your scalp blood flow—and may cause bleeding. A bump to your head may dislodge the grafts or flap.

How Much It Costs

Your cost for **punch grafts** will be between $15 to $30 *per graft*. A **strip graft** may cost about $1000, depending on its size. Some strip grafts consist of short strips, others of long, irregular shapes which makes the surgery more complicated and time consuming.

If you are having a **scalp flap** or a **scalp reduction** the surgeon's fee will vary from $1500 to $3000. With all these fees there will also be an operating room fee: about a minimum of $500 for local anesthesia and light sedation or $2000 or more for general anesthesia for a complex flap. It is impossible to give an average cost for hair transplants because they are done in stages. Which stages are done depends on your hair, your goal, and the extent of your balding. However, a minimum cost would be three sessions of 50 punch grafts, each spaced 4 months apart, costing between $2000 and $5000.

Insurance Coverage

Insurance will *not* pay for this surgery unless you can *prove* that your baldness resulted from a medical condition—for instance, after a burn. Even then insurance reimbursement is unpredict-

Hair Transplant: Recovery-at-a-Glance

This chart represents the *average* recovery times for this cosmetic operation.

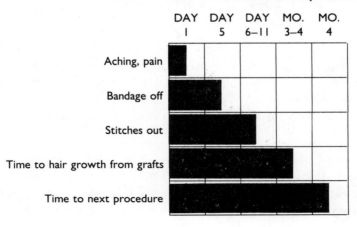

able. You should call your insurance company and find out if they *might* pay. If so, ask what information they need to authorize payment for your surgery. You should submit this information to your insurance company for their approval *before you begin treatment*. If they do approve your hair surgery, try to get a written commitment from them as to the *dollar* amount that they will pay for each stage.

My Assessment of This Procedure

Until we have a drug that brings hair follicles back to life, hair transplant surgery is the only treatment available to correct hair loss. These hair operations are the most common cosmetic procedures in men (cosmetic nose surgery is next). Women also have hair transplant surgery done, but women tend to develop thin hair all over their scalp and thus may not have good *donor* sites for hair transplant surgery.

The best hair transplant results are in people who have dark, curly hair with closely clustered hair follicles in the *donor* sites. Transplants of this kind of hair look thicker because they are curly; the growth is thick, because the follicles are close together and the dark hair shows up against the scalp. (Fine blond hair grafts may not be noticeable against pink scalp.)

Many people with less than ideal hair have successful hair transplant surgery. The **scalp reduction** has helped a lot—it cuts out bald skin, and so reduces the area that needs grafting. Hair transplant surgery requires careful planning with your surgeon because you have so many options. For instance, the same area of baldness might be treated with three sessions of punch hair grafts—as the simplest approach—or with two scalp reductions, strip grafts at the front hairline, and punch grafts behind. For your best result, sit down with your surgeon, tell him what you want and figure out what—given cost, risks and time—will work best for you. Make a plan together. Without a plan, you might have a hundred scattered punch grafts and decide that what you really need is a scalp reduction. You can still have it, but the balding scalp that is cut out might have all the punch grafts in it!

Side Effects and Complications

In hair transplant surgery, the more extensive your surgery, the greater your risk. With a **punch graft**, your risks are few. The hair growth may look unnatural, scattered tufts of hair. This can often be concealed with hairstyling or with further grafting. The scars around the grafts may be noticeable. For this reason the grafts at the front are placed so that hair grows forward and can be combed back over the scars, concealing them. Bleeding around a graft may harm it: It may scab, or it may survive but grow no hair. Still, if you have fifty hair grafts, and a few bleed, you have over 90 percent success.

The larger hair transplant operations have greater risks. A **scalp reduction** could leave a wide scar across your scalp. This is especially likely to occur if too much skin was removed because the tight scalp will pull on the scar and stretch it. A scalp flap may leave a wide scar at the back of your head, making your hair thin. The scar may show through. Also, the tip of the flap, which is farthest from the blood flow, may not heal, leaving a bald scar at the front of your scalp. This may require touch-up surgery to correct.

If your goal is the minimum *risk*, even at the cost of less improvement than you hope, then you will do best with the less risky punch hair graft technique. However, if you want maximum improvement, you might do best to accept the somewhat increased cost and risks of scalp reduction and flaps.

Enrico: A Great Result
Enrico, a handsome middle-aged man, had extensive hair grafting for baldness in the front of his scalp. Over two years, he had 300 hair grafts placed. Enrico had thick curly hair at the back of his scalp, and it grew well when grafted in the bald areas at the front. The scars at the back of his head were covered by hair. He felt that his hair looked great—he had exactly the result he wanted.

Charles: Hurry Up—and Wait
Charles was in his late thirties when he had hair transplants done. He had thin hair, and his hair follicles in the donor area were spaced far apart. He was not an ideal candidate, but his hair was dark, so every hair that grew would work well to correct his baldness. Charles first had two scalp flaps done to re-create his front hairline. His large bald patch on top of his head was reduced next by a scalp reduction.

Finally, the remaining bald areas were filled in with punch grafts. Charles was impatient and persuaded his surgeon to put in these grafts too close together, at the first session. (Each 3 mm graft should be 3 mm from the adjacent graft. A grafting session 4 months later fills in the gaps—otherwise there is not enough blood flow to keep the grafts alive.) As a result, a third of his grafts came off as scabs. Charles had to have no further grafting for 6 months to let his scalp rest. He then had two punch grafting sessions—the first to fill in half of the remaining baldness, and the second to fill in the gaps.

Margarita: Repairing a Scar
Margarita had a brow lift and had an infection that left a bald patch. She waited a year but it did not improve. She decided to have it corrected. Her surgeon first did a "mini" scalp reduction—the bald area was cut out and sutured to narrow the scar. Next, 4 months later, punch hair grafts were placed along the narrow scar. Grafts may not survive in scar tissue because the blood flow is diminished. Two-thirds of Margarita's grafts survived. She was pleased. The bald spot was changed to a narrower scar hidden by hair growing in her punch grafts.

What Other Patients Say

- **Account executive, 33:** "You can't be in a rush for this. I had a good plan worked out with my surgeon and we followed it. I don't have a full head of hair, but I don't feel bald either. I feel normal."

- **Store manager, 45:** "I felt my thinning hair made me look ineffective. I have light hair, but once it grew out, I tinted it so it would show. For a while I looked ridiculous, as though I was sprouting wheat sheaves all over my scalp, but it turned out okay. It made a big improvement in my self-confidence."

- **Politician, 54:** "I wouldn't have had this done, but my campaign manager told me I had to. We live in front of the TV cameras. I took to wearing a hat before I started having hair transplants. The scalp reduction did a lot at one time, which I liked. The punch graft sessions I lived through. I'm impatient. The hair takes too long to grow out to suit me. But it's okay now it's here."

Cosmetic Mole Removal and Scar Revision

What Surgeons Call It

Removal of moles is called mole excision. Cosmetic surgical treatment of scars is called *scar excision* and *revision*. The scars may be referred to as *hypertrophic* (thickened), *contracted* (shortened), or *keloid* (enormously thick).

What Is a Mole?

There are *hundreds* of different skin growths and marks that *you* may think of as a mole or like a mole. For example, you may have:

- Freckles: flat small brown skin stains from sun exposure
- Keratoses: brown, raised rough patches of skin, usually from too much sun
- A port wine stain: a flat red or bright pink discoloration of the skin, present since birth
- A strawberry mark: a raised red "cluster of grapes" like lump in the skin, showing up shortly after birth and diminishing with age

In the Procedures section, I will indicate the treatments for some of the other common skin marks besides the mole.

Moles that you were born with are called *nevi*. However, *most* moles don't develop until you have been in the sun. (The skin color cell is called the *melanocyte*.) Some people never get moles. Others get hundreds. Moles can cause problems because:

- You may think they look ugly.
- The "mole" may not be a mole, but a skin cancer called *melanoma*.
- The mole may be prone to turn into a melanoma.
- Removing a mole can leave a scar which looks worse than the mole.

What Is a Scar?

Scar is the tissue your body makes when it heals. Any cut in your skin other than a slight scrape heals with a scar. Scar consists of cells called *fibroblasts* and the protein they make, called *collagen*. New scars are a disorganized mass of fibroblasts and tangled strands of collagen. A flat, pale, old scar is a paragon of organization, with excess fibroblasts and collagen gone from the scene and the remaining fibroblasts and collagen parallel to each other like soldiers on parade, as described in the chapter on healing.

For reasons we don't yet know, scars on some places on the body, in some people, never reach that final healing stage. And sometimes blotchy brown-and-white skin color will call attention to an otherwise well-healed scar.

Nine Facts About Scars

Most bad scars are red, raised, lumpy, and thick. You usually need to see a plastic surgeon to determine exactly what kind of scar you have and what it needs. Nine little-known facts about scars are:

1. **Time** makes all scars better. You do *not* need to see a surgeon to check your scar 2 days or 2 weeks after an accident, if your only concern is the way it will look "in the end." Wait *6 months* before going for a consultation about the *looks* of a scar. If you go earlier, you are likely to be told to wait until at least 6 months go by.

2. A lumpy scar will flatten if **pressure** is put on it. No one knows exactly why, but it seems that the pressure tells the protein fibers how to line up. If you have a red, lumpy scar on your arm, for instance, a special elastic pressure wrap can be worn to speed your scar's improvement.

3. **Vitamin E** does *not* help healing. Studies show that it *slows down* healing, because it is chemically similar to steroid hormones which delay healing. However, the steroid effect of vitamin E *may* make it helpful *about 6 weeks after surgery* if your scars are red or itchy. Clinically, though, it hasn't been proved to be effective.

4. A *scar* is not a **keloid**. You may be told that your red, lumpy scar is a "keloid." It almost certainly is not. (Technically it is hypertrophic, or overgrown, scar.) A keloid is a scar that *grows*, ending up far longer, wider and thicker than any normal scar. Fortunately, keloids are uncommon. They tend to occur in darker skins, for reasons we don't understand.

5. **Laser treatment** of scars is used if the scar is abnormally red or has many dilated veins around it. Surgeons tend *not* to use lasers on children because they can cause thick scars. For teenagers, lasers are used cautiously, especially in those in the 13- to 15-year-old range. Growth is so rapid at this age that thick or wide scars are more likely to occur. Laser treatment of scars has been most useful when red, dilated veins form on the nose after cosmetic nose surgery, but it may fade redness in any scar. Although lasers are not used to remove moles, they are used to fade port wine stains. Laser treatment may be done in the office. Risks include turning the treated skin a brown color. Also, laser treatment may make scar redness fade only temporarily. Thus laser treatment of a red scar is reasonable only when the redness is disfiguring, and persistent.

6. Hydroquinone is the essential chemical ingredient of **fading creams**, which are used to treat brown discoloration of a scar. (The prescription creams are stronger.) Hydroquinone temporarily stops your skin color cells from making too much of the brown color called melanin. In time—which may be years—the hydroquinone will stop melanin production altogether. I have found these creams most useful shortly after the brown color appears. When used at this time hydroquinone may halt the brown color formation *permanently*. Once the brown color is well established in a scar, hydroquinone will fade the color for a day or less and must be used every day.

7. **Tattooing** may help conceal a discolored scar. This technique has not been used extensively, but with the new medical tattooing instruments it is used for some scars that otherwise had to be lived with. See the section on Eyeliner Tattooing for details of this technique.

8. **Hair transplants** can be used to conceal a scar if in an area that normally grows hair. For instance, after a facelift, the scar above the ear may widen. It is noticeable because the hair is

thin, since no hair is growing in the scar. These scars can be successfully camouflaged by taking hair punch grafts from the back of the head and inserting them into the scar. First, though, the scar may simply be cut out and restitched to see if this simpler technique can't narrow it. (See section on hair transplants for details on punch grafts.)

9. **Scar-concealing makeup** sometimes turns out to be your best treatment for a scar—especially when you are waiting 6 months, a year, or longer while it improves on its own. Lydia O'Leary used to be the only scar makeup, but there now are a number of scar makeups available (scars are smooth, and most ordinary makeup won't stick to scars, although concealer creams may). I recommend a consultation with a makeup specialist. If you rely on your surgeon, he may recommend a makeup that you don't know how to use properly, so you don't use it at all.

What It Will Do

The surgeon can (1) remove the **mole**, (2) make sure it is not cancerous by sending it to a pathologist, and (3) exchange the mole for a scar, that ought to look better than the mole removed.

Scars *cannot be erased.* Surgeons can reshape and restitch scars, but once a scar, always a scar. Your goal is to improve, not remove, the scar. (Sometimes improving a scar will make it appear invisible, but it is still there, if you look.)

What It Won't Do

Surgery can't remove a mole without leaving a scar. And it can't erase a scar.

How Long It Will Last

Permanently. Scars continue to improve all your life. If a mole "returns," it is because it was not completely removed the first time. The surgeon may have been trying to leave a tiny scar, and inadvertently left a fragment of mole behind.

When to Have It

Mole or scar surgery can be done at any time. Moles present at birth have a slight tendency toward developing into melanomas and are often removed in infancy. Small moles may not be removed until the child is old enough to have the surgery with local anesthesia—at least 8 or 9. The same is true for scars. A disfiguring scar may warrant surgery with general anesthesia even in an infant. However, a small scar is often left alone until the surgery can be done with local anesthesia. I recommend against such surgery at puberty, because rapid growth at this age can lead to a thick, unsightly scar. At puberty a mole or scar is best left alone until the growth spurt is finished, unless there is a medical reason to have the surgery. After puberty this surgery can be done at any age and at any time of year.

Where to Have It/Usual Anesthesia

Almost all moles are removed and minor scars revised by surgically cutting them out or rearranging them in an office operating room with local anesthesia. Sedation and/or a hospital or surgery center is used *if* many moles are to be removed at once *or* if the scar surgery is extensive.

How Long It Takes

Mole removal takes about 15 minutes per mole. **Scar revision** depends on the size of the scar and whether it needs only to be cut out and restitched, or whether the skin around the scar must be rearranged as well. A short scar that needs only to be restitched may take 15 minutes. Complex facial scar revisions may take several *hours*.

The Procedures
(Figures 11-42 through 11-44)

Removing Moles

Shaving. Some moles can be shaved off. With this technique, your surgeon first numbs the skin around the mole. Then he slices off the mole from the skin. This technique *does* risk leaving part of the mole behind (moles can go deep, through the skin), but thick scars are less likely to form with this technique. They can occur, however. Also, shaving a mole leaves an indented, pale, circular patch in the skin. Shaving is *never* recommended when the mole might be melanoma, because the pathologist who examines the mole under the microscope *must* examine all skin layers to help your doctor decide how to treat you if you have melanoma. Facial moles are rarely shaved because the indented patch looks worse than a scar. The tip of the nose is an exception. Here scars are often sunken and shaving is often the best treatment.

Shaving is used to remove **keratoses**, the brownish, crusty skin growths that appear from too much sun. Unlike moles, keratoses are only in the outer skin layers, and shaving them off at the skin surface leaves a pink or white patch, but usually no scar.

Other skin growths that are often treated with shaving include:

- Lentigo (flat dark brown spots)
- Warts
- Sebaceous hyperplasia (thickening of small skin glands)

Note: Scraping, freezing, burning, and curetting (digging out) as well as shaving are commonly used for various benign (noncancerous) skin growths.

Excision. Moles are often excised (cut out), especially if they are on the face (cutting makes a better scar) or if they may be malignant. To excise a mole, the surgeon first cleanses the skin around the mole with surgical soap. Then he uses a tiny needle to inject local anesthetic near (not into) the mole, until the mole and the area around it are numb. Then he will cut the mole out, using a tapered, oval incision a bit longer than the mole so that the scar will lie flat when he puts in the stitches. Too short an incision makes the scar puff up at both ends—surgeons call this a "dog-eared" scar. Dog-ears improve gradually—at times completely. A "dog-eared" scar may be made intentionally, if such a scar would be better than one that is too long.

Scar Revision

Scars can be corrected in several different ways.

Steroid Injection. They can be injected in the office with steroid (triamcinclone) if they are lumpy, raised, and red. The steroid thins out the scar tissue by making your body absorb the excess scar. This is usually *not* done until 6 months after surgery because your own healing will also flatten the scar. Steroid may cause too much scar to be absorbed, giving you a wide, purple, sunken, thin scar, just as ugly as the raised, red, lumpy one.

Dermabrasion/Dermaplaning. Scars can also be **dermabraded**, which simply means sanding your skin down. Sometimes surgical sandpaper is used in the office, for a small area of skin. More extensive dermabrasion, for anything other than one or two small scars, is described in the section on Dermabrasion/Dermaplaning. Dermabrasion is used for acne scars, as is a combination of dermabrasion, chemical peel, shaving and **dermaplaning**. Dermabrasion can smooth down rough scars—for instance, those left on the forehead by going through a windshield. It will not help smooth a raised, rough, lumpy (hypertrophic) scar.

Revision. Scars can be cut out, rearranged, and restitched. This is done in the office for a small scar. For extensive scars, surgery is done in the hospital and at times may require general anesthesia or an overnight hospital stay, though not often. Such surgical revision is the most common way to improve a scar. For instance, if you had a mole removed and you were allergic to the stitching material used, you could get a lumpy, ugly scar as a result. You would have no way of knowing that you were allergic to the stitches, unless you had had an allergic reaction to the same kind of stitch before. If this "allergic" scar were still ugly in 6 months, it could be cut out and sewn up with a different suture material. Or, if you had a brow lift and you banged your scar 2 weeks later, your scar would probably separate below the skin even if it didn't reopen. Result—a very wide scar in that area. Since scars don't grow hair, and brow lift scars are in the scalp, you would have a bald patch on your head. Scar revision would consist of cutting the scar out and sewing it up—just don't bump it again!

Scars can be rearranged in very complicated ways—turning straight scars into Z and W and zigzag shapes. This is needed when a scar lies in a bad direction. For example, a long, lumpy up-and-down forehead scar may flatten immediately if it is given a few zigzags to let it move naturally with your forehead expression.

This kind of scar surgery *shouldn't* be needed, except in rare cases, after cosmetic surgery. Why? Your surgeon ought to put the scar in the right place the first time. Such scar surgery is most often used to correct scars from accidents. After cosmetic surgery—or after mole removal—most scars are fine. A poor scar may need to be restitched, or injected with steroid, but will rarely need complicated scar rearrangment.

Surgical Removal of Moles

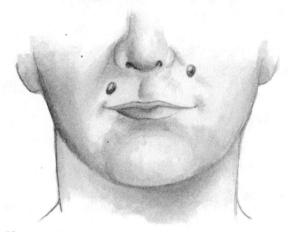

Figure 11-42.
Two common sites for moles are the upper lip and the cheek.

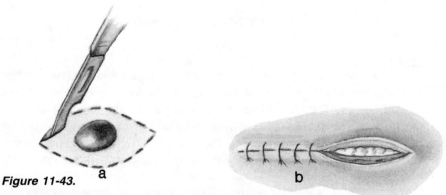

Figure 11-43.
The surgeon cuts out the mole in an oblong piece (a) so that the edges of the incision can be stitched into a straight-line scar (b).

Surgical Revision of Facial Scars

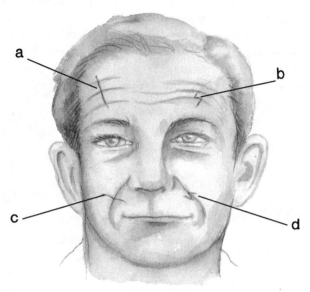

Figure 11-44.

The scar at (a) goes across all the natural brow lines, making it noticeable. A "Z-plasty" of the scar gives it a Z shape (b), zig-zagging it into the natural lines so that it will blend with the natural lines and *move* naturally instead of pulling against them. The scar at (c) goes across the natural fold so that the scar is noticeable. Also, the tightness of the scar will hinder natural movement. The "Z-plasty" (d) zig-zags the scar into the natural line and permits it to blend with the line and move with normal facial expression.

The Process of Recovery

What to Do About Pain

There is usually little pain after mole or scar surgery. The treated area will ache for several hours while the local anesthesia wears off, and for the rest of the day. The day after surgery the *bandage* is a nuisance, but the surgery itself will only hurt at the end of the day when you are tired. Aspirin will take the ache away, but *don't* take aspirin. It will make you bruise and may make the surgical area bleed. Take an acetaminophen (an over-the-counter nonaspirin painkiller such as Tylenol) instead for any mild pain for the first 2 weeks after surgery.

Bandages

Usually a Band-Aid or small gauze pad will do to absorb oozing on the day of surgery and to protect the surgical area. It is more "socially acceptable" than stitches that show. You should wear a Band-Aid or gauze pad over the area at night, so that you don't hurt your wound by tossing or turning. If you are at a desk all day you may want to take the Band-Aid off—especially if it is making your skin itch.

The Healing Process/Caring for Your Wound

The surgical area may be covered with a spot Band-Aid if you had one small mole removed, or you may have a complicated gauze and tape wrapping if you had more extensive surgery. I let my patients bathe and shower normally if they have Band-Aids. After bathing, they remove the wet Band-Aid, pat the area dry, and put on a new one. This helps prevent skin irritation under the Band-Aid. Your skin will itch under the bandage. If your surgeon lets you remove your bandages, let the surgical area dry in the air for part of the day, even if you keep it covered for protection at work or at night. Scabs won't usually form if you have stitches, but a mole that is scraped or burned off forms a scab as part of healing.

About a week after surgery, the scar will itch. This is partly from healing and partly from skin dryness. Once the skin is healed, you can coat an itchy scar with Vaseline or another bland lotion or ointment.

It is important to protect your incision from being bumped. Even when the stitches are out, the wound is weak for weeks. Avoid even a light blow on or near the operated area—even 2 weeks after surgery, the trauma can reopen the incision or widen a scar. A violent blow can have the same effect even 6 weeks after surgery.

Stitches

Stitches on your face are usually out on days 4 to 6. They stay in longer (7 to 10 days) elsewhere on your body. Stitches will stay in up to 14 days over the knuckles and other joints because body areas that move a lot take longer to heal.

Tips

- Certain places on the body are bad scar zones which will almost certainly heal with a red, wide, lumpy, itchy scar—even from "just" having a mole removed. The worst area is your upper back, around the shoulders. After 1 to 2 *years* these scars may flatten, but they will still be wide, perhaps thick and pink. Re-operating won't help.
- Injections of steroid (triamcinclone) will help flatten most of these scars but you may need several office visits for injections 4 to 6 weeks apart.
- Besides the upper back and shoulders, you are likely to have a lumpy, red scar, even if you heal well in other places, in:
    —the midchest
    —the midabdomen
    —the groin just above the pubic hair
    —the lower back
    —the neck, especially under the chin
    —any scar that goes against a natural fold of the skin—for example, an up-and-down scar behind the knee or in the front of your neck.
- Remove a mole only for *medical* reasons in bad scar zone areas—that is, if it may be cancerous. Don't ask a doctor to remove a mole in a bad scar zone because a scar would be prettier—it probably won't be.
- Bad scars in these areas are *normal*; they are not keloids and are not a sign that you heal poorly in other areas.

Back to Work

You will be able to go to work the same or the next day, unless you had sedation. Then, you will be ready for work on days 3 to 6, or when your bandages are removed.

Back to Sports

It may seem silly to stop sports after minor mole or scar surgery, but a blow from a ball or contact sport can disrupt your wound. Such sports are out for 2 weeks, unless you are willing to take the risk of pulling apart your scar. Noncontact sports such as walking, jogging, or swimming are fine. Extensive surgery may keep you away from sports for longer, depending on what was done.

Back to Parties

You can go to parties the day of minor surgery. If you had sedation, you will be tired and may not enjoy the evening. If you had a very large mole removed or major scar revision, you should wait 3 or 4 days, or longer . . . until you feel back to your normal self.

Back to Sex

Sex is like a sport. If you can have sex in such a way as to avoid any bump or blow to the surgery, then go ahead. For instance, if you needed a few stitches on your lower chest, you can probably have sex and still protect the incision from an inadvertent blow. However, scar surgery on your face and on areas likely to be sex contact spots make sex inadvisable for about 10 days, until the wound is healed enough to resist a minor force.

How Much It Costs

Mole removal costs about $150 to $200 for the first mole and about half of that for others removed at the same time. A minor scar revision would cost the same. **Scar revisions** vary tremendously in cost; complex scar revisions can cost from $2000 to $5000, including hospital fees (see Insurance Coverage).

Insurance Coverage

Insurance will almost always reimburse you for surgical **removal of moles**. Even though you may be doing it because you don't like the way the mole looks, there is always a question of a mole being cancerous. However, if you have many moles on your face removed, your insurance may balk at paying.

Your insurance *may* pay for surgical **scar revision**. If the scar is from a car accident, then your car insurance (or the other driver's) may pay. Scar surgery can become expensive; it is important to straighten out the financial details before your surgery. Ask your surgeon to write out for you what he intends to do and how much it will cost. Contact your insurance company and try to get their *approval in writing as to how much they will pay*. Most insurance companies are reasonable. Some will argue that if the scar only looks bad—no matter how bad—then they won't pay.

My Assessment of This Procedure

Moles are removed and scars revised by the thousands every day. Understanding your healing helps you to know when your surgeon did something less than perfect—and when it's your body, not your surgeon, who gets "the blame" for a less than perfect scar.

Sukie: A Dog-eared Breast Scar

I had done a breast reduction on Sukie, a teenaged girl who was a little overweight. I wanted to keep her breast crease scars as short as possible. Otherwise they could be visible. At the sides of her breasts I could not get the scar to lie flat, no matter how I arranged the skin and trimmed the fat under it. I left the scar dog-eared intentionally. I explained this to her, but she thought I had forgotten to finish that part of her surgery. In 6 weeks, the dog-ears were down 50 percent. In 6 months, they were down 75 percent. In 1 year all that remained was a millimeter of dog-eared skin on either breast. I removed these in the office. Sukie needed two stitches. She had a much shorter scar than if I had made her scars perfect at surgery.

Breast reductions, tummy tucks, and facelift incision behind your ear can all leave you with a "dog-ear"—time will fix it for you most of the time.

Teresa: A Wide Breast Scar

Teresa, who was 27, had a breast enlargement done by me. She had a perfect result, except that her scars started out as hairline scars, but over 6 months spread to half an inch wide and turned brown. I thought cutting out the scars and restitching would lead to the same healing. Her scars seemed to be from her healing and not from the surgery. However, she wanted to see what surgery could do. I cut out the scars and sewed them up, using different stitching in case part of the problem had been from the stitches I used the first time. I operated in my office and didn't charge her. The result 2 weeks later was perfect. The scars widened slowly in the next 6 months, despite her use of tape strips to give them support. They were slightly less brown.

She didn't mind the scars and wasn't disappointed. She had just wanted to be sure that there wasn't anything more I could do. This was reasonable.

Colleen: An Upper Lid Scar

Colleen came to me for a second opinion while visiting her granddaughter. She had had upper lid surgery 6 weeks before. Her scars were like a red rope across each eyelid. One was hidden in the natural upper lid crease. The other was swollen and showed above the crease. Colleen told me that her surgeon had wanted to remove her stitches 4 days after surgery, but a snowstorm had kept her housebound for almost 2 weeks. Her surgeon had told her that the scars were so bad because the stitches had been in so long. He told her to wait for 3 to 6 months. If they hadn't improved by then, he would cut them out and sew them up again. He promised her that this would improve them. She wasn't sure if she should believe him, or if he was "covering up" something that he had done wrong. In my opinion, he wasn't covering up. Eyelid skin heals fast, and stitches left in too long are irritating and leave ugly scars. Time and perhaps surgery were almost sure to be the solution for Colleen.

Clark: Complex Facial Scarring

Clark was a lawyer who made the mistake of helping a friend with a chain saw one weekend. The saw jumped, cutting into Clark's lower face around his lips. Of course, he was rushed to the nearest hospital. I was called to sew up the lacerations. Fortunately, Clark had fast reflexes: although he had many cuts, none were deep and no bone or nerves were injured.

Six months later, Clark had some faint scars. But there was also a jagged collection of red, raised scars distorting one side of his mouth.

With Clark under local sedation as an outpatient, I cut out those scars and rearranged them. After surgery, Clark healed well, but he had a sneezing fit from hayfever. This made some stitches bleed and widened a few of his new scars.

Six months after that, I operated again, on those scars, with local anesthesia in the office. I cut out and sewed up the scars that had spread after the sneezing. Also, I rearranged a few scars that still seemed poor. He was pleased with his final result—as was I. His scars from the chain saw accident were permanent and permanently visible—but conforming to natural crease lines so that Clark was no longer disfigured.

Cosmetic surgery puts scars in the best possible places, given the surgery to be done. Unlike Clark's facial scarring from his accident, the surgeon controls the most important part of a scar: *where it is.* Infection or poor healing can make any scar wide or lumpy. Some scars will heal like that, regardless, because that is how you heal—or because the scar is in a bad scar zone.

Lots can be done though to improve a scar, besides merely waiting. Steroid injections—after 6 months or more—will flatten a raised scar, although they won't necessarily improve the color and won't make it narrow. Re-operation on a scar may be worthwhile to be sure that everything surgical has been done to improve it. Techniques like fading creams, tattooing in color, and dermabrasion all may be used, depending on how the scar has healed.

Collagen and Silicone Injections

What Surgeons Call Them

Depending on the material that is being injected, these procedures may be called liquid silicone injections or collagen/Zyderm/Zyplast injections.

What They Will Do

Both collagen and silicone injections aim to fill in depressions in the *skin*. They will not fill in deep depressions, such as "ice-pick" scars from acne. These scars go right through the skin, and the injected material cannot get under them to plump them up. Treatable scars include most chickenpox and acne scars, age lines, frown lines, and scars from an accident that has left a slight depression in the skin.

What They Won't Do

Neither collagen nor silicone will *erase* a scar. The material simply fills out the skin depression that *accompanies* the scar, although the scar may become much less visible. That is because skin depressions appear darker than surrounding skin. A depressed scar that is raised may end up less noticeable.

The Injected Materials

Collagen. The collagen used in cosmetic surgery is the same kind of collagen protein that we have in our skins and that our bodies use to make scar, but it is derived from cattle hide. Trade names include Zyderm and Zyplast. To be sure you aren't allergic to collagen itself or to the anesthetic or preservatives mixed with these products, your doctor will give you a test injection in your arm. If you are allergic, you should not be given more collagen. You must wait *1 month* between the test injection and treatment. An allergic reaction can vary from a rash, a lumpy swelling, or a flu-like syndrome of temporarily aching bones and joints. The cause of these symptoms is not known. Collagen is very safe. Its biggest drawback is that it is *temporary*. Over 1 to 2 years, your body will absorb the injected collagen and you will need "touch-up" treatment or retreatment.

Silicone. This product is much less widely used than collagen. Some studies suggest that skin eruptions or reactions to injected liquid silicone can occur years after it is injected. The problem with silicone is that it is *not* temporary. If it is put in the wrong place, it cannot be removed without cutting out the entire area of skin, because the silicone disperses in and around the skin as tiny microdroplets. (It may be possible to suction out the silicone, leaving only a tiny scar, but this may leave an indentation worse than the original problem.) A doctor with extensive experience with silicone can get good results, but it is technically more difficult to administer and can only be given in tiny amounts in each treatment session.

How Long They Will Last

The improvement from a **collagen injection** will usually last 1 to 2 years. It may last longer—up to 5 years—but such prolonged results are unpredictable and unusual. **Silicone injections** are permanent, which in itself can pose a problem as already explained.

When to Have Them

These injections can be done at anytime for a line or wrinkle. You must wait 6 to 12 months before treatment of a scar from an injury or infection. There is no age limit. Teenagers can be treated, too.

Where to Have Them

These procedures are done in a doctor's office by a cosmetic surgeon or dermatologist.

Conditions That Increase Your Risk

If you have an **active skin infection**, this treatment may make the infection worse. If you have **dark or sallow skin**, or if your skin discolors easily, the injections may cause inflammation that leaves permanent, although faint, brownish discoloration. If you have had **anaphylaxis** (severe shock reaction to a drug) or if you have an autoimmune disorder like rheumatoid arthritis or lupus, you *cannot* receive collagen.

Usual Anesthesia

Local anesthetic is mixed with the silicone or collagen. These treatments do not require sedation. However, if you are very anxious, your doctor may prescribe an anti-anxiety sedative for you to take shortly before your treatment.

How Long They Take

The treatments will take 15 to 60 minutes, depending on how extensive the treatment.

The Procedures
(Figure 11-45)

Before

These treatments are done in the doctor's office. You will come in as for a regular appointment. You will be taken to the treatment room or minor operating room, where your doctor will use purple surgical ink to mark the area(s) to be treated. Your skin will be cleansed with soap or alcohol.

During

Your doctor will use a fine needle (#30—smaller than the finest sewing needle) to inject the collagen or silicone into your frown lines, your acne scars, or whatever area will be treated. He may cool your skin before the treatment with ice or a freezing skin spray to lessen the sting of the needles, but this makes your skin stiff and harder to treat.

You will feel burning or stinging at times as the material is injected. What you feel depends on the area being treated. The frown and forehead lines may be virtually painless. The lip is extremely sensitive—treatment here will be done slowly to minimize your discomfort.

If your skin is bruised by the injections, ice will be put on the bruise immediately, or you will be asked to do so after you leave.

After

I may cover the treated area with a Band-Aid, but never on the lips. Here a Band-Aid always feels and looks worse than the faint redness and tiny dots left by the needle injections. Afterwards, you can go home, or back to work or school, if you wish.

Collagen and Silicone Injections

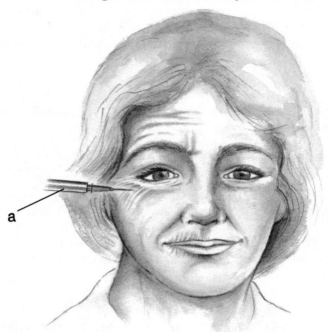

Figure 11-45.

The fine lines of the forehead, between the eyebrows, and around the eye and mouth (seen in the "before" view on the left-hand side) can be filled in with collagen through the use of a needle (a). The "after" view, on the right, shows that the fine lines have been filled in with collagen. Remember, collagen is *not* a permanent treatment.

The Process of Recovery

What to Do About Pain

After the treatment, the local anesthetic will wear off in about an hour. Your treated skin may sting, burn, or throb slightly, but not enough to need medication.

The Healing Process

Your skin will be red or pink where the injections were done. This should fade in 24 hours, or may not occur at all. A few people notice that the redness lasts several days. If bruising occurs, it may last 3 to 10 days, lasting longest in fair skin.

Bandages

Your doctor may conceal the tiny pinpoints left by the needles after treatment, with Band-Aids or tape strips. You can remove these at home and wash the area gently to remove the minuscule dot of blood around each injection. New Band-Aids or tape do *not* need to be applied, unless you want to use them to *conceal* the redness.

Taking Care of Your Wound

You can have this treatment done and return to work. However, if you go home and put ice on the treated area, the risk of redness and bruising is minimized. If you had sedation, it is probably best not to go back to work or to school. You won't be thinking clearly. Men can shave the evening after a treatment, and women can put on makeup.

Stitches

There are no stitches.

Scars

Any needle that punctures your skin leaves a tiny scar. This scar is so small that you may not be able to see it. However, if your skin is dark, you could heal with tiny *white* dots of scar that show up against your normal skin color. This should be temporary, because the normal skin color cells will move into the scar and re-color it. It is possible, although very rare, for the tiny needle scars to show. If this happens after a first treatment, you *might* decide to cancel further treatments.

Tips

- To minimize bruising, keep ice over the treated area for an hour or so afterwards. However, if you return to work it is not practical and is not *necessary*.
- You can go in the sun after a treatment, but wear a #15 sunscreen, or higher. The mild inflammation from the treatment, plus the ultraviolet rays of the sun, can make your treated skin burn, sting, or form brown color in your skin.

Collagen and Silicone Injection: Recovery-at-a-Glance

This chart represents the *average* recovery times for this cosmetic procedure.

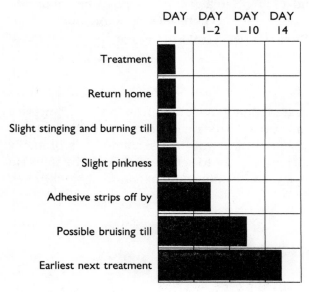

	DAY 1	DAY 1–2	DAY 1–10	DAY 14
Treatment	■			
Return home	■			
Slight stinging and burning till	■			
Slight pinkness	■			
Adhesive strips off by	■■			
Possible bruising till	■■■			
Earliest next treatment	■■■■			

Back to Work

You can go back to work directly from the doctor's office. The redness or the Band-Aids may make you self-conscious. Many people have treatment at the end of one day and go back to work the next.

Back to Parties

You can go to a party the day of treatment. However, alcohol may make the treated area *more* pink. Most people prefer to postpone parties for about 3 days, unless they cover the treated area with makeup and stay away from alcohol.

Back to Sports

Exercise, like alcohol, will make the treated area more pink. However, most people don't care about looking their best during a workout. This need not keep you inactive. The area may throb slightly after exercise for 24 to 48 hours after treatment.

Back to Sex

Sex will make the treated area flush and may make it throb. However, sex will not be injurious. You can have sex the same day.

How Much They Cost

The test injection for collagen costs between $80 and $200. No test is needed for silicone injection. Each treatment will cost between $100 to $300, depending on what material is used, and how much. Injectable collagen comes as Zyderm I, Zyderm II, and Zyplast, the first being the least concentrated and least expensive. If you have frown lines between your eyes, the total cost will be between $300 and $550. You will need a test injection and two treatments—a total of three. If you have extensive superficial scarring from acne, your cost may be $1500, and your treatment may be spaced over several months with five to ten doctor's visits.

The cost of an office treatment is similar for silicone, but there may be twice as many visits over six months or longer.

Insurance Coverage

Insurance will almost certainly *not* pay for silicone, because it is considered experimental or unproven by many doctors and insurance companies. Some insurance companies will pay for collagen in certain cases—for example, for acne *scars* but not for skin furrows or wrinkles.

My Assessment of These Procedures

Collagen Injections

I have used collagen extensively. It is good for filling in frown lines, shallow acne scars, and other fine lines (such as around the lip) if you can accept the fact that it is temporary. It may be a perfect temporary solution for people who have some lines or scars and don't yet want the cost and recovery of an operation or chemical peel. Collagen may correct the problem. At the end of a year, or so, people can then decide between more collagen treatments or surgery.

344 / THE COMPLETE BOOK OF COSMETIC SURGERY

Collagen is *antigenic*; that is, it can react with your body and cause an allergic problem. This is almost always detected by the test injection. However, if a treatment site is inflamed and lumpy for more than a few days—do *not* proceed with collagen until you and your doctor are sure that this is *not* an allergic reaction.

Silicone Injections

Most dermatologists and cosmetic surgeons, including myself, do not use silicone. I have seen only problems from this treatment. However, I do know a few dermatologists who have used it extensively and find that it works for them. Remember, silicone is permanent. Be sure your doctor is skilled in its use before he treats you. If in doubt, get a second opinion.

Side Effects and Complications

Most people find that the worst aspect is the discomfort of the injections. Even tiny needles hurt around the lips. A sedative pill *does* help, but most of my patients feel that the sedative side effects are worse than the pain. The pain stops when the injection stops, but the grogginess from the sedation lasts several hours.

Anything injected into your skin can cause an allergic reaction, bleeding, or scarring. I find collagen preferable to silicone, but its disadvantage is that it is temporary—it is absorbed on average within 2 years.

Remember that *caution* is best, especially with silicone, which has the disadvantage of being permanent. If it is wrong for you, it won't be likely to improve with time.

Fred: Some Lasting Allergy Problems

Fred had lines around his eyes and mouth that he detested. He had a collagen test injection, which appeared totally normal. However, after his first collagen treatment, the treated area and the test area swelled up, becoming firm and red. Fred persisted in his collagen treatments, feeling sure that the redness and swelling were insignificant. They weren't. He had developed an unusual delayed allergy. The redness and swelling returned intermittently for months, until the collagen was absorbed.

Charisse: A Silicone "Bulge"

Charisse had extensive acne scarring with the worst scars being on her cheeks. Her dermatologist recommended silicone injections, which she had twice a month for several years. The silicone filled out the scars a bit, but a firm lumpy bulge formed over her cheekbone, from the silicone droplets plus scarring around each drop. Minor surgery was done to remove the silicone "ball." The surgery left another scar but removed the bulge.

Horace: "Repeats" As Needed

Horace was 50 and claimed that his deep frown lines came from worrying about his job. He wanted a "quick fix" because he didn't have time for more. He had a collagen test injection, and two 20-minute office visits spaced a month apart. The collagen completely filled in his frown lines, and he returned with characteristic thoroughness every 18 months to have the lines touched up with another collagen "fix." Horace thought it was terrific—his kids no longer assumed he was angry when he came home now that the deep frown lines were gone.

Merrilee: Playing for Time

Merrilee had fine lines all around her mouth. She had a fair skin and could have had a chemical peel, but she felt that at 35 she was too young. She opted to have collagen instead. She wanted to see what it could do, hoping it would buy her time until she felt ready to have something more "drastic" done to her face. Collagen lasted in her only a short time—about 9 months—but since she needed only a small amount to fill in her fine lines, it seemed right to Merrilee. "I'll have a peel when I have a facelift," she decided. "This is perfect for now."

What Other Patients Say

- **Systems analyst (female), 49:** "I didn't want a lot done and it [collagen] didn't do a lot, but it did what I wanted. My age lines are softer. They're there, but not to notice. Compared to anything else I could have done, it's cost effective."

- **Business secretary, 31:** "I liked the effect. I didn't like its being temporary."
- **College sophomore (male), 20:** "I had had three dermabrasions for acne and I still had scars. The collagen helped my cheeks a lot. I'm lucky. It's lasted 3 years in me and I can see I'll need some touch-ups, but not yet."
- **Business woman, 71:** "I had everything done to my face. Collagen was the last fine-tuning to fill out lines that I didn't like. Believe me, it's easier than having my teeth cleaned."
- **Computer salesman, 26:** "I bruised. It took my skin so long for my bruising to fade that I decided to have a dermabrasion instead of fool around with collagen anymore."
- **Grandmother, 67:** "I was going to have a facelift until I realized that it wouldn't flatten the lines by my mouth. I have thin skin and the collagen worked almost too well. I had a ridge where it was put in, but when that faded, I was really pleased."

CHAPTER 12

Procedures for the Breasts

Breast Enlargement

What Surgeons Call It
This procedure is technically called an augmentation mamma-plasty.

What It Will Do
The goal of cosmetic breast enlargement is to give you fuller breasts, with a bit more "lift." The surgery can correct slight drooping—for example, the kind that's likely to occur after pregnancy. Your best guide to the improvement you get for drooping is: Are your nipples *below* the line of your breast crease? If so, breast enlargement with implants isn't likely to correct your droop enough. (See the section on Breast Lift.)

As far as size is concerned, the surgery can make you as large as you want to be—eventually. Most women want to be one or two cup-sizes larger. But if your goal is to go, for instance, from a small B to a DD, the operation alone can't do it. Your skin needs to stretch, and this happens in stages. An expandable implant is placed and is inflated over 4 to 6 weeks, by injecting water into it to gradually stretch the skin. Your surgeon will do this in his office.

What It Won't Do

This operation will not change an unsatisfactory breast shape. Some women have breasts that are droopier, more pointed, or more tubular than others. Minor variations may not be worth trying to change, because it may not be *possible* to perfect a slight variation in breast shape. However, misshapen breasts can be improved with surgery to cut the breast and stitch it to hold the new shape. This can be done *at the same time* as a breast enlargement, but breast enlargement alone changes only your size—making you larger, rounder, and fuller.

How Long It Will Last.

Permanently. Your breasts may diminish in size—after pregnancy, with weight loss, or at menopause. However, your implants will not. So, even if your breasts become smaller, they will not be as small as they were before your breast enlargement.

When to Have It

You can have this surgery once your breasts have finished developing. If you plan to have children and want to breast-feed them, postpone your surgery. After breast augmentation, you *can* breast-feed, but you shouldn't, because you have a high chance of developing mastitis (breast infection). If an infection develops, you won't be able to breast-feed for fear of infecting your baby. What's more, your implants may become infected or develop capsules (hardening of the tissue around the implant).

Where to Have It

Breast augmentation is usually done on an outpatient basis in a doctor's office operating room *or* a surgery center operating room *or* a hospital operating room. (It is rare to stay overnight, even if you decide to have general anesthesia.)

Conditions That Increase Your Risk

If you have **breast-fed a baby** within a year before surgery, the breast enlargement surgery *can* stimulate your breasts to form milk. This is painful although temporary (a few days to a week after surgery). Drugs that stop milk formation are available, but they cause nausea and stomach cramps. You won't necessarily have this problem, but you *may*.

If you have an **autoimmune arthritis** (there are various kinds—if you have arthritis, ask your doctor what kind) you should probably not have this surgery. Recent research suggests that a few women develop arthritis after a breast enlargement. It appears that their body's reaction to the silicone implant stimulates an underlying tendency to this disease. Treatment is removal of the implant.

Bleeding after surgery is rare. But if you have a **bleeding tendency** or if you have to take aspirin or any medicine that makes your blood slow to clot, your risk of internal bleeding around the implant after surgery is increased. If this happens, an urgent second operation must be done to stop the bleeding and drain off the blood.

Usual Anesthesia

Breast enlargement is most often done with local anesthesia with sedation. Some patients prefer general anesthesia because they are afraid of pain during surgery. General anesthesia seems to slightly increase your risk of bleeding because it relaxes your blood vessels. Local/sedation may make this operation tolerable (you may not remember the pain or may have none). But when the surgeon pulls up the breast (see The Operation) you'll feel a heavy pressure, which one patient described as "an elephant sitting on my chest." Local/sedation is much less expensive than general anesthesia, and the recovery time is shorter. For example, you can go back to work a week sooner. Nevertheless, if the extra cost and recovery from general anesthesia are *not* a consideration, many patients would prefer it. (See What to Do About Pain.)

How Long It Lasts

Breast enlargement surgery usually last 1½ to 2 hours.

About Implants

The basic implant is an oval or round ball of *semi-solid soft silicone* in a *solid silicone envelope* (Figure 12-1). It weighs about

8 ounces. The average implant would fill a soup bowl, but they come in all sizes. Thicker envelopes are now being used in many implants since silicone gel can leak through the thin envelopes of the older implants.

Some implants are made of **silicone covered with polyurethane**. They are called "fuzzy implants" because the polyurethane coating makes the surface of the implant rough, whereas silicone is smooth. The polyurethane lets your body tissue grow into it. Fuzzy implants have problems. Getting a polyurethane implant out, once you have grown into it can be a major operation. Infection is more common. This type of implant was very popular a few years ago but is now much less commonly used.

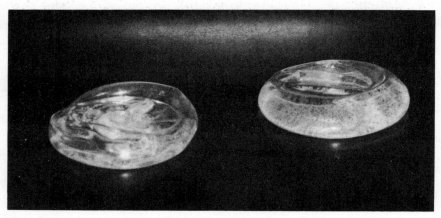

Figure 12-1.

Breast implants used in breast enlargement, and reconstruction after mastectomy. The implant on the left is double-lumen (walled). Notice the air-filled outer envelope that is filled with water at surgery. On the right is a silicone-only implant. It is a 230cc implant, which would be a full C cup, compared to a 150cc implant on the left, which would be a medium B cup.

Water-filled implants are a silicone envelope that the surgeon fills with water during the operation. Because these implants have a valve to allow them to be filled, they can deflate, or the water can leak out. They are the least expensive implant—a pair may cost $150, as opposed to $500 or more for a pair of silicone-filled implants. Thus, the cost may make the risk of deflation seem worthwhile. If a water-filled implant does deflate, it should be removed and replaced within a few days. Otherwise, your implant pocket will shrink, and instead of replacing the deflated implant, which is a simple office procedure, your surgeon may have to re-create the pocket, which would be like having the operation redone.

Implants with **double-walled envelopes** were developed for postcancer breast reconstruction but are now also used for cosmetic breast enlargement (Figure 12-1). These implants are more expensive (by $200 or $300) than many of the silicone-filled implants. Around a standard silicone implant, they have an outer or inner envelope that can be filled with water. The newest such implant is expandable and can be made larger or smaller using a needle to withdraw or inject water. If steroid drugs are used to try to prevent a capsule from forming, they can be put in this outer envelope. (More on steroid drugs shortly.) Some studies suggest that the outer envelope makes the formation of capsules less likely. However, the outer envelope rim can rub and thin the overlying skin. Because of this, such implants are usually placed behind muscle, not under the breast where the implant is nearer the skin.

Placement of the Implant

Your cosmetic breast implant may be placed between your breast and the muscle behind it. Or, it may be placed *under the muscle*, between the muscle and the ribs. You and your surgeon will discuss the pros and cons, which are:

- Placing the implant under the *muscle* seems to decrease your risk of a capsule (firmness of your breast from scar shrinkage, after surgery). This is probably because your chest muscle constantly presses on the scar and keeps it stretched. *But*, capsules are only *less* likely and can still occur. (Risk seems to be between 8 and 12 percent versus 10 and 30 percent, according to various studies.)
- A capsule around an implant that is under the muscle can only be treated by re-operation.
- Placing the implant under the muscle is a more painful, extensive operation and tends to require general anesthesia. There is more postsurgery pain, and recovery takes 2 weeks.

- Placing the implant between the breast and the muscle is the less painful, less extensive operation, but it carries a higher risk (up to 30 percent) of capsule formation.
- If you develop a capsule and the implant is between the breast and muscle, it can be treated by pressure on the breast. This pops the capsule inside like popping a balloon. This is done in the office but only works *temporarily*. Breast firmness returns within 3 weeks to 6 months.
- You and your surgeon should discuss capsules before surgery.
- Every plastic surgeon has his own way of dealing with capsules. What works best for my patients is to put the implant between the breast and the muscle, and then have the patient exercise (see Exercise section below) for 6 months after surgery, to keep scar tissue stretched and reduce the risk of capsule formation. Other surgeons put the implant under the muscle and/or teach their patients to massage their implants after surgery, instead of exercising. I have not found massage to be useful. It is embarrassing for most women to do, and few women do it for long.

There are three possible incision sites: in the crease under the breast, in the lower half of the areola (the colored skin around the nipple), and in the axilla (armpit). The most commonly used incision is in the breast crease. It is hidden by all clothes and is not visible when you stand without clothes. The other advantages of this incision site are that it is near to most of the blood vessels so bleeding is easily controlled. Also, it lets the surgeon see the entire space behind the breast easily. However, this scar tends to be wide (about half an inch) and at times pink or pinkish-brown.

The advantage of the incision around the areola is that it tends to heal with a thinner, finer scar than that in the breast crease, and it is concealed by the color of the areola. However, the surgery is more difficult for your surgeon to do, and if you heal with a poor scar, it is visible on your breast. This is very troubling for those few women who develop bad scars in this area.

The incision under the arm has become very popular on the West Coast. It probably is the preferred incision if you plan to go topless on the beach. However, it can leave an indented or wide scar—which will show in all sleeveless clothes. Also, it is more difficult for your surgeon. Since the incision is farther from the blood vessels that tend to bleed, bleeding is harder to control. Finally, this incision is under the arm, and it is somewhat difficult to make the implant pocket far down on your chest. There is a risk that your implant will lie too high or may shift up toward your arm. None of these problems makes the underarm approach unusable, but they do make it the least preferred incision for most patients as well as most surgeons.

Using Steroid Drugs

Steroids are a group of natural hormones manufactured in your adrenal glands. They stop the formation of scar tissue, but they also inhibit your natural resistance to infection and your normal healing. Some surgeons will put steroids in or around a breast implant to try to prevent a capsule from forming. However, these steroids can also make your scar, over months, stretch and redden. They can even make the breast weaken, becoming droopy. And they increase your risk of an infection.

Using steroids around a breast implant is neither "right" nor "wrong." I don't use them, because I don't think that the benefits outweigh the risks. Ask your surgeon to discuss the pros and cons with you. There is no way to *prevent* a capsule; steroids are used to try to *decrease the chances* of getting one.

The Operation

(Figure 12-2 through 12-4)

Before

You and your surgeon will already have decided on the kind of implant, whether or not he will use steroids, and where he will make the incision. You will probably have your surgery as an outpatient, with local anesthesia with sedation. You will have had nothing to eat or drink after midnight the night before your surgery. You will come to the operating room about an hour before your surgery and you will change into your hospital gown. You will probably go to a preoperative area to have an IV placed in your arm so that you can be given a solution of dextrose and/or saline to prevent dehydration during surgery. You'll receive

Breast Enlargement

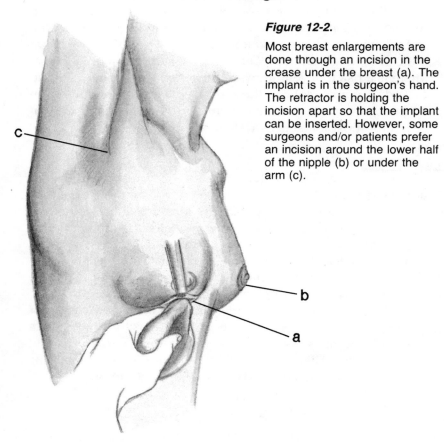

Figure 12-2.

Most breast enlargements are done through an incision in the crease under the breast (a). The implant is in the surgeon's hand. The retractor is holding the incision apart so that the implant can be inserted. However, some surgeons and/or patients prefer an incision around the lower half of the nipple (b) or under the arm (c).

some presurgery sedation, by mouth, by injection, or through your IV. Your surgeon will probably see you and mark where the incisions will be. You will probably receive a dose of antibiotics before your surgery to decrease your risk of infection, although it is not known if this is effective or necessary.

You will then be taken to the operating room. On the operating table, a safety strap is put across your knees, sticky pads are put on your chest to monitor your heart, and a sticky pad is put on your hip under your gown. This is a grounding pad so that surgical cautery can be safely used. (Surgical cautery means using an electrical heat device to seal off bleeding blood vessels.)

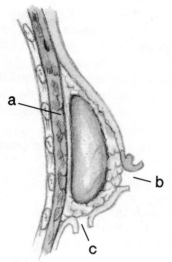

Figure 12-3.

Most breast implants are placed as shown here: *on top of* the muscle (a), behind the breast. Also note the two (of three) possible incisions: the one around the nipple (b) and the other under the breast (c).

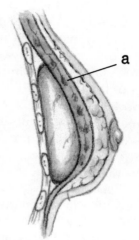

Figure 12-4.

Here the implant has been placed *under* the muscle (a). Note how there is nothing between the ribs and the implant.

If you are having general anesthesia, you will now be given anesthetic through the IV, and you go to sleep. You will remember nothing more.

If you are having sedation, you will be given a test dose of sedation to see how you react. Your chest will be washed with soap, and sterile surgical drapes will be put over your body and around your chest. You will not be able to see the surgery being done. Your surgeon will give you more sedation until you are dozing, and he then will inject local anesthetic around the incision site and the breast to numb it. No injections are done into the nipple itself. You may remember the injections, but not the pain of the injections.

During

Your surgeon will operate on one breast first. He will make a small incision through the skin and the fatty layer beneath it until he reaches the muscle. If he is putting the implants between the breast and the muscle, he will lift the entire breast off the muscle by cutting all the fibers that attach it to the muscle. This is called "making the pocket." He will look inside, through the incision, using an instrument that lifts up the breast and has a light at the end, so he can see inside. He will cauterize any bleeding. You *may* feel the sting of the cautery. You may feel pulling when your breast is lifted. Once he has cut all the fibers to make the pocket, the surgeon may put the implant in, or he may then make the pocket on the other breast and put both implants in at the end of the procedure.

If your surgeon is putting the implants under the muscle, he will form the pockets slightly differently. He will first cut through the skin and fatty tissue and through the muscle, down to the ribs. He will use an instrument to strip the muscle from the ribs. This may hurt if you are under sedation, but with this technique you are more likely to be asleep.

If you are sedated, you may feel pressure when the implants are put in their pockets. This feels like a weight on your chest. At the end of your surgery, your surgeon will put in the stitches. If you had the implant put under the muscle, your surgeon may put in a small plastic tube, called a drain, in between two stitches. This lets blood under the muscle drain out. Drains are rarely used if the implant is under the breast. The surgeon will then apply the bandages. Your breasts may ache by the end of surgery if you are under sedation.

After

When you go to the recovery room, if you had sedation, you will probably sleep for 30 minutes or more. You are usually awake enough to go home in 2 or 3 hours. It may take a little longer to wake up if you had general anesthesia.

The Process of Recovery

What to Do About Pain

After your surgery you will probably have little pain. Your breasts may ache the first day. They will certainly ache if you go bra-less in the first 2 weeks after surgery. You can eventually go bra-less, but not until you are healed.

A few patients will develop an intense burning in the nipple, from bruising of the nerves to the nipple. This may require pain medication for a day or so, and may persist for 2 weeks.

After surgery, if you develop swelling and sudden *pain* in one breast, this often means that you have internal bleeding around your implant. *If this happens, call your doctor!*

The Healing Process

The surgery makes your own breast tissue swell, so your new breasts will often look too big at first. Some swelling will go down in 2 weeks. The rest will be gone in 6 weeks.

Bandages

Your incision is small, about 2 inches long. I put tape strips over the stitches to support the incision and to keep the stitches from sticking to your bandage. The only other bandage is a piece of gauze over the tape strips.

My patients buy two inexpensive front-fastening bras, without underwire or padding, in their new cup size and one chest size larger than they need. (Your whole chest will be slightly swollen. A too-tight bra will hurt.) They wear the bra day and night for 2 weeks, except for changing into a clean bra or bathing. Some surgeons wrap the whole chest in elastic bandages. This is not wrong, but I think it is unnecessary, and uncomfortable!

Taking Care of Your Wound

You can bathe, but you have to keep the bandage/bra dry for the first week. Even going bra-less to bathe in that first week can make your breasts ache. After a week, your breasts are healed enough for you to bathe and shower as usual, putting the bra back on afterwards.

Stitches

You may have outside stitches or pull-out stitches, or both. The outside stitches are visible on top of your skin. These are regular stitches. A pull-out stitch lies under your skin with a piece showing at either end of your incision. Pull-out stitches are less irritating to your skin, so they can stay in for 2 weeks. However, they are less precise. You may have regular *and* pull-out stitches.

Scars

Depending on whether your incision was in the breast crease, around the nipple, or in your armpit, you'll have a 1½ to 2 inch scar in one of these three places.

Your scar will be pink and firm for the first 6 weeks. After that it may not change, or it may widen slightly over the next 6 months. Around 6 months, scars begin to fade. If the scars widen—which they do most often, especially in the breast crease—they may fade as time goes by, but they won't become narrower.

Tips

- If you want to be sure that others will *not* notice the sudden change in your breast size, wear loose tops and dresses for a few weeks before and for a month after surgery.
- Before surgery, buy two front-fastening bras, one chest size larger than usual and in the larger cup size you will be, with no underwire. Once your bandages are off, expect to wear a bra day and night for 2 weeks.
- Surgery will make your breast skin decrease its natural oil production, and feel dry. Rub body cream into the breast skin, gently and well away from the stitches, twice a day for 2 weeks after your surgery.

Exercise for Capsule Scars

A major problem after breast enlargement is that the thin layer of scar tissue around the silicone breast implant tends to shrink (*all* scar tissue tends to shrink—it can contract, like muscle). The result is that the shrinking scar, which is called a "capsule," makes the space for the implant too small—hence your breast feels firm, even hard. New scar tends to lose its "shrinkability" after 6 months. Thus, for 6 months after surgery exercising your chest muscles helps keep your new breasts soft by keeping the scar stretched. Swim, work out with Nautilus or a rowing machine, and/or lift light arm weights two to three times a week. Jogging, aerobics, dance *won't help;* you must stretch your chest muscles *against resistance.*

Back to Work

If you return to work in 5 to 7 days, you will feel groggy and *tired* from the effects of the sedation you were given during surgery. If you wait 10 to 14 days, you should feel completely rested. It won't *hurt* you to go back to work after 5 to 7 days, though.

Back to Parties

It will be 2 weeks before you have energy for a party. Your breasts will be too sensitive for anything but slow dancing for *another* 2 weeks.

Back to Sex

Your breasts will be too sensitive for sexual manipulation for about 2 weeks at least. Sex at 2 weeks should be done cautiously without touching your breasts, if they are sore.

How Much It Costs

Your surgeon's fee will be between $1800 and $2500. The cost of a pair of implants will be $400 to $800. The cost of your anesthesia will range from a minimum of $800 for sedation to as much as $3000 for general anesthesia.

Insurance Coverage

With *rare* exceptions, insurance will *not* pay for this operation. If the size of a breast has been changed by medically necessary surgery, or if your breasts have been damaged by trauma or infection, your insurance company *may* pay for your surgery. You should find out if your insurance will pay *before* you have your surgery. It is worth paying your surgeon for extra photographs and for a report *before* surgery so you can consult your insurance company ahead of time. If your insurance company tells you it will pay, be sure to get the verdict *in writing*, including how much they will pay for the surgery, the implant, and the anesthesia. A verbal "We'll pay" is worthless when you try to collect afterwards!

Breast Enlargement: Recovery-at-a-Glance

This chart represents the *average* recovery times for this cosmetic operation.

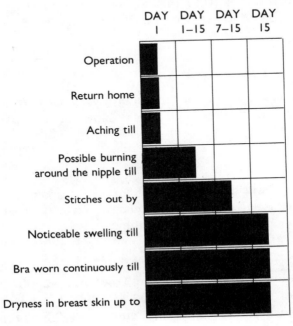

	DAY 1	DAY 1–15	DAY 7–15	DAY 15
Operation	■			
Return home	■			
Aching till	■			
Possible burning around the nipple till	■■			
Stitches out by	■■■			
Noticeable swelling till	■■■■			
Bra worn continuously till	■■■■			
Dryness in breast skin up to	■■■■			

My Assessment of This Procedure

For years, breast enlargement has been the *most common* cosmetic operation performed. You will probably be aware of some pressure during surgery, if you have sedation anesthesia. Once your surgery is over, you have little pain to contend with—your recovery from the sedation is usually *almost* all you need to deal with. You must accept the risk of forming a "capsule"—the firmness of the breasts that occurs after enlargement 10 to 30 percent of the time. This is not always bothersome, but capsules are difficult and often impossible to correct.

Side Effects and Complications

Side Effects

The side effects of breast enlargement include breast or nipple sensitivity, feeling too big until the swelling goes down, and scars that are less than perfect: wide or pinkish-brown. The surgery may make part or all of your breast numb for weeks, or even as long as 6 months. On rare occasions, numbness may last well over a year, or even be permanent.

Surgery may decrease your nipple response to sexual stimulation for several months, but it almost always returns. In fact, some women find that their nipples are more responsive, not less, during the healing phase, for reasons that aren't clear.

Complications

Possible complications from breast enlargement include bleeding, infection, or complications related to the implant. Silicone is a very safe substance—it does not damage your body. But if an implant is defective, for instance, and leaks silicone gel after the operation, the result is not harmful to you, but you will have an irregular, lumpy-looking breast, and the silicone may lodge in nearby lymph glands. Treatment for this complication is simple—removal of the gel (it sticks to itself and is pulled out like a string of taffy) and placement of a new implant. Some implants are guaranteed by the manufacturer, so that if an implant ruptures in the first year after surgery, the implant is replaced free.

Infection is very rare; it occurs less than 1 percent of the time. However, an infection usually means that your implant must be removed. The breast cannot fight off the infection with the implant in place. After 3 to 6 months, the implant can be put back in place. If only one side is infected, your breast sizes will be lopsided during the waiting period.

It may be possible to treat an infection, without removing the implant, if your implant is under the muscle. However, treatment involves surgery to wash out the infection around the implant. After surgery you'll need 6 weeks of intravenous antibiotics—although with modern techniques you do not need to be in hospital for this. Some women will opt to have the implant removed and later replaced rather than to go through all this trouble. An infection is rare—but so discouraging—that it helps to know what lies ahead if you are unlucky enough to get one.

Clarissa: A Mind of Her Own

Clarissa, a businesswoman in her thirties, had a breast enlargement. She was a very independent woman and not used to listening to advice—mine included. The first day after surgery, she removed her bra and soaked in a hot bath, despite my instructions to the contrary.

One breast hurt and swelled right after her hot soak, so she called me. But she decided to stay at home rather than come to see me, fearful that I would suggest re-operation (which I might or might not have done). I did tell her that the hot soak had led to internal bleeding and the swelling was from a blood clot around her implant. (Hot water makes blood vessels expand and blood clots loosen.)

When Clarissa did come in to see me—at the end of a week— that breast had a bulge the size of an apple where she had bled. A blood clot forms a thick hard shell around it within a few days, and the body starts to absorb the blood. So, I knew that with the (relatively) small amount of bleeding she had had, her body had already started to replace it with scar tissue. (If she had bled more, re-operation would still have been necessary.)

Since surgery was unlikely to help her now, I advised her to swim every day for half an hour and to lift arm weights on alternate days to try to diminish the scar that was replacing the blood clot. If this didn't succeed, she would need re-operation in 6 months to re-move the unsightly scar. Exercise worked—Clarissa was an accomplished athlete. After 6 months, her breasts were soft and the lumps were gone.

Kathy: A Calculated Risk

Kathy, an accountant, had an increased bleeding risk because she took medication for arthritis. She was flat-chested and wanted breasts, even with her increased risk. The day after her surgery Kathy had painful swelling of one breast, until it was three times the size of her other breast. It hurt. Such severe bleeding must be surgically drained. Kathy had surgery that same day to reopen the incision, wash out the blood, and put back the implant. This second operation left her very tired, and the bleeding made her much more bruised, but 6 weeks after surgery both breasts had healed well. Kathy was extremely pleased, as she had predicted she would be.

Nancy: A Between-Job Change
Nancy, a bank manager, had breasts that were a small B cup. Being tall with broad shoulders, she wanted to be fuller breasted. She had been offered a job in another bank and decided to have surgery between her old and new jobs. I put in implants that would make her a small C cup, which was what she wanted. She confided to me later that she thought I had made her too big and had been afraid to ask me about it, but it was only the swelling, as I had warned her before surgery. Nancy went back to her regular exercises, which included swimming, 2 weeks after surgery. She was thrilled. No one noticed that she had had surgery but she got more compliments on her figure at her health club.

Ashley: A Recurring Capsule
Ashley was 23 when she had her breast implants done. When one breast got firm, she came back to see me. The firm breast looked normal and didn't hurt Ashley, but the firmness made it uncomfortable for her to sleep on her stomach, especially around her period. She definitely did not want any surgery to correct this. I explained to Ashley about popping the capsule. This is done in the office, but there is a slight risk of damaging an implant or causing bleeding— both of which could lead to an operation she didn't want. She decided to try it. She lay down. I put my hands on her chest around the breast and squeezed. Ashley gave a startled "Oh" and said, "I heard it." She was right—if the capsule is round, it can be heard (faintly) when it pops. Ashley sat up and felt her breast. It was soft again. Capsules re-form after being popped—the usefulness of "popping" depends on how soon the capsule reappears. Ashley's came back every 6 months for 2 years and then disappeared. That breast stayed a little firmer, but now she could sleep on it.

Priscilla: Correcting Asymmetrical Breasts
Priscilla was 18 and fairly miserable with the way her breasts looked. One side was a B cup and one was an A. This was a maldevelopment, but the cause was not clear. Priscilla had breast enlargement done on both breasts. She wanted her small B to be a slightly fuller B. By

*having implants placed in both breasts, she would be more sym-
metrical because implants would fill in the upper part of both breasts.
Priscilla had her surgery under general anesthesia. She went home
the same day. She could not believe that her breasts looked so much
better—and that she could now fill in both bra cups. She wore a
bathing suit in public for the first time that summer!*

What Other Patients Say

- **Housewife, 30:** "My husband was opposed to this. He said he
  liked me the way I was, but I wanted it. I'm thrilled. I feel that I
  look like a woman for the first time. I had *nothing* to start with."
- **Lawyer, 38:** "I had sedation and I kept right on working, but
  from my home, after the surgery. At work, you can't tell I had it
  done—I wear blouses and jackets all day. But you sure can tell
  in a cocktail dress. I think it's great."
- **Saleswoman, 26:** "I developed a capsule: One breast is firm
  and I don't like it, to be honest. It aches during my period. But
  there's no way that I'm having them taken out, and they don't
  bother me enough to have another operation."
- **Executive secretary, 32:** "I like to go to the beach and I used
  to feel ashamed of how I look. I enjoy myself more. I've forgotten
  about worrying about me."
- **Mother, 29:** "My doctor made me huge, for whatever hangup
  he had in his head. I went right back and had him take them
  right out again." (Women usually have implants removed because the implants are *much* too big.)
- **Social worker, 35:** "I had postsurgical bleeding from blood-
  thinning medication. I was scared out of my mind when I had
  to go back to the operating room the day I bled. It was like I
  thought I was crazy to ever have done this, but I really wasn't. I
  had thought about it a lot. I'm really pleased to look so good. I
  have capsules on both sides but I hate exercise so I had expected
  to get them."
- **Ballerina, 19:** "I did not want to be too big. I turned out just
  right. Now I don't have to worry about my tutu flapping!"

Breast Lift

What Surgeons Call It

The technical term for a cosmetic breast lift is mastopexy.

What It Will Do

A cosmetic breast lift removes stretched breast *skin* but not breast *tissue* and lifts your nipple up to a normal position. Your breast size is unlikely to change. Your breast *shape* is changed.

What It Won't Do

A breast lift will not make your breasts larger; for that, you need a breast enlargement, which can be done at the same time. Also, it will have no effect on your chest muscles. It is a *skin* operation.

How Long It Will Last

This operation is usually permanent. However, if you gain, then lose, a lot of weight, or if you get pregnant, your breast skin will stretch. Then, when your breasts revert to their original size, the skin will be loose. Some women have weak skin and find that their uplifted breasts slowly droop again. This tends to be more common in women with full breasts and those who had a breast enlargement along with the mastopexy. In time, all breasts droop—although usually only slightly.

When to Have It

A breast lift can be done whenever your breasts have drooped. However, if you plan future pregnancies, have your surgery *after* all your babies. Also, it's best postponed till *after* weight loss, if you are plump and think you may diet successfully. Breast uplifting can be done in teenagers—some women have droopy breasts at a very young age. It may run in their family. For them, if their breasts droop noticeably, it's still worth correcting—knowing that in the future, for instance after pregnancy, additional tightening may be needed.

Where to Have It

Breast lifts are usually performed on an outpatient basis with local/sedation in a doctor's office operating room *or* an outpatient surgery center *or* a hospital's outpatient operating room.

Conditions That Increase Your Risk

Breast scars from previous surgery may diminish the breast blood flow and increase your risk of poor healing. If you've had **previous breast infections** you have a higher risk of an infection after surgery. An infection may cause poor scars which may need touch-up surgery. If you have **breast-fed** in the 6 to 12 months before surgery, you *may* begin to lactate again shortly after surgery. *If* this happens, you may require medication to stop the lactation.

Usual Anesthesia

Local anesthesia and sedation is usual for a breast lift. General anesthesia may be used if your breasts are so stretched that an excessive amount of local anesthesia would be needed. Breast lifting and breast enlargement are often done together. If the breasts will be lifted and enlarged at the same time, general anesthesia is more likely to be used. The amount of local anesthetic needed is more likely to exceed a safe dose for you.

How Long It Takes

This operation will take between 1½ and 2 hours to do.

Placement of the Nipple

The placement of your nipples is a most important part of a breast lift or breast reduction. Watch your surgeon as he marks where your nipples are to be moved. He will use a combination of three methods to determine and cross-check the nipple position. All three result in about the same placement:

1. Normally, the nipples lie 19 to 22 centimeters from the bony notch in a woman's neck. This is about 10 inches, but your surgeon will measure the distance in centimeters.
2. Your nipple position after surgery should be at approximately the level of your breast crease. *If the surgeon marks it well above*

your breast crease, point this out to him. A nipple that's been placed too high can be moved and sewn to a lower place on the breast—*but* it leaves unsightly scarring behind. Don't be shy about asking your surgeon about this—it's your body!

3. Finally, the nipple should be roughly halfway between your elbow and your shoulder. Your surgeon uses this as a double-check.

Your surgeon may do the necessary surgical markings (in purple ink) in his office the day before your surgery. If not, he will make them just before the operation, in the preoperative area or operating room. You have a right to privacy. If your surgeon does not suggest it, request that he consider doing the markings beforehand. I do my nipple markings the day before surgery whenever possible. This method is less embarrassing for a patient. Also my patients can go home and check their markings in the mirror. Besides, this lets me check the markings with a fresh eye the morning of the surgery. "Measure twice, cut once" is the best guide to breast markings.

The markings are done while you sit or stand. It is almost impossible to choose a proper nipple position when you lie down because the breast falls to the side, and the proper nipple position can't be judged.

The Operation
(Figure 12-5)

Before

You will arrive about an hour before surgery, having had nothing to eat or drink since midnight the night before. You will change into a hospital gown and go to a preoperative area. If your surgeon has not already done the nipple markings (see previous section), he will do them at this time.

An IV will be started in your arm so that you can be given a solution of sugar (dextrose) and/or saline to prevent dehydration during surgery. If you are having general anesthesia, your blood and urine will be tested, unless this was done the day before. (Lab tests are not always done before local with sedation; they *are* always done before general anesthesia.)

You will be given some sedation, by mouth, by injection, or

through your IV. You may also be given an IV antibiotic. You will then be taken to the operating room. If the room has windows, shades or screens will cover them to protect your privacy. Once you are on the operating table, sticky pads are placed on your chest to monitor your heart, and a sticky pad is placed on your leg under your gown as a grounding device to make surgical cautery safe to use. (Surgical cautery is using an electrical heat device to seal off bleeding blood vessels.) If you are having general anesthesia, you will now be put to sleep by an injection in your IV. If not, you are given further sedation. Your chest is washed with surgical soap, and sterile drapes are put around

Breast Lift

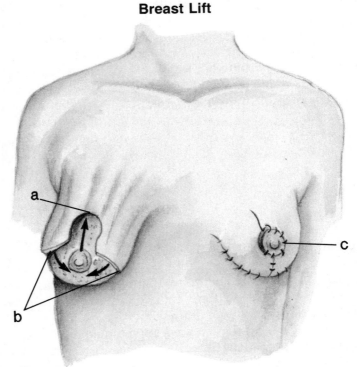

Figure 12-5.

In a breast lift, the nipple is moved up to a higher position (a). The excess skin is removed and the edges of the incision brought together, to lift the breast (b). At (c) nipple is being sewn into position with the skin sewn up around it.

your body and around your breasts. Your face is shielded with drapes so that you cannot watch your surgery.

Next your surgeon injects local anesthetic into the skin, between the breast crease and the nipple, around and above the nipple, and into the new nipple site marked on the skin.

During

Once the skin is numb, the surgeon cuts off the skin above the nipple, below the nipple, and from on either side. The preoperative markings allow your surgeon to determine how much excess skin to remove.

Once the excess skin has been removed, you may hear a buzzing sound as tiny blood vessels are cauterized to seal off areas of bleeding. Next the nipple is stitched in its new position. Other stitches will bring the skin together under the nipple and in the breast crease. In some cases, a surgeon will cut into the breast tissue to change its shape or to move the nipple.

Once all the stitches are in, the surgeon will operate on the other breast. Then your skin is washed and dried. Tape strips are put across the incisions, and you are put into a surgical vest, wrapped with bandages, or fitted into a bra with a few layers of gauze over your breasts.

After

At this point you should be quite awake if you had sedation. You will go to the recovery room for an hour or two—and will wake up here if you had general anesthesia. From there you go home. Someone must take you home and look after you. Your job is to go to bed and rest.

The Process of Recovery

What to Do About Pain.

After surgery, your breasts will ache. You may hurt the first night, but you will usually have little pain after that. However, if you remove your bra or bandage, you will immediately notice that your breasts ache—a sign that they need support.

The Healing Process

If you had local anesthesia with sedation, you will be tired and sore for about a week. If you have general anesthesia, you will still be a bit tired after 2 weeks.

Your soreness will usually be gone in a day or two, but it will be about 2 weeks before you can take off your bra and not ache. Your breasts will be slightly swollen. You may be numb in patches, or both breasts may be entirely numb for a week or more. Your nipple may be numb, or it may be oversensitive and sting from time to time. Most or all of these sensations are gone in 2 weeks.

Bandages

This varies from one surgeon to another. Yours may put you in a snug elastic surgical vest (hot and itchy) or wrap you with elastic bandages (hot, itchy, and tends to fall apart). Or he may use a bra—the best solution. I have my patients buy two cheap front-fastening non-underwire bras, one cup or chest size larger than usual (to allow for the postsurgical swelling). The bras work as a bandage. Whatever your surgeon uses, you will have gauze and tape strips directly over the stitches to protect them. Keep gauze over the incisions at least a week after the stitches are removed, so that the bra does not rub the incision. Tape strips are kept across the incisions for as long as possible to keep the scars from stretching. Ideally this would be 6 months (the period during which scars tend to stretch). The limiting factor is your skin, which may become so irritated that tape must be discontinued.

Taking Care of Your Wound

There is little that you must do for your surgical wounds after mastopexy. I let my patients bathe, wearing their bras, during the first week. They can change into a clean bra every day and if the bra gets wet. My patients bathe and shower without a bra during the second week, as long as the incisions don't ache.

You may have a skin patch that heals slowly and forms a small scab. Keep a gauze pad over it, put a dab of antibiotic ointment on it after bathing, and wash with water (no soap). It will heal in a week or so.

Stitches

You will probably have three kinds of stitches.

1. The deepest layer, which you won't see, will be absorbed by the body. (Sometimes they aren't absorbed but work their way out through the skin.)
2. A "running pull-out" will run under your skin and come out at either end of the incision. It is pulled out 2 to 3 weeks after surgery.
3. The traditional stitch—a loop over your skin with a tiny knot—is removed between days 6 and 11. Surgeons call these "interrupted sutures." They line the skin up perfectly. The other types of stitches supply support and strength while you heal.

Scars

Your scar will vary with the surgical technique used. There is always a scar around your nipple and one from the nipple down to and along the breast crease. Your scars will become thick and red for about 6 weeks after surgery. They will gradually fade, becoming pale and flat within 6 to 18 months. Some scars, especially in younger women, are itchy, red, and lumpy for even longer.

Tips

- You probably won't need new bras. Your breasts will not be smaller, just rounder, firmer, and "up."
- The surgery will dry your breast skin. Have a large jar of skin moisturizer ready to rub gently on upper breasts, even while stitches on the lower half are healing.
- Don't count on going bra-less for *months*. Your breasts will need support to minimize the risk of scars stretching.

Back to Work

If you had local/sedation you can go back to work at the end of a week, but you will be *tired*. If you had general anesthesia, 1 week is too early—you will wear out during the day. After 10 to 14 days, you will feel fairly rested and able to resume work without a struggle.

Breast Lift: Recovery-at-a-Glance

This chart represents the *average* recovery times for this cosmetic operation.

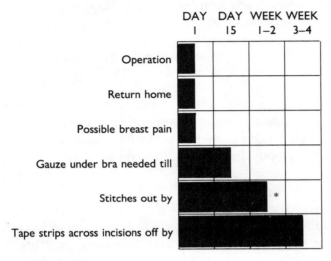

	DAY 1	DAY 15	WEEK 1–2	WEEK 3–4
Operation	■			
Return home	■			
Possible breast pain	■			
Gauze under bra needed till	■■			
Stitches out by	■■■	*		
Tape strips across incisions off by	■■■■			

*Depending on type of stitch.

Back to Parties

You should wait 10 to 14 days before you go out for the evening. Even then, you may be too tired to enjoy yourself. Besides, your incisions will be likely to ache at the end of a day. No dancing, except slow dancing, for 3 weeks. Not only will your breasts hurt and swell, but they may bruise or bleed in spots. They aren't strong yet.

Back to Sports

You can limber up at the end of a week, but stretch your *legs*, not your chest, to avoid pulling on the incisions. At the end of 2 weeks, you can swim, jog, and do exercises—slowly, at a third or less of your normal rate. Between 3 to 4 weeks, you can resume all sports. Highly competitive sports like soccer or basketball are best avoided for up to a month.

Back to Sex

You should avoid sex for 1 week after surgery. The stimulation to your breasts—even if they are not touched—will make them swell. Even a minor blow to your breasts can hurt and cause widening of the scar as late as 2 to 3 weeks after surgery.

During the second week, you may cautiously resume sex but:

- Keep your bra on.
- There should be *no* breast contact.
- There is still a small risk. It would be best to wait another 7 to 10 days.

By the fourth week after mastopexy, you can have sex with your bra off—assuming that you are healing without complications. Your breasts may be numb and you may not want them manipulated for another week.

How Much It Costs

For the breast lift alone, your surgeon's fee will be between $1500 and $2500. The hospital fee will range from $800 to $1200 for local/sedation, up to $3000 or more for general anesthesia and an overnight stay in hospital. If your breast lift surgery is combined with a breast enlargement, your surgeon's fee will be about $1000 more, plus the implants which will cost up to $500. General anesthesia is more common when the two operations are done simultaneously, and even with local/sedation your hospital cost will be at least $1000.

Insurance Coverage

Insurance will *not* pay for a breast lift except in very rare cases. For instance, if you can prove that extreme breast drooping is causing serious irritation and infection in the breast crease, insurance *might* pay a part of your cost. Don't count on it. If you want to find out, call your insurance company. Take the name of the person to whom you talk and explain the problem. They may say "no" right then. They may review your case. If so, your surgeon may need to send in a report (costing $30 to $100) and photographs of your problem. It will take between 2 to 8 weeks for an insurance company to give you an answer. When they do, *try to get in writing the dollar amount that they will pay you, before the surgery.* Otherwise your company may say that it will pay "appropriately" and decide that this means $100—after the operation!

My Assessment of This Procedure

A breast lift is an excellent operation. The results can be dramatic. The scars are unavoidable, so *slight* droopiness may not be worth correcting, especially if your scars tend to be red and lumpy.

Side Effects and Complications

A breast lift operation involves only the skin, so the complications and side effects tend to be limited compared with the breast operations—enlargement and reduction—that go into or under the breast.

Side Effects

You *can* breast-feed after this operation. The nipple is not severed from its milk duct attachments in most cases. Also, since only the skin around the nipple is cut, nipple feeling is rarely damaged. (Cutting the breast below the nipple can damage the nerve of feeling to the nipple, so surgery is done cautiously here.) Complete numbness would be expected to be from temporary swelling. Normal skin feeling tends to return by about 6 weeks after surgery, although patches of numbness may persist for months. Sexual responsiveness also should return (or may not be affected at all). Your breasts may be somewhat less—or more—responsive to sexual stimulation for 6 to 12 months after surgery, while residual swelling remains.

Complications

This is a skin operation, so serious **bleeding** is rare, although bruising can be quite severe.

If **infection** occurred, it would be treated with warm soaks and antibiotics. The scar in the infected area might become wide or lumpy and require minor scar revision under local anesthesia in 6 months or later.

If you decide to have a breast *lift* when you really need a breast *reduction*, your breasts may droop again, by their sheer weight. You can expect your surgeon to tell you if a lift is the wrong operation for you, but it does no harm to ask him directly.

Don't expect more from this operation than it can deliver. If your breasts are flat on top but full below, the mastopexy is not likely to improve that. You probably need a breast enlargement as well to fill out the upper breast.

Some women want their breasts *very* uplifted. If this is done, you risk having the breast drop down while the nipple stays high—stranded too far up your breast. Your nipple should normally lie near the level of your breast crease, and coaxing your surgeon into too much lift may ruin your result. Be restrained in your goal.

If you have any problem after this operation, it's likely to be **scars**. About 10 percent of women have lumpy and/or wide scars. This *may* be the way you heal, but a minor scar revision in the office, under local anesthesia, may help to find out. This would be done 6 to 12 months after the surgery.

Rhonda: An Inherited "Droop"

Rhonda had droopy breasts, like her mother and sisters. After three children, Rhonda's breasts sagged below her navel. She was only 30. She had a mastopexy with general anesthesia and stayed in hospital one night because she lived 50 miles away. She healed without any complications. All Rhonda's scars were fine white lines. She wished she'd known of the operation when she was 18—her breasts had been almost the same then as they were 12 years later.

Penny: A Problem with Stitches

Penny was in her early thirties and worked in a day care center. She had moderately droopy breasts which made her look and feel old. Her husband didn't mind—she did. Peggy had a mastopexy under local anesthesia with sedation. She went home the same day. Her body did not absorb all the absorbable sutures, some of which came to the surface of the skin and had to be removed. This occurred in the first month after surgery and required several extra office trips. The scar between her nipple and breast crease became wide and brown. A year later we decided to try to correct this. I cut out the scars and restitched the skin, using a different kind of suture material than before. Penny's final scars in these areas were better—but about half the width of the original ones. She was content.

Amy: A Lift Plus Enlargement

Amy was a hospital worker in her midthirties. Her breasts were droopy and flat on top. She had always wanted larger breasts. Amy had breast enlargement and breast lift surgery simultaneously, done with local anesthesia and sedation. Amy went home with a friend that day, and she had no complications. Her breast swelling subsided within a few weeks. She was delighted with her new breasts and with her fiancé's reaction: he had not approved of her having the surgery because she looked fine to him, but afterwards he was as pleased as she was with how she looked.

What Other Patients Say

- **Political pollster, 42:** "I feel 20, I am 40, and my breasts looked like 100. Now they look the way I feel."
- **College sophomore, 19:** "I felt dumb having this surgery but my breasts looked so weird that I hated sharing a room in the dorm. I hid to dress or bathe and I felt self-conscious. I don't like my scars but my breasts look normal, so I don't mind living in the dorm this year."
- **Housewife and mother, 31:** "My husband told me I was nuts, but I wasn't about to go back into the job market after three children without having my breasts fixed. I had sacrificed my body for my family, so I deserved it. They look fine, although they'll never be perfect. Actually the big difference is inside. I feel better about me."

Breast Reduction

What Surgeons Call It

The technical terms for this procedure are breast reduction or reduction mammoplasty.

What It Will Do

Cosmetic breast reduction aims to give you smaller, more attractive breasts and relieve you of the backache, shoulder ache, and breast crease irritation that large breasts cause. In addition, it may relieve you of the self-consciousness that some women may feel from having too large breasts.

Breast reduction surgery cuts out excess breast skin and breast tissue. If your skin is stretched *and* your breasts are large, you need a reduction. If your breasts don't seem too big but are limp and stretched, you are more likely to need a *mastopexy* or breast lift. If your chief problem is stretched skin, you may even need to have your breasts enlarged as well. If you think this is your situation, consult the previous sections on breast lifting and breast enlargement.

What It Won't Do

You won't be able to pick out your new breasts from pictures in books. If you look at 100 breasts, each will be different. For example, if your upper breasts have little fullness and most of your breast "hangs down," this operation can fill out the upper portion somewhat, but it's not likely to give you "*Playboy* centerfold cleavage." That particular upper fullness is almost always from a silicone breast implant. Breast reduction surgery will make your breasts smaller—indeed, it can remove almost all of your breast—and your breast shape is improved, but not necessarily to the point that you look good enough to go topless. (You can go bra-less—if your breasts are made small.)

You won't be able to breast-feed after a breast reduction. The nipple is usually not totally cut from the breast, but so many ducts attaching the nipple to the breast are severed that breast-feeding is impossible.

How Long It Will Last

Breast reduction surgery has permanent results, but your breasts can still change size. Your breasts may get *smaller* if you lose weight or go off the Pill. Breast size usually decreases after pregnancy and after menopause. Your breasts may get *larger* if you gain weight, go on the Pill, or develop cysts in your breasts. Some surgeons say that if you lose weight after breast surgery, your breasts won't diminish. *Not true*—unless your breasts are largely made up of glandular tissue and not fat tissue. It is true that if you have very large breasts, are overweight, and *lose* weight, but don't have surgery, your breasts may still be a problem: flabby, droopy from dieting but still too big for your slimmer shape.

When to Have It

This operation can be done once your breasts stop growing. For some girls with *very* large breasts, it can be done before breast growth is complete, to make life tolerable. Then a second can be done later, if the breasts, when fully developed, are again too large.

Where to Have It

Your operation will be done under general anesthesia in a hospital operating room. You will need to stay in hospital several days after surgery.

Conditions That Increase Your Risk

If you have had recent **breast infections**, such as mastitis while breast-feeding, or a breast abscess that had to be drained, you have an increased risk of infection in the wound or the breast itself after surgery. To *minimize* your risk, let your doctor know what bacterium (germ) caused the infection, or ask him to call the doctor who treated you to find out. That way, you can be given preventive antibiotics for that germ.

Also, if you are very **overweight** you have an increased risk for infection after *any* operation. We think this is because fat-filled cells have relatively less oxygen delivered to them than empty fat cells, cutting down the body's effectiveness in washing away bacteria that have lodged in them. The more fat there is in these cells, the less effectively the body fights infection.

Finally, for women with **very large or stretched breasts** (for example, a 42DD or larger, or breasts stretched so that the nipple is at hip level) the surgery is prolonged and there is much healing to be done. Thus, for women with these problems, the risk of infection or poor healing is also increased.

Usual Anesthesia

General anesthesia is always used. You will be asleep for surgery.

How Long It Takes

Your operation will last between 2 and 4 hours. Bleeding prolongs any operation. If you have tiny blood vessels that don't bleed during surgery, the surgery will be short. If you have unusually large or long breasts, or large veins that bleed briskly, then surgery *may* take over 4 hours.

Nipple Placement

The placement of your nipple is one of the most important parts of a breast reduction. Watch your surgeon as he marks the position where your nipples are to be moved. He will use three methods to determine and cross-check the nipple position.

1. Normally, the nipples lie 19 to 22 centimeters from the bony notch in a woman's neck. This is about 10 inches but your surgeon will measure the distance in centimeters.
2. Your nipple position after surgery should be at approximately the level of your breast crease. *If the surgeon marks it well above your breast crease, point it out to him.* A nipple that's been placed too high can be moved and sewn to a lower place on the breast—*but* it leaves unsightly scarring behind. Don't be shy about asking your surgeon about this—it's your body!
3. Finally, the nipple should be roughly halfway between your elbow and your shoulder. Your surgeon uses this as a double-check.

The markings are done while you sit or stand. It's almost impossible to choose proper nipple position with you lying down, because the breast falls to the side. Your surgeon will draw a circle around your nipple and areola and a similar circle higher up on your breast, to mark the new nipple position. He will draw a short line below either side of the nipple for the nipple "pedicle"—the strip of breast that contains nerves and blood supply—and then triangles on either side of the lower breast, where the excess skin and breast will be removed.

Your surgeon may do the necessary surgical markings (in purple ink) in his office the day before your surgery. If not, he will make them in the operating room or the preoperative area, just before the operation. You have a right to privacy. If your surgeon does not suggest it, request that he consider doing the markings beforehand. I do my nipple markings the day before surgery whenever possible. This method is less embarrassing for a patient. Also, my patients can go home and check their markings in the mirror. Besides, this lets me check the markings with a fresh eye the morning of surgery. "Measure twice, cut once" is the best guide to breast marking.

The Operation
(Figures 12-6 through 12-8)

Before

Breast reduction surgery is always done under general anesthesia. You will come to the operating room about an hour before surgery, having had nothing to eat or drink since midnight the night before. Patients who were admitted to the hospital the night before surgery are taken to the operating room on a stretcher, although many women now come in for surgery from home. If you've come from home, you'll change into a hospital gown. Then, you go to a preoperative area, where an IV is placed in your arm so that you can be given a solution of dextrose and/ or saline to prevent dehydration during surgery. The IV will also be used to give you an antibiotic and some of the anesthetic. You may be given preliminary sedation and an antibiotic in the preoperative area.

Once you are in the operating room, you will be positioned on the operating table with a safety strap across your hips, sticky pads on your shoulders and back to monitor your heart, and a sticky pad on your thigh under your gown as a grounding pad to make the surgical cautery safe to use. (Surgical cautery means using an electrical heat device to seal off bleeding blood vessels.)

Most surgeons ensure their patient's privacy, even when asleep, by covering windows in the operating room.

You will then be given intravenous anesthetic to put you to sleep. Once you are asleep, a tube will be inserted through your mouth and anesthetic gases mixed with oxygen will go directly into your lungs.

Your chest is washed with surgical soap and sterile drapes are put around your chest.

During

Your surgeon will operate on one breast first, then move to the other side of the table for the operation on the other breast. The procedure for both breasts is the same.

First, the surgeon shaves off skin from the area where the nipple will go. He cuts around the areola (dark skin around nipple) and then cuts from here to the breast crease. He takes off only the outer skin between the nipple and breast crease, leaving intact the deeper tissues with blood vessels and nerves that supply the nipple. Thus the nipple remains attached to your breast. Wedges of excess skin and breast are cut out on either side of the lower breast. Bleeding is stopped with cautery.

After cutting out these wedges, your surgeon will contour the breast by taking more breast tissue until he is satisfied that the shape and size are right for you. He will then put in three "tacking" stitches to give himself a rough idea of how your breast looks.

- One stitch attaches the nipple to its new position.
- A second stitch closes the skin under the nipple.
- A third stitch closes the gap between breast skin and breast crease.

The surgeon will probably walk around the operating table, looking at the breast from different angles, to decide whether he needs to do any more cutting to improve the size and contour. Once he is satisfied, he will sew your nipple into its new position with fine thread (usually nylon). He will also do deep stitching and surface stitching to support the breast while it heals. In effect, your surgeon takes your breast apart and sews it back

Breast Reduction

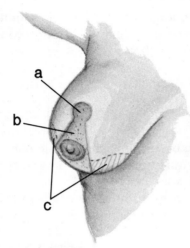

Figure 12-6.

The new position for the nipple is at (a), and the stippled area (b) indicates where the skin will be shaved above and below the nipple. This allows the nipple to move up without being cut entirely off the breast. The striped areas (c) show where excess skin and breast tissue will be cut away, to be discarded.

Figure 12-7.

The excess breast has been cut off and a stitch is pulling the nipple up into its new position (a). With the excess skin and breast gone, a stitch is placed (b) to pull the skin together underneath the nipple. The deep layers of skin, still attached to the nipple (c), will lie buried on either side under the skin, which is sewn up over them.

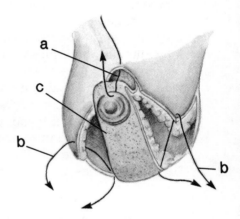

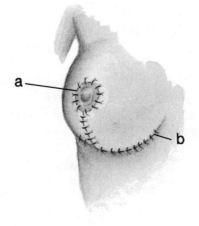

Figure 12-8.

The nipple (a) is now sewn completely into its new home. The skin on the sides (b) is sewn together, reshaping the now-small breast.

together. Although the trend is to use the smallest possible incisions, the "smallest possible" will still seem large to you.

At the end your surgeon may place a small plastic drain between some stitches if your tissues tended to bleed. Tape strips are put across the stitches.

Free Nipple Grafting

The above technique is used on 90 percent of breast reductions. Sometimes, if your breasts are extraordinarily long or large (for example, a 48F or a nipple stretched 12 inches down from the breast crease) the standard technique can't be used. The nipples in such large breasts don't have enough blood flow to survive being moved so far. In this case, the nipple must be taken off *completely* (without a pedicle) and sewn in a new place like a graft. The rest of the procedure is the same.

After

After the surgery is done, your chest is washed with water to remove the surgical soap. Gauze bandages are put over the breasts, and your chest is either wrapped with elastic wraps or you are fitted into an elastic surgical vest. The breathing tube is removed, and you are taken to the recovery room. Here you will wake up and then be taken by stretcher to your hospital room, after about 45 minutes. You may feel cold and you may be slightly nauseated.

The Process of Recovery

What to Do About Pain

You will *hurt* virtually all day the first day after surgery—and possibly the second day. The pain is not so bad when you lie still, but if you move, sit up, laugh, even take a big breath, it will hurt. Pain is tiring, and until this phase is over, you will feel exhausted. You will need narcotic painkillers by injection. (This is *one* reason you stay in hospital.) These drugs tend to make you groggy and nauseated, but they help you rest.

· You will probably need narcotic pain pills on and off even after you're home—for as long as 10 days. Once the first few days of pain are over, most people are comfortable except for an hour or so at the end of the day, when their breasts start to ache or throb. Your first postsurgery menstruation may be more painful than usual, because the hormonal stimulation will make breasts swell, pulling on the surgical incisions.

Motion—even walking—in the first few days and car rides will be painful as late as the fourth or fifth day. You will react by hugging your arms across your chest, to support your breasts. This phase may last a week or 10 days.

The Healing Process

A breast reduction operation will leave you tired, because of the general anesthesia and because of the extent of the surgery. You will come back to your surgeon's office about 5 days after you leave hospital and once a week for the next 2 or 3 weeks. You will be able to buy some new bras after 2 weeks, but you will still be swollen. Wait to buy the rest of your new bras until 6 weeks after surgery. From time to time you will have sharp shooting pains, even weeks after surgery. These last only a second and indicate that nerves are recovering.

Your breasts will be bruised for the first week, turning yellow in the second week after surgery. Your breasts will probably be completely numb for many weeks. This is discussed under Side Effects and Complications. Many people think that this surgery will make their shoulders stiff because that is what happens after a mastectomy for breast cancer. The two operations are completely different. This operation has no effect on arm and shoulder motion.

Bandages

I use an elastic surgical vest on my patients for the first 2 days after surgery. This zips up the front and has Velcro shoulder straps and can be removed without *your* moving. After a day or two, I replace it with one of my patient's too-large bras, with the underwires cut out. This is more comfortable than the vest, which is hot and makes the skin itch. Many surgeons do this. Others use an Ace bandage around the chest or gauze and tape over the incisions. You may be kept in a surgical vest for a week or longer—but only by a male surgeon!

Taking Care of Your Wound

Wearing your own bra avoids tape on your skin. The bra holds the gauze bandages over your stitches in place. You must wear the bra day and night, so you can't shower, but can bathe, as long as you keep the bra dry. If your bra gets wet, gently take it off and put on a dry one. One week after surgery you can remove your bra to shower or bathe, and you can shave under your arms. (Before then you are too sore to shave efficiently under your arms, but you can try. An electric razor is best.)

Your stitches stay in for 2 to 3 weeks. Stitches can get wet during bathing. Pat them dry afterwards. Not every surgeon will permit this—ask your surgeon what he recommends.

The undersurface of your breasts heals slowly. You may have one or two patches where the skin forms a small open sore. Using medicated gauze and antibiotic cream may help such an area to heal. Cleanse the area with half-peroxide and half-saline solution. (Saline is salt water. You can buy it, or make it by dissolving a tablespoon of salt in a quart of water and boiling it for 15 minutes.) Such areas will be healed 3 to 4 weeks after surgery. Until then, keep a gauze pad between you and your bra so the area doesn't stick to your bra. Drains are removed before you leave the hospital, and usually on day 3.

Stitches

Separate stitches ("interrupted sutures") around your nipples are usually removed between days 5 and 7. Other stitches are removed in 10 to 14 days. Pull-out stitches (ones that run *under* your skin, surfacing only at the ends of a scar) are pulled out after 2 to 4 weeks, depending on how you heal. You will have inside stitches. These are meant to dissolve ("absorbable sutures"). However, your body may reject these stitches, especially ones near the skin. If this happens, a tiny white dot or blister first appears in your incision and in a day or two a tiny pinhole opens. Your surgeon will probe delicately into the pinhole and remove the stitch, which lies *directly* under it. You may feel frustrated that you "can't get healed," but the problem is temporary. Most such stitches are rejected within a few weeks.

Scars

Your scars will vary with the surgical technique, but you will have a scar around the areola. This scar will continue down to the crease under the breast and in the breast crease itself. The areolar scar tends to be flat but wide, but it may be raised, pink, or a hairline scar. A "broad" scar in this area would be about a quarter-inch wide. The scar *from* the areola to the breast crease is almost always flat but wide—a quarter-inch or occasionally a half-inch wide. The scar in the breast crease is thicker near the center of the chest and flattens at the side of the breast.

These scars are designed to be as inconspicuous as possible and are largely concealed by the breast crease, except around the areola. Since the nipple is placed at the level of the crease, even the scar from the areola to the crease will be on the *undersurface*.

Scars are your *biggest* concern with this operation, because scars are *unpredictable*. One patient may have fine, white hairline scars after 3 months. For another patient with the same operation, all the scars may be raised, lumpy, and red even a year later. The scar progression in most people is:

- Scars red and lumpy in the first 6 weeks
- Scars beginning to fade to a paler pink and to soften and flatten from 6 weeks to 6 months
- Scars flat and white, pale pink, or brown by 1 year.

Some scars may be unsatisfactory even at a year and require minor corrective surgery or steroid injections to soften them.

If your scars are going to widen, it will usually be apparent within 6 weeks. Once a scar widens it will *not* become narrow again, no matter how much it improves in other ways.

Various methods are used to keep breast scars from spreading. Vitamin E cream will *not* help—if anything, it may make them widen slightly. Supporting the incisions with tape for 6 weeks *may* help, but it often is so irritating to the skin that many women cannot use tape. Wearing a bra day and night for 6 weeks or even 6 months has also been recommended. So far, I am not convinced that any of these methods work, but the second two are harmless and worth a try.

Tips

- *If you are on the Pill*—and *if* it enlarged your breasts—go *off* the Pill at least 6 weeks to 3 months before surgery, if you can. Otherwise your surgically reduced breasts may be too small if later you stop the Pill.
- *Before* surgery ask your surgeon about donating your blood for yourself, if he hasn't mentioned it. You can catch infections via blood transfusions. Transfusions are not commonly needed for breast surgery, but if you can donate your blood, it can be *held for you* in case you need it at surgery.
- If you are overweight, try to lose weight before surgery, for your own sake. But you do *not* have to be your ideal weight for surgery, although your risk of an infection is lower if you are not obese.
- Do *not* buy your new bras before your surgery. Your breasts will be swollen and you will have surgical bandages over them, so you will still need a large bra temporarily. Your old bras will now be fine—loose-fitting and comfortable—but remove the underwires. (To do this, cut the fabric over the underwire. Slip the prong of a fork under the exposed wire and pull.)
- You can buy two interim bras about 2 weeks after surgery, when you are still swollen but too small for your old bras.
- Buy your final bras 6 weeks after surgery.
- About 1 year after surgery, you may need to buy other bras. Your breasts will retain swelling for months, and their shape will slowly change, so you *may* find that you prefer a different style.
- Your breast skin will be dry because the surgical trauma to your breasts decreases the oil production of the breast skin. Buy some body cream and rub it gently into the breast skin twice a day— staying away from bandages and stitches, of course.

Back to Work

You can return to work or school 2 weeks after surgery, but you will feel tired, so don't arrange *anything* else for your first week back. If you return to work or studies after 3 weeks, you will have more stamina, but you may not have this much time. Expect your breasts to be sore at the end of the day, for the first 2 weeks.

Breast Reduction: Recovery-at-a-Glance

This chart represents the *average* recovery times for this cosmetic operation.

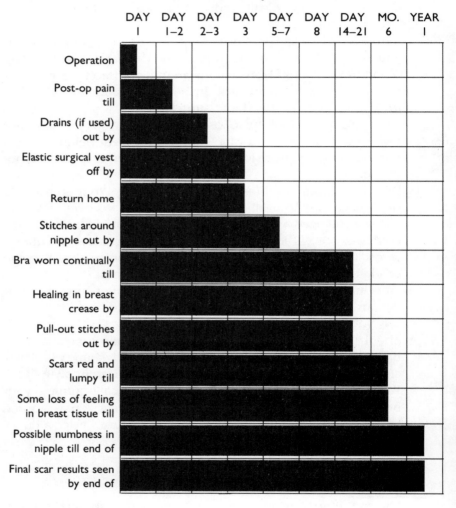

	DAY 1	DAY 1–2	DAY 2–3	DAY 3	DAY 5–7	DAY 8	DAY 14–21	MO. 6	YEAR 1
Operation	■								
Post-op pain till	■■								
Drains (if used) out by			■						
Elastic surgical vest off by				■					
Return home				■					
Stitches around nipple out by					■				
Bra worn continually till							■		
Healing in breast crease by							■		
Pull-out stitches out by							■		
Scars red and lumpy till								■	
Some loss of feeling in breast tissue till								■	
Possible numbness in nipple till end of									■
Final scar results seen by end of									■

Back to Sports

After 2 weeks, you can resume sports, but you will lack your presurgery stamina, so start slowly. You will need a support or athletic bra for the first month. A few patients save the surgical vest and use it when they exercise for the extra support it gives.

"Resuming sports" does *not* mean that you start with an advanced aerobics class or a five-mile run. It means bending and stretching exercises, workouts on a bicycle, or a slow swim in the pool. If you play tennis, you can work out with the ball machine for 15 minutes or rally at the baseline with a friend. Runners can start with a walk, then shuffle into a slow jog for 10 or 15 minutes. You need another *2 to 4 weeks* to build back to your usual pace.

Back to Parties

After 2 weeks, you can enjoy an early dinner party or a brief cocktail party. You won't be up to a late night or dancing for at least 3 weeks.

Back to Sex

You should not even consider sex for 3 weeks. Sexual excitement will make your incisions swell and your breasts ache. At 3 weeks, if you are healed, you can have sex with minimal or no breast contact. It takes 6 weeks before breast manipulation is comfortable. Remember that many breast nerves have been cut during surgery. Your breasts may be numb or sexual stimulation may be unpleasant temporarily, until the nerves heal.

How Much It Costs

Your surgeon's fee will be roughly $2500 to $4000. Your hospital fee will be about the same: $2500 to $4000, which includes the hospital room, the operating room, and the anesthesia.

Insurance Coverage

Breast reduction surgery is both cosmetic and reconstructive. It is cosmetic because it changes how you *look* but reconstructive because it corrects physical problems: the shoulder pain from the pull of heavy breasts, skin rashes in the breast creases, and upper and lower back pain. This is the reason that insurance often pays for this surgery. Insurance will *not* pay because of your doctor's "say-so." Insurance pays by the *weight* of breast tissue removed. It sounds like a butcher shop, but your surgeon hands over the excess breast tissue which he removes to the circulating nurse so that she can weigh it! Most insurance companies will reimburse you if at least 200 grams of breast tissue are removed from each breast. Very roughly, 200 grams of tissue is a bra cup size. Some insurance companies do not pay unless 400 grams or more are removed.

Your surgeon may be able to estimate how much tissue he expects to remove. Since the breast is partly fat (which is light) and partly glands (which are heavy), remember that this is an *estimate*. A surgeon can remove a larger piece of breast from one person yet have it weigh *less* than another's—if the first breast is largely fat and the second largely glandular tissue.

Try to get a decision *in writing* from your insurance company stating (1) how much tissue they require to be removed before they pay and (2) how much they will reimburse you. You must pay in advance for the surgery. If your insurance company will only pay $2000 of a surgeon's fee of $3500, you need to know that in advance. "Reimbursement" does not mean "payment in *full*." If so little tissue is removed that your insurance company does not pay for the surgeon, chances are they will not pay for the hospital, either! This is exactly what to do:

- First, call your insurance company. Talk to a *person* and deal with that person, not a computer. Ask them what they need.
- You will probably have to ask your surgeon to send them a report, including the amount of tissue he expects to remove and the surgical insurance code.
- The insurance company may require photographs of your breasts—your face shouldn't be included.
- Your insurance company should tell you the *dollar* amount of reimbursement in *writing*. An occasional insurance company will decide after surgery that it doesn't want to pay after all. If the company has committed itself in writing to pay you, you are protected.

My Assessment of This Procedure

Breast reduction is one of the very best cosmetic operations available. Surgery removes the emotional and physical burden of too-large breasts, and the nuisance of never finding clothes that fit. Thus it is rare to find a patient who isn't happy with her result, assuming she was realistic about what it could do and where the scars would be.

Side Effects and Complications

Side Effects

The scars are the most common source of dissatisfaction, at first. Time, minor scar surgery or steroid injections to soften the scars may be needed. The next most important side effect is the possible reduction in or loss of nipple and breast sensitivity. The nipple is cut free from many nerves when it is moved to a new position. These nerves slowly regrow, but nipple feeling may not return for months. If your nipples are unusually sexually sensitive, this extra sensitivity may be gone permanently after surgery. If your large breasts don't have much sexual sensation at the nipples—it seems to come more from the whole breast—the loss of sexual nipple feeling may not be such an obstacle to surgery, but breast feeling may also diminish.

Surgeons rarely discuss these sexual effects with you, because it is embarrassing and because few scientific studies have been done. Some women keep *all* nipple feeling. (I had one woman of 20 who had no numbness anywhere in her breasts after surgery.) But as a rule your breast skin may be numb in areas for 6 months. There may be a temporary loss of all sexual response in the nipple for up to a year, or such a slow return of feeling (years) that the sensation seems permanently lost. (A surgeon who promises no change in feeling, sexual or other, from his "special technique" is misleading you. Studies have shown that even breast enlargement, which is a lesser operation than reduction, causes prolonged changes in feeling in a few women.)

Complications

A possible complication is poor healing of the nipple, caused by swelling and decreased blood flow. As a result, a nipple may blister and scab, healing with patches of scarring or discoloration. This is *rare* with our present techniques but is more likely if you develop an infection.

Gertrude: Happy Results and Fast Healing

Gertrude, a college student about 15 pounds too heavy, was scheduled for breast reduction surgery. Her breasts were a 40DD, so she couldn't fit into a size 12, her proper dress size, unless she found a dress with a loose, unfitted top. In high school, boys had made sexual comments about her large breasts. This hadn't happened in college, but the painful memories stayed with her. The night before surgery, her mother called me in distress. A friend had confided her experience with breast reduction—dreadful scars and no return of feeling in the nipples. After weighing the benefit of surgery against these possible side effects, Gertrude decided to go ahead with surgery, despite her mother's panic. She breezed through her operation, feeling that her one day of pain was "no problem." She went home in 2 days.

When Gertrude came back at the end of the week to have her stitches removed, she sported a tight tank top, looking very pleased with herself. Her mother was convinced that the decision had been right for Gertrude. Her skin feeling was back to normal in 6 weeks. Her scars matured unusually early, and even at 6 weeks it was clear that they would be narrow, flat, and pale pink, blending so well with her surrounding skin that they barely looked like scars.

Judy: "I Can See My Waist!"

Judy was in her thirties, a nurse, and 50 pounds overweight. She had always had huge breasts, far too large, even for her weight. She wore a custom-made bra. Her breasts covered her pubic area and were so large that she could not see her waist, except in a mirror. She had considered it a sign of weakness to "lean" on surgery and had lived with her breasts. However, when a disturbed man at work started annoying her with phone calls about her breasts, she took action against him and also decided she would take surgical action for herself.

Judy had to have a nipple graft. Her nipples could not survive the two-foot move upward except as a thin free graft. Her operation took longer than most, and she stayed 5 days in hospital. Her first comment on coming to the office was, "I have seen my waist." Her nipple grafts healed. She could feel nipple touch, but not sexual responsiveness, 6 months later. Manipulation of the breasts was sexually stimulating, however, and she had had little sexual sensation in her nipples before surgery. Her scars were fine white lines 6 weeks after surgery.

Cecily: "Just Right" After a Diet

Cecily had breast reduction surgery during her college Christmas vacation. She was a 38DD before surgery and wanted to be a B. She was tall and hoped to lose 10 pounds, but felt she couldn't because she was so preoccupied with her breasts that she could not concentrate on dieting.

Cecily was delighted with her results, but a little disappointed that she "ended up" with a 36C cup. I explained that I had tried to take into account her future weight loss, and that her breasts had contained much fat as well as glandular tissue. Cecily came back to see me one year later. She had lost the weight and wanted to show me that her breasts were "right" after all—she was a 34B.

Everyone wants her breast size to be perfect, but what is perfect for you this month, may not be perfect in 3 years. If you are on the Pill, are overweight, and/or have not had children and plan to do so, your breasts should be kept on the full side of what you can live with. Some women have had very nice results. Then, after a diet and/or a pregnancy, they have found that their breasts were too small.

Mia: First Reduction, Then Enlargement

Mia was in her forties when she had a breast reduction. Although her size a year after surgery looked good, she found it too small to live with. She had lost 5 pounds and after that, plus her surgery, she didn't feel like herself any longer. Mia had another operation—this time a breast enlargement! She was quite happy with the results. Fortunately for Mia, the breast enlargement could be done through the original breasts reduction scars.

Holly: Problems With Scarring

Holly was 30 when she had her breast reduction. Three weeks after her surgery, all of her scars were red and lumpy. I prescribed a steroid cream, and she used that and vitamin E. Her scars worsened for the next 3 weeks and then did not change for 9 months. At that time, I injected her worst scars with steroid. This only softened them. So, I re-operated, under local anesthesia in the office, without charge, and cut out the scars, stitching them up with a different suture material. I thought that perhaps her scar problem was from an allergy to the first sutures. Revising the scar in this way helped a lot—her scars had yet another healing period, but at the end of 2 months they were softening, and by 6 months they were soft, flat, and faintly pink.

What Other Patients Say

- **Grandmother, 59:** "I wish my doctor had told me to do this years ago. I know my mother did. I feel comfortable for the first time since I can remember."
- **High school student, 18:** "I feel normal. I didn't care if I had no breasts. I was sick of getting stared at by my brother's friends."
- **Mother of three, 36:** "I thought I'd change my clothes but I didn't. What did change is the way I behave. I don't stoop. I don't sit with my arms around my chest. I hold my head up. I go bra-less around the house and I feel sexy, but it wasn't easy at first. My scars were hideous for months."
- **Policewoman, 23:** "I was the only woman in my family with large breasts. I guess the men liked the way I filled out a uniform, but I was tired of feeling beat up by my own body by the end of the day. My back was killing me. All that is gone. I did lose my breast feeling almost completely for a year, but I knew that was a risk. I can wear dresses, because I'm the same size top and bottom, and I can buy fancy bras. I love it."
- **Teacher, 39:** "My sister just had it done. I've always wanted it but I was scared and I hurt after surgery for at least a week. My husband thought it was high time I did it. It made sex better for us because I always considered my big breasts unattractive for my body."

Breast Reduction for Men

What Surgeons Call It

Men sometimes develop a condition in which their breasts have a female appearance. This is called *gynecomastia,* and the operation to correct it is called gynecomastia reduction.

What It Will Do

Gynecomastia surgery aims to give you a flat (or flatter) chest with no suggestion of female breast formation.

What It Won't Do

This operation will not necessarily give you a good-looking chest. If your skin is very stretched, it may look *more* stretched and loose after surgery. (The excess can be cut out, but the scars will be visible.) Nor can this operation give you a flat chest if, for instance, you are a weight-lifter with thick pectoral muscles. These muscles can become so large that they may make the chest stick out around the nipple. Gynecomastia surgery won't remove this muscle. Also, the operation may leave ridges or depressions on the chest skin and slight asymmetry when you compare one side to the other. These changes improve with time but may not vanish completely.

How Long It Lasts

This operation is permanent. The tissue under the skin, around your nipple and chest, is removed, so it can't come back.

When to Have It

A rapidly growing **teenager** should *not* have this surgery if the chest fullness is slight, because this fullness is temporary and will go away on its own in a year or so.

A man who is **overweight** and planning to diet should either try to lose the weight or decide he can't. The surgery is somewhat easier if you lose weight, improving your chances of a good result. Also, being somewhat fat increases your risk of infection.

A man who **drinks heavily** or **smokes marijuana** heavily should get help for this problem first. Your health is more important than your appearance. These chemicals may cause gynecomastia and also interfere with the anesthesia and/or your healing, making surgery unsafe for you. If you don't want to discuss a chemical dependency with your surgeon or your family doctor, there are chemical dependency programs at many hospitals or private institutions. Your local medical society may be able to refer you. However, it is best to be frank with your surgeon and let him determine the medical severity of *your* problem. (I have had several patients who considered themselves alcoholics, but who drank only one or two drinks a day, and others who had "no problem" but drank a case of beer a night.)

The *average* man with gynecomastia is unlikely to be fat or to have a chemical dependency. For you, as long as your teenage growth is over, the surgery can be done at any time.

Where to Have It

Gynecomastia reduction is most often done in a surgery center or a hospital when general anesthesia is needed. For a young man with minor fullness under the nipple, the surgery can be done with local anesthesia and sedation, and making a doctor's operating room a third choice.

Conditions That Increase Your Risk

Men who are overweight tend to have a greater risk of poor healing with any operation. Also, removing large amounts of fat from under the chest skin may leave the skin loose—this is difficult to remove without leaving unsightly scars on the chest. Of course, high blood pressure, a bleeding tendency, or severe diabetes will increase your surgical risk, here as for any operation.

Usual Anesthesia

For minor gynecomastia, local anesthesia with sedation may be sufficient. For patients with more severe gynecomastia, general anesthesia is needed.

How Long It Takes

A gynecomastia operation usually takes 1½ to 2 hours.

The Operation
(Figures 12-9 through 12-11)

Before

You will come to the operating room about an hour before your surgery and will change into a hospital gown. You will have had nothing to eat or drink the night before unless you are having *minor* surgery, in which case you may have been permitted a liquid breakfast. For general anesthesia, you may have had—or may now have—a blood test and a urine test. These are often not done when local/sedation is being used.

Next, you are taken to a preoperative area, where an IV is placed in your arm so that you can be given a solution of dextrose and/or saline to prevent dehydration during surgery. (Sometimes patients go directly to the operating room, and the IV is started there.) Before then, your surgeon will see you. He may mark your chest with purple surgical ink to guide him during surgery, or he may do these when you are on the operating table. (The markings are less crucial than the intricate markings needed for female breast operations.)

You may be given an injection or two before you go to the operating room, to sedate you. Once you are on the operating table, a safety strap is fastened over your hips and sticky pads are placed on your chest to monitor your heart. Also, a sticky pad may be placed on your thigh. This is a grounding pad to make surgical cautery safe to use. (Surgical cautery means using an electrical heat device to seal off bleeding blood vessels.)

If you are having general anesthesia you will now be put to sleep by a drug given through your IV, then kept asleep with anesthetic gases that are mixed with oxygen and given through a tube in your throat. (If you are having local/sedation, you will now be given sedation to make you very drowsy.) Your chest is now washed with surgical soap, and sterile drapes are put over your body and around your chest. Your chest is *not* shaved.

During

If you are having local/sedation, your surgeon will now inject local anesthetic into one side of your chest. He may do this even if you are asleep, because the epinephrine in the local anesthetic will diminish your bleeding. If your surgeon is using fat suction to help correct your problem, he will first make a tiny incision, just large enough to push the long, hollow suction tube under your skin. This tube is used like a vacuum cleaner to remove any fat deposits that are contributing to your chest excess.

Suction can't be used to remove breast, or fibrous, tissue which is not soft, like fat, so your surgeon must make a semi-circular incision just inside the brown areola of your nipple. He will cut the nipple free from the tissue beneath it and, working through this small incision, free the skin from your chest muscle so he can reach the tissue underneath. He will then cut the excess fibrous tissue from the muscle. This is a lot of surgery through a small incision. Your surgeon will use a headlight to see inside. If you are awake, you may see the light flash against the wall if he looks up. The cut blood vessels are cauterized. You may feel a sting when the cautery instrument is used, if you are not asleep.

After cutting out the excess fibrous tissue, your surgeon may do further fat suction. Some surgeons leave all the fat suction for the end. If your problem is from overgrowth of fibrous tissue and *not* from fat, he may use *no* suction.

The surgeon may sew up the first incision, or he may leave the stitching of both incisions to the very end. You will have a drain—a small plastic tube under the skin to drain away any fluid that collects under your skin. This may come out through your incision or through a separate tiny incision on the side of your chest. When both sides are stitched closed and the drains are in, your surgeon will wash the surgical soap from your chest. He and the assisting nurse will put a bulky gauze dressing over your chest, taping it in place or—more often—holding it in place with an elastic wrap.

After

You are next taken to the recovery room. You should be able to go home within 2 hours. Someone will need to take you home. Once you're home, you should go to bed and rest. You will probably sleep because of the sedative drugs you have received.

Reduction of Enlarged Male Breast

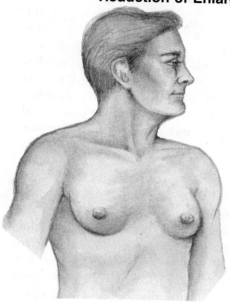

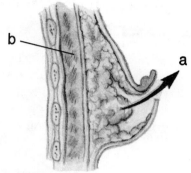

Figure 12-10.

The incision lifts up the nipple (a). Note that the excess tissue and fat above the muscle (b) is being removed.

Figure 12-9.

Enlarged, feminine-looking breasts in a man.

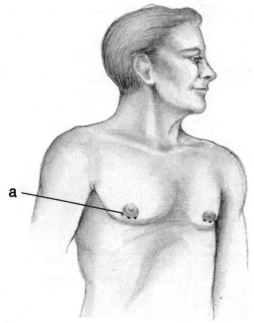

Figure 12-11.

The scar, indicated by the broken line (a), lies along the areola (colored skin around the nipple).

The Process of Recovery

What to Do About Pain

Your chest will be sore. Severe pain is rare. It may mean that there is bleeding, infection, or a problem with the bandage— perhaps a drain or tape pulling on your skin. You should call your doctor if you develop pain, especially if you also develop a fever or swelling on one side under the bandage. (When in doubt, call—don't wait.)

The Healing Process

Your recovery depends largely on the anesthesia and the extent of your surgery. A young man who has had a minor gynecomastia reduction with local/sedation might feel fine after 5 days. A man of 50 who needed extensive surgery and general anesthesia might only *begin* to feel normal after 2 weeks. Some men have so much excess chest tissue that surgery removes *more* tissue from them than from many women having breast reduction! In general, after gynecomastia reduction and general anesthesia it will be 7 to 10 days before you can work—and then you will feel tired.

Bandages

The chest skin is surgically lifted off the underlying muscle, so a bandage is needed to press the skin down on the chest wall. You will be wrapped with bulky, wide Ace bandages around your chest and over your shoulders. Or, you may only have gauze and heavy elastic tape across your chest. This bandage *looks* better, but the tape can pull on your skin and blister it. This hurts. Chest binders are also available. These are more comfortable but more expensive. Whatever the bandage, it stays on for 5 to 7 days.

Taking Care of Your Wound

You will not need to care for your wound. Your surgeon will check and replace your bandage after a few days. After the bandage is removed (day 6 to 8) a layer of gauze over your nipples will keep the stitches from sticking to your clothes. You may remove the gauze and tape to shower or bathe and replace it afterwards.

You need no bandage once the stitches are removed, other than surgical tape strips over the incision for a week to protect against its being accidentally pulled apart.

Stitches

Your stitches will be removed around days 8 to 11. If you have inside stitches that support the skin, your outside stitches may be removed as early as day 6.

Scars

Your scar will go halfway around the outer edge of the areola— the pink-brown skin around the nipple. The areola usually heals with flat, fine scars—although not always. The *color* of the areola also helps conceal the scar.

At times, gynecomastia can be removed with fat suction only. If that is done, the scar is very short, also at the outer edge of the areola.

Tips

- Your skin will be dry after surgery. Keep a jar of hand cream or body lotion to rub onto the chest skin once your bandage is removed.
- Avoid sun exposure to your chest for 6 months, or use a high number (15 or higher) sunscreen on your skin. Otherwise the operated skin may become permanently dark or pink.
- You may feel too self-conscious for several months to bare your chest. Your scars need time to fade, and swelling may make your chest skin noticeably wavy. For men who work out or run—start wearing a shirt several weeks before surgery. This prevents questions after surgery that could embarrass you.

Back to Work

After correction of minor gynecomastia, you can work within a week. If you had more surgery, count on 10 days, minimum, out of work.

Back to Parties

You won't enjoy a party until 10 to 14 days after surgery. Even then, a late party, especially after a tiring day, will leave you exhausted and your chest aching. Don't count on fast dancing for 3 weeks. This will make your chest hurt.

Back to Sports

You should do *no* sports for about 2 weeks. The skin on your chest is trying to heal, and movement may make the chest swell, ache, or bruise. However, after 10 to 14 days you can start to get into shape by long walks, swimming with a kickboard, or working out with an exercise bicycle. After 3 weeks, you can resume all sports except contact sports. Football, soccer, ice hockey, and other sports that risk a blow to the chest are best avoided for a month.

Back to Sex

Same as back to work—5 to 7 days for minor surgery, up to 2 weeks if more was done.

Reduction of Male Breast: Recovery-at-a-Glance

This chart represents the *average* recovery times for this cosmetic operation.

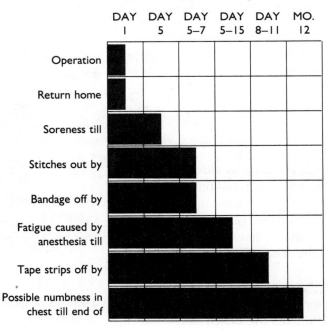

	DAY 1	DAY 5	DAY 5–7	DAY 5–15	DAY 8–11	MO. 12
Operation	██					
Return home	██					
Soreness till	████					
Stitches out by	██████					
Bandage off by	██████					
Fatigue caused by anesthesia till	████████					
Tape strips off by	██████████					
Possible numbness in chest till end of	████████████					

How Much It Costs

Your *total* cost might be as low as $1500 for a minor correction. At the other extreme, a man with gynecomastia as severe as a female breast enlargement might face a cost of over $3000 for the surgery and $3000 for the anesthesia! On average, the surgery will cost $1500 to $2500, and the anesthesia will cost $700 to $1500.

Insurance Coverage

Insurance will usually pay, but don't *assume* that yours will. Talk to your insurance company several weeks *before* your operation and try to get a *written* decision as to the *dollar* amount that they will reimburse you for the surgery. Otherwise, your insurance may "approve" the surgery but pay only a fraction of your cost.

My Assessment of This Procedure

This is an excellent operation, especially now that fat suction is available for additional contouring. Gynecomastia surgery is often the *only* way for a man to rid himself of "breasts," and there is no need for a man to live with that.

Side Effects and Complications

Side Effects

The most common side effect of male breast reduction is that the chest skin is numb—perhaps for up to a year. During surgery, your skin is cut off from the tissue beneath, and thus all the nerve branches to your skin are also cut. The feeling *usually* returns completely but not always. While the nerves recover, your skin may feel prickly or scratchy. These sensations eventually go away, but in the meantime any touching of your chest may not feel normal.

Scars from gynecomastia are rarely a problem, but they may pucker and indent. A man who likes to work outdoors without a shirt or who likes the beach may feel self-conscious enough to have such scars cut out and restitched 6 months after surgery. This will usually improve the scars.

A ridge may form under your chest skin at the outer edge of the gynecomastia. You may *feel* the ridge—or it may even be visible. It will almost always go away: as the swelling in the inner tissues subsides, the ridge flattens, but it may last a year. In a few men the ridge is so noticeable that they cannot go shirtless until the ridge subsides.

Complications

The commonest complication is blood or fluid collecting under the chest skin. The surgery is done through such a small incision that slight bleeding may be overlooked during surgery. Or, bleeding may begin hours later. Even without bleeding, the deep tissues may produce a blisterlike fluid that takes time to absorb. A blood clot may be so small that it can be drawn off with a needle in the doctor's office. However, a large blood or fluid collection means that your incision must be reopened and the blood or fluid drained, either in the office or, in rare cases, in an operating room. You can bleed as late as 5 days after surgery—so "no sports" is important.

Raymond: The Wrong Kind of Incision

Fifteen years ago, Raymond, a young engineer, had had a gynecomastia operation done by a surgeon not trained in plastic surgery. The surgeon removed the excess tissue perfectly, but used a 6-inch incision across each breast. This left a long, wide, clearly visible scar on each side of the chest. Needless to say, Raymond felt that the surgery hadn't helped—he still couldn't go shirtless. This almost certainly would not *happen today, but if a surgeon suggests using a long incision across your chest—get another opinion!*

Luke: A Family Problem

Luke was in his thirties and happily married with a large family. He had had enlarged tissue under both breasts since he was a teenager. Luke had an uncle with the same problem. Luke was about to change jobs and thought it was a good time to remove his "breasts," which had always bothered him. Luke had his surgery under general anesthesia, as an outpatient. Luke went home the same day. He had no complications and was delighted with having his chest look the way "it ought to." His wife hadn't been bothered by his appearance, but she was happy when he was pleased with his surgery.

John: Some Temporary Swelling

John, a young construction worker, was single but had a steady girlfriend. John had enlarged tissue under each breast. It had appeared when he was a teenager, but it had enlarged during a time when he smoked dope regularly. His appearance bothered him because he didn't want "breasts" and because it reminded him of an unhappy time in his life that he wanted to forget. John had gynecomastia surgery under local anesthesia with sedation, as an outpatient. After his surgery, a ridge of swelling formed on one side. This kept him from going without his shirt for 3 months, until the ridge subsided. He was pleased with his result. Shortly after surgery, he decided to get married.

Peter: A Major Reduction

Peter was in his teens when he got really fat. Over the next 20 years he gained and lost vast amounts of weight. Finally, he conquered his weight problem, for good. He was left with sagging skin on both sides of his chest and residual breastlike fat deposits. Peter required extensive surgery to remove a great deal of excess skin and tissue—more than would be removed from most women. Peter developed a hematoma (blood clot) on one side that had to be drained in the office. Also, his chest skin still sagged. However, he wasn't bothered enough to undergo more surgery, and he was pleased to look like a man again.

What Other Patients Say

- **High school senior, 18**: "The surgery was easier than I thought it would be. I was more tired from the anesthesia than I expected—even though I was warned about that."
- **Mother of a college freshman, 19**: "He used to be so embarrassed that he wouldn't even let his Dad see him without wearing a shirt. The surgery changed the way he feels. Thank you!"
- **Business executive, 39**: "I felt self-conscious *before* the surgery but I wasn't prepared to feel so self-conscious *after* the surgery. It took me 6 months to get up the nerve to go back to the pool. I *felt* people would look at me."
- **Construction worker, 27**: "I had to go back to the doctor a couple of times to have fluid drawn off. That was a drag, but it

didn't hurt. My skin was completely numb. Otherwise it was no big deal except that I hated not being allowed to lift weights for 2 weeks."

- **High school senior, 17**: "Nothing was worse than thinking a girl would think I had breasts. I look fine, but I didn't care how I looked as long as I didn't look female anymore."
- **Car salesman, 24**: "I had a blood clot on one side. It had to be drained with a needle. I couldn't feel the needle because my skin was numb, but I hate needles. That part was worse than the surgery but it doesn't seem that bad now that it's over."
- **Chemical engineer, 56**: "I should have had this done 10 years ago. It never bothered my wife, but it bothered the heck out of me."

Breast Reconstruction After Mastectomy

What Surgeons Call It

The *general* name for these procedures is postmastectomy breast reconstruction. So many different *specific* operations are used to reconstruct the breast that listing them all would simply be confusing. The major categories of reconstruction are:

- **Implant placement**: A synthetic implant is placed under the chest muscle to create a breastlike fullness.
- **Muscle flap**: Muscle, with or without skin attached to it, is moved from the back, chest, or abdomen to reconstruct the breast. A synthetic implant may be used under the muscle.
- **Skin expander**: An inflatable device is placed under chest skin and muscle to stretch it so that it will accommodate a synthetic implant.
- **Nipple reconstruction**: The nipple is rebuilt, using skin from the chest, groin, or earlobe, and/or by using tattooing to "sketch in" the nipple on the chest skin.

Note: In breast reconstruction, placement of the implant under the chest muscle is similar to what is described and illustrated in the section on Breast Enlargement. Contouring of the remaining breast (including repositioning of the nipple) is similar to what is described and illustrated in the sections on Breast Reduction, and/or Breast Enlargement. Please refer to those chapters as well.

What It Will and Won't Do

Every plastic surgeon who does breast reconstruction would like to re-create the breast to perfectly match your remaining breast. But this is not yet an attainable goal. At present, we must be satisfied with building a breast mound similar in *size* to your other breast, although often quite different in shape, with less of a breast crease and less nipple projection. The new breast should fill out most of a bra, but the front may not be completely filled and you may need to add a small pad of foam or cotton. Some patients get far better results than this—almost matching the other breast. Other patients get worse results—a size and shape far different from the other breast.

Some surgeons believe that you should postpone reconstruction until after your mastectomy, so that you will compare your new breast to "no" breast rather than a normal appearing breast. Not everyone agrees, but the controversy illustrates that breast reconstruction, although miraculous compared with 10 years ago, *cannot* yet be expected to build you a breast that looks and feels normal.

How Long It Lasts

Breast reconstruction is permanent. Your implant may change in size slightly in time. Most reconstructive implants have an outer pocket of saline (salt water), and if this is absorbed, the implant may need replacement.

When to Have It

If your reconstruction will use your chest tissues plus an implant, the easiest time for you will be reconstruction at the time of the mastectomy. However, a mastectomy is often done within days after a biopsy shows cancer. This may not leave you time to not only psychologically prepare yourself for a mastectomy but also consult with a plastic surgeon, decide on your options, and coordinate the combined operations (mastectomy plus reconstruction) with two surgeons and the hospital.

Timing depends partly on what *you* want, and partly on what your mastectomy surgeon feels is right, given your medical problem. However, *many* women find it reassuring to consult a plastic surgeon before their mastectomy so they know what lies ahead, even if reconstruction won't begin for months. On the other hand, some women don't want a reconstruction until years after a mastectomy. The same reconstructive surgery can still be done. Perhaps techniques will even have improved. So you don't necessarily lose by waiting!

Where to Have It

Breast reconstruction usually requires two or more operations. The first, which is usually the longest, is done in a hospital under general anesthesia and may require an overnight stay. The subsequent operations are usually for nipple reconstruction and adjustments in the size or shape of the new breast. These can often be done on an outpatient basis with general or local/sedation anesthesia. Thus they may be done in a hospital, a surgery center, or a doctor's office operating room.

Conditions That Increase Your Risk

If you have had radiation treatment for your breast cancer, the irradiated skin is likely to be stiff and unable to stretch enough to accept the usual silicone breast implant. An expandable implant may be used to stretch the skin, or a flap may bring non-irradiated tissue onto your chest. Radiation also makes you more susceptible to postsurgery infection. The radiation combined with the reconstruction may lead to malfunction of the lymph glands under your arm, making it swell.

Chemotherapy (drug treatment for the breast cancer) will make you temporarily more susceptible to infection and poor healing. For this reason, reconstructive surgery is not usually done until the chemotherapy treatment is finished and your white blood count indicates that your immune system has recovered so that surgery is safe.

The mastectomy scar is usually horizontal or oblique (angular), but it may be vertical. If you had a lumpectomy, the scar may be small, but it may leave the breast misshapen. Your reconstructive surgery must adapt to such scars. For example, a vertical scar may make additional incisions necessary that would not be needed if the scar were horizontal.

Usual Anesthesia

Your anesthesia will almost always be *general* for the first stage of reconstruction. For subsequent operations, you may be able to have local/sedation instead of general anesthesia.

How Long It Takes

The duration of surgery varies. It may take 4 hours or more to move a "flap" of skin and muscle to the chest. On the other hand, a nipple reconstruction might take as little as 1 hour.

The Operation

There are too many different techniques of breast reconstruction for me to describe them all here. The first-stage procedure described here is the submuscular implant placement—the most common technique used. I'll also describe a common way to reconstruct the nipple.

First Stage: Submuscular Implant

Before. You will arrive for your operation an hour before surgery, having had nothing to eat or drink since midnight the night before. You'll change into a hospital gown before being taken to a preoperative area. An IV will be placed in the arm *opposite* the mastectomy if possible, to avoid swelling from the IV in that arm. The purpose of the IV is to give you a solution of saline and/or dextrose to prevent dehydration during surgery and also to provide a means of administering sedation and other drugs (if necessary).

Your surgeon will see you and will probably mark the incision areas with purple surgical ink. He may also wait until you are asleep to mark them. You will be given antibiotics and probably sedation through your IV before going to the operating room.

Once you are lying on the operating table, a safety strap will be fastened across your hips, and sticky pads will be placed on your chest to monitor your heart. A sticky pad will also be placed on your leg under your gown to serve as a ground to make the surgical cautery safe to use. (Surgical cautery means using an electrical heat device to seal off bleeding blood vessels.)

Next, you will be given an intravenous anesthetic such as pentothal to put you to sleep. Once asleep, you breathe anesthetic gases mixed with oxygen. Your chest will next be washed with surgical soap, and sterile drapes will be placed over your body and around your chest.

During. Your surgeon will probably inject a little epinephrine to diminish any bleeding before cutting into the mastectomy scar
near your arm. Once he has cut through the skin, he will cut
through the muscle layer and lift it off the ribs using scissors, a
blunt metal pusher, and at times his fingers to detach the muscles from the ribs.

He will also use a lighted instrument to look under the muscle to see which fibers to cut and to find areas of bleeding to
cauterize. He will not lift the muscle off the ribs on the upper
chest or under your arm, or else the implant may shift into these
areas, giving your new breast an odd shape.

Once the muscles are lifted up your surgeon may put in the
implant right away, or he may use "sizers" to make sure it will
fit correctly first. If your skin won't stretch enough for him to put
in a large enough implant, he may put in a tissue expander. This
is like an implant, but it is filled with water and has a little plastic
valve through which he can inject more water (in the office, after
surgery) until your skin has been stretched enough for the appropriately sized implant to be placed. (If your surgeon plans to
use an expander, he will have discussed this with you before
your operation.)

The implant is made of silicone gel—just like a cosmetic
breast implant. However, the reconstructive implants tend to be
larger and shaped so that your new breast will project forward
—which is not needed in cosmetic breast enlargement.

Once your implant is in place, your surgeon will put in stitches
to sew up the muscle—taking care not to puncture the implant.
(If this happens it doesn't harm you, but the implant must be
removed and replaced with an undamaged one.) Finally, your
surgeon will stitch the skin together. If you have been bleeding,
he may put a small plastic tube under your muscle to drain out
blood from around the implant. Usually this is not necessary.

Next, your chest is washed off with water. Tape strips are
put across your incision and then a gauze bandage is placed.
You may be fitted with a surgical bra or wrapped in elastic
bandages—or one of your own bras may be used as a bandage.

After. You will be taken to the recovery room. Once you are awake
—about 45 minutes—you will be taken to your hospital room.
Usually, you only need to spend a night in hospital. At times you
can go home the same day.

Second Stage: Nipple Reconstruction

If the size and shape of your breast need no further adjustment, your second stage can be done in 6 weeks. This is unusual. More commonly, your surgeon will want you to wait about 6 months so that you can heal and your skin can recover enough to allow further adjustments in your breast to be done in addition to the nipple reconstruction. Your nipple reconstruction may be done under local/sedation anesthesia or under general anesthesia.

Before. You would arrive for your surgery as you did for the first stage, and the same preoperation steps would be done: an IV, the heart monitor, the cautery pad, and so on.

Then, once you are asleep or sedated, your chest is washed with surgical soap and so is your inner thigh, up at the top of your leg, near the groin. The graft for the nipple is taken here. (The inner thigh skin will darken to a color similar to the areolar skin around the nipple.) Next, this area, and also the area on your chest where the nipple will be placed are injected with local anesthetic.

During. Your surgeon will remove some skin from your chest to make a raw surface to place the graft. He may roll the skin up in strips to build a central mound for nipple projection. Once this is done, he will cut out a piece of skin from your inner thigh—about 3 or 4 inches long and 2½ inches wide.

Your surgeon will take off all the fat on the deep surface of the skin graft so that new blood vessels can quickly grow into it and nourish it. Otherwise, parts of your graft might fail to grow. Then he will trim the graft to fit the new nipple area and sew it in place with fine stitches, usually of nylon. He will stitch the incision in your thigh. The skin is loose and can be pulled together even after removing a large piece of skin.

A bulky dressing such as fluffed-out gauze or foam is put over the graft to keep it in place while it heals. The first 5 days are crucial: if a graft is not alive after 5 days, it must be replaced with a new graft. (This is *rare* in nipple reconstruction.)

If your breast needed touch-up procedures at this same operation, your surgeon may do them before or after the nipple reconstruction. If a scar needs to be cut out and restitched, he may do it at the end. However, if you need a different reconstructive implant, he may do that before he makes the nipple to avoid disrupting the nipple graft when he removes and replaces the implant.

Bandages. Once your surgery is over, your chest is washed with water, and tape strips are put across the incisions, except for those on the thigh, where tape won't stick. These are bandaged with gauze and tape or gauze and an elastic wrap. Gauze is put over the chest incisions and held in place with an elastic bandage around your chest or a bra—a surgical one or one of your own.

After. If only a nipple reconstruction was done, you may be able to go home the same day. However, if you had extensive touch-up surgery, you will probably need a night in the hospital.

The Process of Recovery

What to Do About Pain

The operation to build the breast mound leaves you tired and sore. You will have several days or even a week of discomfort and intermittent pain. When you have surgery to reconstruct your nipple, the new nipple will not hurt, but the inner thigh, where the skin is usually taken, will be sore and tight for a week, or more.

The Healing Process

For your **first operation**, you will need 4 to 6 weeks' recovery if you have a *flap* to rebuild your breast. If your own chest tissues are enough, you should allow 2 to 3 weeks' recovery, to get over the effects of general anesthesia. For the **second surgery**— unless major changes have to be done—you will need 1 to 2 weeks to recover if you had only local/sedation.

Usually you need to see your surgeon twice in the first week after you leave the hospital and about once a week after that for several more weeks.

Taking Care of Your Wound

You do not need to care for the incisions on your chest, except to keep them covered with gauze. You will have to care for the incision made on the inner thigh for the nipple graft. This area can be washed and *gently* patted dry or dried with a cool hair dryer. Pantyhose will tend to make it itch and to heal slowly, so you should wear no hose or wear stockings for the first 2 weeks.

Stitches

The stitches on your chest will stay in for a week to 10 days. The stitches in your thigh stay in for 10 to 14 days. The stitches around the new nipple may be removed as soon as day 6.

Scars

You will have the mastectomy scar across your chest. If your reconstruction requires a flap (not described), you will also have a scar on your back or your abdomen—wherever the flap is taken. However, if your reconstruction is placement of an implant using the chest tissues only, you will have no *additional* scar, only the mastectomy one. Fortunately, the mastectomy scar usually lies where your new nipple will be placed. Thus, your reconstructed nipple will cover the midportion of the mastectomy scar, covering part of it up.

Tips

- A woman who is about to have a mastectomy may find it helpful—and comforting—to talk to a plastic surgeon about breast reconstruction before the mastectomy.
- There are many ways to reconstruct a breast, and you may become confused. Don't be embarrassed to return two or three times to talk things over with your surgeon.
- Your reconstruction *may* be done at the same time as the mastectomy, depending on what your mastectomy surgeon recommends.
- As a general rule, the smaller the breast, the easier your reconstruction, so your plastic surgeon may recommend reducing the size of your remaining breast, if it is very large.
- If you are a perfectionist, surgery may leave you disappointed. The goal of breast reconstruction is for you to wear a bra without an outside "filler." Although at times reconstructed breasts practically match the remaining breast, this is not (yet) common.
- Your new breast should be similar in size and shape to the remaining breast. You should be able to wear a bra or sportswear without embarrassment.

Back to Work

You will lose about 10 to 14 days after your **first operation**. You may lose a month or more from work if you have a flap. If your first operation is done with your mastectomy, you will lose only the time (4 to 6 weeks) for recovery from the mastectomy.

For the **second operation** if the surgery is done with local/sedation on an outpatient basis, you may be able to work after a week. Your leg will still be sore if the graft for the nipple was taken there.

Back to Parties

You should allow yourself *2 months* if you required a major flap for the **first operation**. You should allow at least a month if your first operation was done with general anesthesia following a course of chemotherapy. The combination of mastectomy, chemotherapy, and general anesthesia for reconstruction will leave you too tired to enjoy a party for quite a while.

If your **second operation** is done 6 months after the first, the usual interval, you can probably enjoy a party 2 weeks after the second operation unless extensive revision and general anesthesia were needed.

Back to Sports

If your first operation was done with the mastectomy or required a *major* flap, then you cannot exercise for about 6 weeks. It is important for you to conserve energy—not burn it up in exercise. However, you will begin exercises to loosen up your arm right after your mastectomy. It will tend to be very stiff.

If your **first operation** was done 6 months after the mastectomy, especially if you had no chemotherapy *and* if the surgery does not involve a major flap, you can begin limbering-up exercises after 10 to 14 days. By 2 weeks you may be able to begin swimming a few laps or working out with an exercise bicycle. After a month, you can exercise fully, although not at your usual speed. That will take another 2 weeks to build up strength and endurance.

Breast reconstruction leaves most women too tired to exercise much at first. Thus you are unlikely to hurt yourself with exercise because you heal before you feel energetic.

Breast Reconstruction After Mastectomy: Recovery-at-a-Glance

This chart represents the *average* recovery times for this cosmetic operation.

FIRST OPERATION
(Not a major flap)

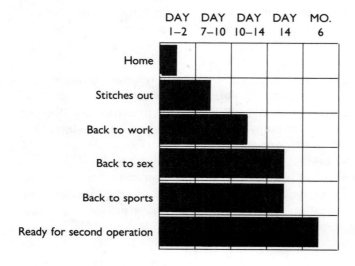

	DAY 1–2	DAY 7–10	DAY 10–14	DAY 14	MO. 6
Home					
Stitches out					
Back to work					
Back to sex					
Back to sports					
Ready for second operation					

SECOND OPERATION

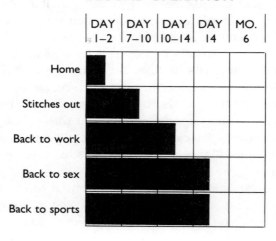

	DAY 1–2	DAY 7–10	DAY 10–14	DAY 14	MO. 6
Home					
Stitches out					
Back to work					
Back to sex					
Back to sports					

For the **second operation**, if you had only minor revision and a nipple graft, you may be ready to limber up after 1 week—and be back to full exercise 2 weeks later.

Back to Sex

Surgery can reconstruct your breast, but it will not restore normal sensation. Your new breast will not be sexually responsive. The skin may be completely numb for months after your mastectomy, and it may become temporarily numb again after the first reconstruction operation.

After your **first reconstruction operation**, sex depends on the operation: after a flap taken from your abdomen, sex may be off limits for a month while the abdomen heals. However, if your reconstruction used only the chest tissues, you may be able to resume sex after 2 weeks. However, your chest muscles may still be sore. If so, the chest-muscle contraction during sex may make them hurt, so put off sex another week to let them heal.

After your **nipple reconstruction**, the scar on your thigh will slow down your return to sex. This incision heals slowly and will *hurt* if you resume sex too early—two weeks at the earliest, but for most women closer to 3.

How Much It Costs

If the **first reconstructive operation** of your breast uses chest tissue, the cost may be from $1500 to $2500 for the surgeon's fee. The cost of the hospital will be about the same. If a major flap is done, your surgeon's fee may be between $3000 and $6000. Your hospital charges may be equally high, since the more complicated operation requires more operating room time and a longer hospital stay.

Your **second operation** may cost as much as the first if extensive revisions are needed. However, reconstruction of a nipple done with local/sedation may cost as "little" as $2000 *total*.

Insurance Coverage

Insurance *almost always* pays for breast reconstruction, although an occasional lesser-known insurance company may deem the operation(s) medically unnecessary and refuse to pay. However, knowing what your insurance will cover takes careful pre-surgery planning. For instance, your insurance should approve your nipple reconstruction *before* your first operation as part of your total reconstruction. Otherwise, your insurance may consider nipple reconstruction alone "nonessential" and refuse to pay.

Contact your insurance company with your policy in your hand and review with them what your insurance covers. For instance, if you had a lumpectomy and radiation and your breast shape is odd now, do they consider corrective surgery cosmetic or reconstructive? Once you have decided what reconstruction to have done, ask your surgeon to prepare an insurance report, including all planned operations and his *estimated* fee. Have him include the possibility of additional unexpected surgery. This avoids having your insurance refuse to pay for a larger implant because a change in implant size wasn't specifically listed on your surgeon's report.

Your insurance company should tell you in advance the *dollar amount* that they will pay. Some insurance companies are wonderful; they pay the full amount for your reconstruction. However, other insurance companies may refuse to pay or create enormous paperwork to discourage you from collecting insurance reimbursement. Unless you *know* your insurance company will treat you well, settle all insurance questions before your surgery.

My Assessment of This Procedure

Breast reconstruction was virtually unheard of as recently as the mid-1970s. The majority of women having a mastectomy today opt for reconstruction. However, it is not *necessary* to have your breast reconstructed, and some women simply don't care to go through the operations. A woman whose husband or sex partner is truly not bothered by the mastectomy may decide against it. Women for whom reconstruction is easy are small-breasted women for whom a reconstruction can be quite simple. A woman with a very large breast who had radiation after the mastectomy may face not only an extensive flap reconstruction but also unusually extensive surgery to "match" the new breast and the remaining one.

Side Effects and Complications

Side Effects

Major complications are rare after breast reconstruction; you are more likely to find that the surgery has not achieved the results you would ideally like to see. You may notice that your new breast is harder than your other breast, or lies slightly higher, or that in a V neck dress your cleavage is not symmetrical. These may be improved by further surgery. You may require one or two further operations to get results that are satisfactory to you. Reconstruction of the breast is still being worked out—new techniques are developed every year. If you've had to put a bulky prosthesis in your bra every morning just to keep the bra from riding up on your chest, you may be quite satisfied with less than perfect results.

Complications

Any of the complications that can occur with cosmetic surgery can occur with breast reconstruction—bleeding, infection, poor healing, bad scars, but infection is the major concern. An infection in your new breast is likely to be more serious than an infection elsewhere. First, you have an implant under your tissues, and if the infection settles here it may need to be removed. Second, treating the infection *without* removing the implant may require surgery to drain the infection, plus *intravenous* antibiotics for 4 to 6 weeks. You can receive antibiotics as an outpatient—even when intravenous—so you need not be in hospital all that time. But, an infection is going to greatly delay your healing. It may not be possible to treat it successfully without removing the implant. Though infections after breast reconstruction are uncommon (perhaps 2 to 3 percent of cases) they are serious. Also, since you have had a mastectomy, an infection may lead to prolonged swelling of your arm, even if you've had no swelling before.

Shirley: "Perfection or Nothing"

Shirley was 30 and single when she had a mastectomy. She was a professional woman and had high expectations of herself and others. She decided that she wanted her breast reconstructed—but that it would have to match her remaining breast to be worthwhile. Otherwise, she saw no point in bothering with reconstruction at all. Shir-

ley consulted three different plastic surgeons. Each one told her the same thing: that her new breast was highly unlikely to match her other breast, and that her goal was unrealistic, given what surgery can do at this point. Shirley had no trouble with her decision—if it wasn't perfect, she didn't want it. She used a bra prosthesis instead.

Barb: A Double Mastectomy

Barb was middle-aged, married, and about 100 pounds overweight. She had had both breasts removed—one for cancer, and the other for a serious premalignant breast tumor. Breast cancer ran in her family. She had been large-breasted and was quite depressed with how she looked after mastectomy. Barb's mastectomies had left her with bulges under her arms and over her chest where the fat kept her skin from lying flat. Her first operation placed an implant on each side of her chest and suctioned away the fat to smooth out the bulges. She was pleased, but the implants were too small for her. At her second operation, Barb had larger implants placed. Her nipples were reconstructed, and tissue was shifted up from her abdomen to create more of a crease for her new breasts. Barb was pleased. She felt normal once again. She could forget about her distressing mastectomy and get on with her life. She looked normal in clothes and a swimsuit. In fact, she began to exercise for the first time in years and shed a few pounds as well.

Polly: "I Feel Normal Again"

Polly had a mastectomy about 10 years before she considered a reconstruction. She raised her family but split up from her husband after her children were grown. She decided she would like to begin dating to find a new man in her life, but she felt embarrassed about her appearance. A flap of skin and muscle from Polly's back had to be used in her reconstruction because her operation had been a radical mastectomy. Her new breast was smaller than her other one, and the flap skin didn't quite match the color or texture of her chest skin. Back skin is different. Still, Polly was not troubled by that. She didn't mind having to explain her situation to a man she was having sex with—she just wanted to look as good as she could before she reached that point. She was surprised to find how happy she felt when she walked into a store to try on clothes without the risk of a saleslady seeing the prosthesis in her bra. She had always hated them feeling sorry for her. She wanted to feel normal—and after her reconstruction that was how she felt.

What Other Patients Say

- **Young mother, 30**: "I was devastated by my mastectomy. I felt mutilated. Fortunately my breasts were very small. I not only had a reconstruction, I had the other side enlarged. It made me feel I was still attractive."
- **Woman, 60**: "I thought I was too old to care about this. My husband accepted everything, but I couldn't. It sure doesn't look like the breast I lost but I'm not planning to go topless. I just wanted to wear a nightgown without feeling like a ship listing to starboard."
- **Career woman, 45**: "I knew I was going to have a reconstruction and I insisted that my surgeon have a plastic surgeon start working on me before I was off the operating table. If there had been women surgeons 20 years ago, this operation would have been developed a lot earlier. I wasn't wasting my time waiting for reconstruction when we could get started right away. Perfect it's not, but compared to nothing, it's fabulous."

CHAPTER 13

Procedures for the Body and Legs

Major Cosmetic Abdominal Surgery ("Tummy Tuck")

What Surgeons Call It

The technical description of this surgery is abdominal lipectomy with repair of diastasis recti, resection of lipocutaneous excess, and repair of umbilical or abdominal hernia. All those medical terms mean that the surgeon will remove excess skin and adjacent fat, tighten loose or weak muscles, and repair a hernia if there is one. Hernias are usually seen only after multiple pregnancies or major abdominal surgery.

What It Will Do

This operation removes excess skin and as much excess fat as possible from your abdominal area, and tightens your abdominal muscles. The trade-off is a repositioned navel and some scars. If your *only* problem is that you have lost a lot of weight and have a fold of excess skin in your lower abdomen, you may not need the full operation. Cutting off the excess skin may be enough. This operation is described more fully in the following section on the "Mini Tuck."

What It Won't Do

The tummy tuck will *not* remove stretch marks unless they are in the lower abdominal skin, which is cut off at surgery. Stretch marks are in your skin and to date there is no treatment for them. This operation will not make your hips or bottom smaller; that requires diet or fat suction (see the section on Liposuction). The surgery will tighten your abdomen and, depending on your muscle tone *and* on the fat inside your abdomen as opposed to under the skin—will give you a flatter, or even a flat, abdomen. It won't make your skin drum-tight, and it won't eliminate the natural skin folding that occurs when you bend over. That fold is found in virtually everyone over 30. Exercise and dieting will flatten your stomach even more after surgery.

How Long It Will Last

This operation is permanent to a great extent. The fat and skin that are removed do not return. However, the tightened muscles can stretch again, especially if you gain much weight or become pregnant. This is why surgery is preferably done *after* your weight is stable and/or you have had your family.

When to Have It

The right time for this operation is after the *cause* of your stomach-stretching is gone: when you have had your babies, lost your weight, had your abdominal surgery. Preferably it's done when you are in fairly good shape, physically.

If you have this operation and get pregnant again, it may not completely undo the operation—but it will undo some of it, leaving your skin and muscle noticeably stretched, even if not as bad as before the surgery.

This operation is *uncommon* in young people, but that's because they rarely have lived through the pregnancies, weight loss and/or surgeries that create the need for this operation. A young person whose skin and muscles were stretched certainly *could* benefit from a major tummy tuck.

Where to Have It

A tummy tuck is a major operation which is done in a hospital operating room on an inpatient basis. You will need to stay in the hospital for several days after surgery.

Conditions That Increase Your Risk

If you have had **phlebitis** in the deep veins of your legs, you have at least a 10 percent chance of developing phlebitis again, because it tends to occur after abdominal surgery and when you are kept in bed. Phlebitis can also occur after this surgery, if you have never had phlebitis before. If you have phlebitis now, your surgeon will postpone surgery until it is properly treated. If it is not treated, phlebitis of your deep leg veins can cause a blood clot to break loose and travel to your lungs. This condition, known as pulmonary embolism, causes trouble with breathing and can be fatal.

Smoking increases your risk of phlebitis besides increasing your risk of poor healing from the surgery. If you are a pack-a-day smoker or more, you should make a *huge* effort to stop smoking for the week before and the week after surgery.

Abdominal **scarring** from past surgery (for instance, an appendectomy, gallbladder operation or a Cesarean delivery) reduces the blood flow to your abdominal skin. Although the surgery can certainly be done when you have extensive scarring, scars that go *across* your abdomen, rather than up and down, cut off so much blood supply that your skin may not heal after surgery. Your surgeon may have to modify the operation to avoid new scars and additional damage to the skin blood flow.

Usual Anesthesia

This operation is done with general anesthesia.

How Long It Takes

Your tummy tuck may take between 2½ and 4 hours, depending on how much you bleed and whether or not you have hernias that need to be repaired. Extensive hernias in your abdomen may make your surgery take even longer.

The Operation

(Figures 13-1 through 13-3)

Surgical Markings

Before the operation, the surgeon may want to mark the incision lines on your abdomen with purple surgical ink. You will need to stand up so that the areas of your body fall in the right position. When you lie down, your abdominal skin shifts slightly. What looks like the center of your abdomen may be off to one side. Thus, surgeons will often do markings in the office or in the hospital room the day or evening before surgery. Otherwise, the markings are done in the preoperative area the morning of surgery.

Your surgeon will need to mark the incision line that will go in the natural skin fold in your lower abdomen. He will also mark the excess skin, your navel, and the midline of your abdomen. He may also mark your ribs and the areas where your muscles are stretched. He may mark where excess fat is to be suctioned at the side of your abdomen. These markings are not critical, though, because these areas can be readily marked with you on the operating table.

Unlike breast reduction, for which the markings must be done before surgery, an abdominal correction *can* be done without presurgical markings. But, omitting this step makes a minor misjudgment more likely, leading to later touch-up surgery— for example, to revise a scar or to remove more skin. Thus, even if your surgeon doesn't *plan* to do your markings before you are asleep, it is best for you if you tell him that you want him to do these markings before you go to the operating room.

Before

You will come to the preoperative area, either from home or from a hospital room having had nothing to eat or drink since midnight the night before. An anesthetist will meet you, and an IV will be placed in your arm so that you can be given a solution of dextrose and/or saline to prevent dehydration during surgery. You might be given a little sedation by mouth or injection or through your IV. Your surgeon will see you, and if he has not yet made his surgical markings, he might do them now. He might also wait until you are asleep in the operating room to do some of them.

Once you are in the operating room and settled on the table, a safety strap will be put across your legs and sticky pads will be put on your chest to monitor your heart. Then you will be put to sleep with a drug given through your IV. Once you are asleep, a tube is put down your throat so that oxygen and anesthetic gases can be given directly to your lungs. The nurses will put a tube in your bladder and a sticky pad on your hip to make the surgical cautery safe for you. (Surgical cautery means using an electrical heat device to seal off bleeding blood vessels.) Elastic stockings are placed on your legs to decrease the risk of phlebitis by supporting the deep veins in your legs. Your abdomen is then washed with surgical soap, and sterile drapes are put around your abdomen.

During

If you have much fat under your abdominal skin, your surgeon starts by making the incision around your navel and suctioning out some of the fat. This involves shoving (it is not delicate) a two-foot long hollow metal tube under the skin into the fatty layer beneath and pushing the tube back and forth to pull the excess fat loose and suction it out. (See Suction Lipectomy.) If he is not doing fat suction of the abdomen first, your surgeon will start with an incision right above your pubic mound. Your pubic hair is not shaved.

The surgeon cuts through the skin and fatty layer so that he can separate the deep layer of fat from the muscle all the way to your navel. Then he will cut the navel free from the surrounding skin and continue freeing the skin and deep fat from the muscle, right up to the ribs. Once the skin is free, the surgeon makes sure that all the bleeding vessels are sealed with cautery or tied shut (ligated) with thread. Your abdominal muscles will now be in full view. Usually, your surgeon will tighten them by putting in many stitches right down the middle from the ribs to the pubis, pulling the stretched muscles back together. However, the muscles around the navel are not closed tightly, since doing so might cut off the blood supply to the navel. A hernia around the navel will be sewn shut. Hernias through other muscle layers or scars are also sewed closed. The skin is then pulled taut and the excess cut off. Fat may now be suctioned from the sides of your abdomen to make it even with your new, tighter abdomen.

Finally, stitches are put in to sew your incision closed. A new hole is made in the middle of the abdomen skin for your navel, which is sewn to this new opening. Long thin plastic tubes called drains are slipped under the skin to take out any fluid that collects. The soap is washed off your abdomen, the bandage is put on, and your operation is over.

Variation in Technique. In some patients, stretched muscles and excess skin occur only up and down the middle of the abdomen. Everything else is tight. Usually, this happens from one or more pregnancies in which the babies were carried so that only the center of the abdomen was stretched. This skin/muscle problem can be corrected by a vertical incision from rib to pubis to cut out the excess skin here. A vertical incision makes the muscle easier to stitch. However, the long vertical scar cannot be hidden and may be unsightly. This technique removes only the excess skin in the center of the abdomen, not skin hanging over the groin. It is not the standard operation but is used in certain cases.

"Tummy Tuck"

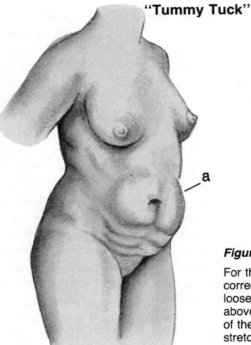

a

Figure 13-1.

For the *major* abdominal cosmetic correction to be necessary, the loose skin and muscle must extend above the navel (a). The protrusion of the abdomen is partly from stretched muscle and partly from excess fat.

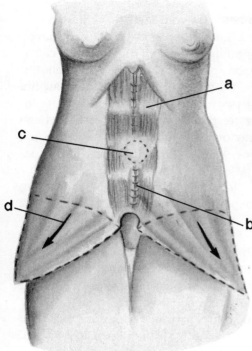

Figure 13-2.

During a tummy tuck the loose rectus muscle (a) is tightened all the way up to the ribs. Stitches (b) are placed to pull the muscle tight. The dotted circle (c) shows where the new opening for the navel will be made. The excess skin (d) is pulled down and will be cut off. Note that the old opening for the navel may be pulled as far down as the incision above the pubic mound.

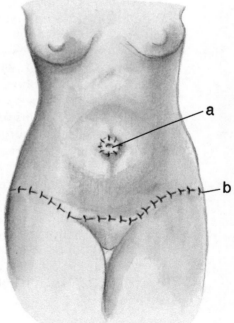

Figure 13-3.

The navel is sewn to its new opening in the skin (a). Note that the scar for this operation (b) is a long one.

The Process of Healing

What to Do About Pain

You will *hurt* after your surgery, and you will need narcotic pain-killers by injection for at least 1 day. The nurses in the hospital will administer these. Most people need to take narcotic pain-killers in pill form one or more times a day for 2 weeks. These drugs may make you groggy or fuzzy-headed, so many people take them only near bedtime, when pain usually is at its worst.

The Healing Process

You will be kept in your hospital bed ("on bed rest") for 1 or 2 days after surgery. You can move around, but you will hurt, so you won't move much.

You will be fed through an IV for 18 to 48 hours after your surgery. The anesthesia will make you nauseated, and until all nausea is gone you shouldn't eat—vomiting will not only hurt but could pull loose some internal stitches.

Because this operation tightens your abdominal muscles, you will feel tight and may walk slightly stooped for 2 to 3 weeks. Once the muscles heal, you will be able to walk straight in comfort again. You will not be comfortable lying flat in bed. A small pillow under your knees will take the pull off your abdomen if you are a back-sleeper. When you sleep on your side, your legs naturally flex. Your abdomen will be too sore for you to sleep on your stomach for 3 or 4 weeks after surgery.

You will have drains under the abdominal skin to keep fluid from collecting. Your surgeon or a nurse removes these after 1 or 2 days. They *may* hurt as they are pulled out from under your skin.

You will have a tube (called a catheter) in your bladder during surgery to keep your bladder from filling up and making it hard for the surgeon to contour the abdominal skin. After surgery, the tube is usually kept in your bladder for 1 or 2 days, until you are allowed out of bed to the bathroom.

Your abdominal skin will be bruised and the bruises travel down to your hips. You will be purplish the first week, yellow the second.

The general anesthesia used for this surgery may make you tired and draggy for 6 weeks.

Once you are home, 3 to 5 days after surgery, you will spend much time resting or sleeping. You will be able to get up and dress, go to the bathroom, and bathe, but you won't have much energy to do it. For instance, just brushing your hair in the morning seems like a big project. After you dress, you need a nap to recover. If you have stairs at home, come downstairs and spend the day on the sofa, rather than going up and down stairs, until about day 6. You need someone to help you at home, *not* because you need lots of special care, but because you will recover much faster if you use your energy to recover rather than burning it up answering the phone and fixing your meals. You will gradually get your energy back, but this is one operation where you will be surprised by how long, not how short, your recovery is.

Bandages

Your surgeon may use any of several methods:

- A layer of gauze held in place with a layer of plaster to contour it to your skin—the plaster is not wrapped around you, but put on top of your abdomen.
- Elastic bandages, wrapped around your lower chest and abdomen
- Gauze over the stitches and a supportive girdle, body stocking, or Velcro binder to keep it in place. (This is the simplest and is replacing the bulkier methods of bandaging. It is what I use now.)

Your bandages are changed on the first or second day after surgery, and your drains are removed. After that bandages will be changed only if they are stained or if you bathe or shower. You need to wear a layer of gauze under a girdle or binder to keep the stitches from sticking to the fabric.

Once your stitches are out, you still may want to wear gauze over the incision for a week or so, if it is sensitive. Wear loose clothes because your abdomen will be swollen, and pressure from clothes will make it uncomfortable. The gauze may visibly bulge under snug skirts or slacks, so wear loose clothing.

Taking Care of Your Wound

Once you are home, you can change the bandage yourself. Simply discard the layer of gauze and put another layer over your stitches, holding it in place with panties or shorts under your girdle, binder, or body stocking.

Most surgeons will let you shower, but not soak in a tub until all stitches are out.

Stitches

You will probably have three kinds of stitches. **Inside stitches** stay inside, holding your muscle and deep skin layers together while you heal. A **pullout stitch** will run in the deep skin layers, starting at one end of your incision and coming out the other end. It may stay in 2 or 3 weeks. Finally, your skin will be aligned by individual stitches (called "interrupted sutures"). These show on the surface of your skin, and their pressure on your skin can leave permanent cross-hatch marks. So, these stitches are removed early—about 7 days after surgery.

Scars

All your scars will be red and lumpy for weeks. Your newly placed navel may be larger or smaller and rounder than your original navel. If the navel scar shrinks or stretches, your navel may look odd, compared with before. You may need minor surgery, to correct this (6 months after surgery).

You will have a horizontal scar in your lower abdomen, just above the pubic hair, going from hip to hip. This is a long scar. Stand in front of your bedroom mirror to show yourself the true length that this scar will be. A long scar here can be hidden by sports clothes. However, your abdomen is not a "good" scar area. Scars here take a *year or two* to fade and flatten. They also tend to widen, to a quarter- or half-inch width. If you have an allergic reaction to your stitches or an infection after surgery, your scars may be improved by cutting out and restitching 6 to 12 months after the surgery. However, most abdominal scars simply reflect your natural healing, and scar surgery will not improve them. Steroid injections 6 to 12 months after surgery may soften hard or lumpy scars, but they will also increase the chance that your scars will stretch even wider. A perfect hairline scar in this area is lovely and can occur, but don't *expect* to be so lucky.

Tips

- A tummy tuck is a big operation. If you are in good physical condition, the anesthesia, bed rest, and abdominal pain are much easier to tolerate.
- Your physical preparation should include exercises or sports that strengthen the abdominal muscles (swimming, dance, rowing). If these muscles are strong, they will heal faster and painlessly.
- Also, if your lungs are in good condition (*don't* smoke—*do* exercise), you will cough less and heal faster after your surgery.
- Trauma from surgery will make your skin produce less natural oil. Thus your skin will be dry and scratchy. Rub lots of body cream gently on your abdomen (away from the stitches) once the bandages are off.
- You will need help at home after your surgery—ideally for 2 weeks after the hospital, but at least for 5 days.
- The surgical swelling will make your waistline thicker temporarily. You may not be able to wear snug slacks or skirts that fit *before* surgery for 2 or 3 months, afterwards.
- Women can quickly reduce the surgical swelling and keep it down by wearing a girdle or elastic body stocking for 6 weeks after surgery. The support also makes you more comfortable.
- Men can get the same result from an abdominal binder. These are bulkier than women's support garments. They can be bought in a pharmacy or a surgical supply store. They are an elastic wrap, like a very wide belt, worn under your clothes and held on with snaps or Velcro.
- Exercise will decrease the swelling—muscle motion from exercise pumps the fluid that is causing the swelling out of the muscle and skin.

Back to Work

You may return to work between 3 and 6 weeks after a tummy tuck. Take into account *how* you get to work. If you have a five-minute quiet ride, 3 weeks may be reasonable. If you face an hour of subways, buses, and/or stairways, you may not physically tolerate an early return to work.

Go back to work at 3 weeks only if you *must*. You will feel tired and may have to leave work early for the first week. Even if you feel you *must* get back to work at 3 weeks, remind co-workers that you *may* not be able to do it.

Major "Tummy Tuck": Recovery-at-a-Glance

This chart represents the *average* recovery times for this cosmetic operation.

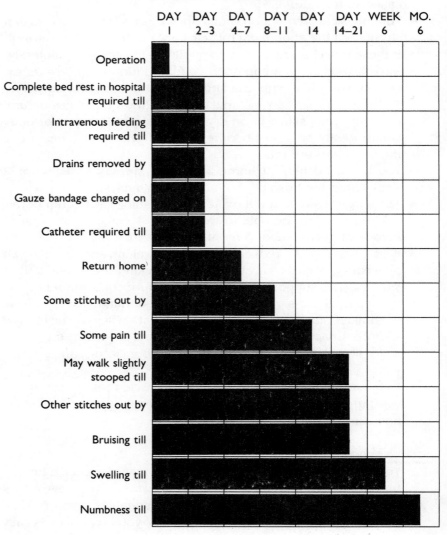

	DAY 1	DAY 2–3	DAY 4–7	DAY 8–11	DAY 14	DAY 14–21	WEEK 6	MO. 6
Operation								
Complete bed rest in hospital required till								
Intravenous feeding required till								
Drains removed by								
Gauze bandage changed on								
Catheter required till								
Return home								
Some stitches out by								
Some pain till								
May walk slightly stooped till								
Other stitches out by								
Bruising till								
Swelling till								
Numbness till								

Four weeks after surgery, you can work unless a long commute or a complication makes this out of the question.

After 6 weeks you are ready, but after a busy day you may be more tired than normal.

Back to Parties

A quiet, early dinner 3 weeks after surgery would be enjoyable. A cocktail party that keeps you standing or a dance will not be fun, until 6 to 8 weeks.

Back to Sports

Two weeks after surgery you can start short walks. At first this "walk" may be once down the block. You may be able to do stretching exercises or a slow, short swim in a warm pool. Cold water may make your abdominal muscles cramp and ache.

If you have never exercised regularly, start now. Exercise reduces your swelling and tones the muscles that surgery has tightened.

After 4 to 6 weeks you can work your way back to your previous exercise regimen. Allow yourself another month to get back to your presurgery condition. No contact sports until 2 *months* after the operation.

Back to Sex

Your stomach will hurt. You will not enjoy sex for about a month after surgery. Sex before 3 weeks could pull a segment of your incision apart, cause new bruising, or tear an inside stitch.

How Much It Costs

Your surgeon's fee will range from $3000 to $5000. The hospital fee will also be from $3000 to $5000—more for a long hospital stay. This cost would include anesthesia and operating room costs as well as the postsurgical hospital care.

Insurance Coverage

A tummy tuck is considered *cosmetic*. Insurance *may* cover some or all of the surgeon's and hospital fees in some cases. It varies from one company to the next. Insurance *may* pay if you have had abdominal operations or pregnancies that have caused a major abdominal muscle weakness; for example, when you lie down and lift your head, intestinal contents form a bulge between weak muscles in your midabdomen.

Insurance *may* pay if your abdomen has excess skin that forms a deep fold over your pubic area, and if the fold is so hard to keep clean that skin rashes and infection develop under it.

Find out exactly what your insurance company will pay for before your surgery, please! Allow yourself 6 weeks to get an opinion. It can be done in two weeks, but only if your insurance company and your surgeon's office cooperate.

- Contact your insurance agency.
- Deal with *one* person.
- Have your surgeon send them all the information they need including photographs.

Your surgeon will charge you for preparing the report and/or for duplicating photographs. (The cost ranges from $30 to $60.) But, if insurance agrees to reimburse you, the modest cost for the insurance report is well worth it.

Get your insurance company's decision in writing and *get a dollar amount for what they will pay.* An insurance company that tells you in writing, that they "will reimburse the full amount allowed for this operation" has told you *nothing!* Such a letter may be followed by a letter after surgery saying that "this surgery is not allowed." Even a letter stating the dollar amount can mean a long wait until you are reimbursed. For this reason, almost all surgeons require full payment in advance, regardless of insurance coverage.

My Assessment of This Procedure

A tummy tuck is a *major* operation. It should not be equated in recovery or risks with such cosmetic operations as eyelid, nose, face, brow, breast, and arm lifts. These are done with local/ sedation anesthesia on an outpatient basis and your recovery time depends as much on how presentable you *look* as on your physical condition.

There is a 3 to 6 week recovery period after a major abdominal lift. If you want to fit it in during a one-week vacation, it can't be done. A serious infection or phlebitis following this operation might delay your recovery a week, two weeks, or longer. If your only complaint is a skin fold when you bend over—skin less tight than is "ideal," or if you have a little pouch in your lower abdomen from a little too much fat, this operation is *too drastic for you.*

Instead you might lose weight, spot-exercise your abdominal muscle, or consider a mini-tuck (see the next section).

This operation will vastly improve an abdomen with stretched/damaged muscle, much loose skin, and hernias. It is *not* the "touch-up" correction to make an abdomen gorgeous enough for a bikini.

Side Effects and Complications

Side Effects

Tummy-tuck surgery will make your abdomen skin dry and will leave you tired for weeks from the anesthesia. It leaves swelling in your abdomen that time (up to 6 months) plus exercise will correct. The skin on your abdomen will be completely numb for 6 weeks or longer. The feeling returns over 6 to 12 months. About 6 weeks after surgery, the tightness from the muscle stitching is gone. However, your scars have only begun to flatten, soften, and fade. You may wait over a year before they are in their final state. The navel scar may shrink and need minor surgery 6 to 12 months after your operation.

Minor Complications

Being disappointed with the results of the operation might be considered a minor complication. Although a tummy tuck can produce dramatically good results, it is best reserved for those people who have a fairly dramatic problem to begin with. Otherwise you may find that the pain, discomfort, and time involved with this surgery are out of proportion to your less-than-perfect abdomen.

Major Complications

Major complications that can occur include bleeding and infection, poor healing, and phlebitis—formation of blood clots in the deep veins of the leg.

Serious internal **bleeding** causes blood to collect under the skin of the abdomen. The bleeding must be stopped and the blood drained. For you it means 3 or 4 extra days of convalescence and lots of bruising.

Infection can require drainage of infected fluid and antibiotics. A severe infection could keep you in the hospital for days, or it could damage the blood vessels that nourish your abdominal skin, leaving you with worse scars than anticipated. However, the worst complication is a **blood clot** in your leg after surgery. By itself this is not a big problem—your leg swells; you need medication to stop the inflammation and elastic stockings to support your leg. However, if a leg blood clot should break loose (this happens about 1% of the time, if phlebitis is treated promptly), it would travel from your leg to your lungs, cause serious breathing difficulty and require emergency x-ray tests of your lungs, and even surgery to block other clots from reaching your lungs. This is *rare*, but you might not think a lung problem could arise from a cosmetic abdominal operation, so it is important to know about this risk.

Simon: Working Hard for Successful Results

Simon was 30. Two years before, and 6 months after losing the last of his 100 pounds of excess fat, he had had his gallbladder removed. After the gallbladder surgery, a blood clot developed in his leg. The surgical scar and his case of phlebitis increased his risk of complications. Nevertheless he decided to have cosmetic abdominal surgery to remove the excess skin and to repair the muscle looseness from his gallbladder operation. Simon had a higher than normal risk for phlebitis. I told him so, but he told me not to worry. He felt he would do fine with his tummy tuck.

Simon was right. He was out of bed, joking about feeling "tight as a drum" on the second day after his operation. He was in the hospital 5 days—and went back to work—at 3½ weeks. He insisted on this because he was too bored to stay at home. He had a year of unused sick leave, and didn't feel pressured to get back to work.

His wife said that since his weight loss Simon found it impossible to rest, and that he might as well go back to work. He was in terrific physical condition because exercise had played a large role in his weight loss. He was thrilled with his result. He wore a trouser two sizes smaller because it no longer had to accommodate his flabby skin. His abdomen still had slight bulge, but the muscles were tight and he could feel them pulling—for the first time since his gallbladder surgery—when he did sit-ups 4 weeks after his tummy tuck. His scars were fine white hairline scars. Simon gave me all the credit. Actually it was his youth, energy, positive outlook, and good healing that led to his rapid recovery.

Dorothy: Golf and Poolside Lounging

Dorothy was 50. She had had three children and had lost 15 pounds over the past year by cutting out dessert. The stretch marks on her abdomen did not bother her. She had very poor abdominal muscle tone, and exercise had not helped it. Her muscles were too stretched to pull when she exercised. Her weight loss and her pregnancies had left loose, stretched muscle and skin all over her abdomen. It formed a fold above the navel and another below. She also had droopy breasts.

Dorothy had tummy-tuck surgery. I stitched her flabby muscles, removed the excess skin and suctioned out her abdominal fat around her waist. I also did a breast lift.

Dorothy had no complications and went home on the fifth day after surgery. Within 2 weeks—when her swelling was not yet gone—she was a size 12 instead of a size 14. (This benefit is not predictable—and not the norm.) Dorothy had intended to go back to work a month after her operation, but even though her sales work in a jewelry store was not physically demanding, she discovered that she was too tired to go back that soon. She went back after 6 weeks, spending the last week with a friend out of town. Dorothy had lumpy scars, for the first 9 months. They then softened just enough to encourage her.

Dorothy had expected the surgery to radically change the way she dressed, but it didn't. She did take up golf. Instead of shopping on weekends, she was out on the links with her husband. Dorothy bought herself a bathing suit for the first time in years and was lounging by the pool. She couldn't decide which operation—breasts or abdomen—had given her the courage to do this. "My boys are the funniest," she said. "One of them calls me 'gorgeous.' I'm not, but I love it, because it means he's noticed!"

Peggy: Infection and a Wide Scar

Peggy was 39 and divorced. Two pregnancies and repeated diets and binges had stretched the skin and muscles on her abdomen. She was fatigued at the end of the working day—her abdomen felt achy. She was not in good physical shape. Peggy hated exercise, and she was still 30 pounds overweight. She wanted surgery, though she knew it wasn't going to make her thin or fit. She smoked and told me—honestly and cheerfully—that she would try to cut down, but would make no promises.

Peggy had her tummy tuck and I found her happily, but a little guiltily, smoking a cigarette the day after her surgery. For whatever reason—and it's easy to blame her smoking, but that may not have been the cause (her surgery was long, and she was still overweight which increased the risk of infection)—she got an infection. This kept her in the hospital for 2 extra weeks. (She never complained, and she never stopped smoking.) Part of her incision had to be opened wide to drain the infection, and she did not believe that it would ever heal. It did—but it took a month after her leaving the hospital.

Despite all these setbacks, Peggy was delighted with the surgery. The flap of skin that had made her feel "like a freak" was gone. Her weak muscles were snug, so she didn't ache in her lower abdomen. In fact, she felt so much better about herself that she demanded and got a promotion. She reluctantly agreed that exercise was unavoidable and began to walk to work.

Pam: A Modified Tuck Was Enough

Pam was thin and had never been fat. She was in peak physical condition, being a dance instructor. She had had three children, and each pregnancy had been carried high in the center of her abdomen. The pregnancies had stretched the muscle that runs up and down the abdomen. (It's the muscle that pulls you up for sit-ups.) When Pam tried to sit up, her muscles did nothing, and she simply bulged in the middle of her abdomen. Pam had lots of loose, wrinkled skin up and down her midabdomen, but none over her groin.

She needed—and had—the modified tummy tuck, with a vertical scar. Since her problem was limited to the midabdomen, this was the only way to get rid of the excess skin. We did know beforehand that Pam tended to form thin, white scars.

Pam wanted her surgery as an outpatient, which was not reasonable. But she was out of bed the first day and home on the third. She was in a leotard at her 2-week office visit—she wanted me to see no bulge when she did a port de bras forward in second position!

What Other Patients Say

- **Mother of two, 33**: "I'm overweight, but I always bounce back fast. I did. The operation really helped—I don't have that elephant fold of skin in front any more. I would like to be skinny, but I know that surgery can't do it all."
- **Man, 40, after weight loss**: "My stomach can exercise now. Before the muscles flopped around. I used to wear swim trunks on the beach and people would stare at me. Now they don't look. I kind of miss the attention but I like not feeling a freak anymore."
- **Teacher, 33**: "My problem wasn't the worst, just everything bulging out. The surgery makes a world of difference inside. I don't feel embarrassed with my body anymore when I take a bath or get dressed. I don't have to hide, mentally, from my looks."
- **Transportation engineer, 29**: "It was a lot of surgery. My belly button used to be an outie, and now it's an innie. I don't like my scars. I hurt for days. I look better but definitely not perfect."
- **Mother of five, 38**: "When you've had five children, nothing bothers you. I loved being in the hospital—no dishes to do. My scars aren't good yet, but my stomach seems pretty near to before I had babies, but it's too long ago to be sure."

Minor Cosmetic Abdominal Surgery ("Mini-Tummy Tuck")

What Surgeons Call It

The technical name for this is modified abdominal lipectomy with repair of inferior diastasis rectus and resection of lipocutaneous excess. These medical terms mean repairing the lower abdominal muscles and removing excess skin and fat from the lower abdomen.

What It Will Do

The "mini-tuck" aims to give you a flatter, tighter lower abdomen with less bulge. It is only for problems in the lower abdomen (below the navel).

What It Won't Do

This operation will not necessarily give you a flat stomach or an abdomen that you want to display in a bikini. It is unlikely to change your clothing size. It will *not* remove stretch marks, which are ruptures in the deep layers of the skin. If your stretch marks are in the skin that is removed, they come out. But unless they lie in this lower abdomen, they will be pulled downward somewhat, but not removed.

How Long It Will Last

This operation is permanent, but if you become pregnant or gain a lot of weight (for example, 20 pounds) or have extensive abdominal surgery, some or all of the muscle-tightening will be lost and your stomach may bulge again.

When to Have It

You should have a mini-tuck *if* your problem is limited to the lower abdomen, below the navel, and *when* the cause of your stretching has ended: when you don't plan another pregnancy, when you won't be gaining weight again (you hope), or when the surgery that damaged the muscle is not likely to be needed again.

Where to Have It

This depends on how much (or how little) will be done. A *few* mini-tucks are done on an outpatient basis with local/sedation, or even on an outpatient basis with general anesthesia. Outpatient procedures may be done in a hospital operating room *or* a surgery center operating room *or* a doctor's office/clinic operating room.

If the surgery requires an overnight hospital stay, it will naturally need to be done in a hospital operating room.

You may be able to go home the day of your operation—and usually will if only the excess skin and fat are removed. If the muscle is also repaired and fat suctioned, you usually need at least one night in the hospital.

Conditions That Increase Your Risk

Heavy smoking (one pack or more a day) will increase your risk of infection. Smoking also will make you tend to cough after general anesthesia, and a bout of coughing increases your pain and may pull out or loosen stitches. Having previously had **phlebitis** (blood clots in the deep veins of the legs) slightly increases your risk of phlebitis from this operation—not nearly to the extent that a major abdominal "tuck" does, though, because you will be up and about sooner. If you have phlebitis *now*, your surgeon will postpone your surgery. The medicine you are taking greatly increases the risk of excessive bleeding during surgery.

Scarring in the lower abdomen increases your risk of poor healing: each scar cuts off *some* of the blood flow to your abdominal skin. If you have *extensive* lower abdominal scarring, this operation may not be possible for you. Instead, you may need a major abdominal "tuck" to remove all of the scarred skin.

Usual Anesthesia

If your operation will only remove the excess skin and fat, it may be done with local anesthesia and sedation.

If muscle repair is needed, or if fat is going to be *suctioned* out, as well as cut out with the skin, then *general* anesthesia is required.

How Long It Takes

A mini-tuck will take your surgeon 1 to 2 hours to do. The longer time is needed if all three procedures—cutting away excess skin and fat, muscle repair, *and* fat suctioning—are required. Also, if you tend to bleed a lot, your surgery may take longer to stop the bleeding.

The Operation
(Figures 13-4 through 13-6)

Before

You will arrive for your surgery about an hour before the operation, having had nothing to eat or drink since midnight the night before. You will change into a hospital gown before going to a preoperative area. An IV will be placed in your arm, so that you can be given a solution of dextrose and/or saline to prevent dehydration during surgery. Sedatives and anesthetic will also be given through the IV. A blood-pressure cuff may be put on your other arm. Your surgeon will see you, and if you are having general anesthesia, an anesthetist will see you. Blood and urine samples may be taken if this was not done before. You will probably be given sedation in the preoperative area. Your surgeon may mark the incision areas in purple surgical ink, or he may wait until you are asleep. Your pubic hair will not be shaved.

Once you are in the operating room and on the operating table, a safety belt strap is placed across your hips. Sticky pads are put on your chest for the heart monitor and another sticky pad is put on your hip or thigh. This is a grounding pad to make the surgical cautery safe to use. (Surgical cautery means using an electrical heat device to seal off bleeding blood vessels.)

Unless you are having local/sedation (unusual), you are now given an injection through your IV to put you to sleep. Once you are asleep, a tube is put down your throat to deliver a mixture of gas and oxygen directly to your lungs to keep you asleep. Your abdomen is washed with surgical soap and sterile surgical drapes are put over your body and around the surgical area. (If you are only having sedation, you are given enough sedation to make you doze, and the lower abdomen skin is injected with local anesthetic.)

During

The surgeon will perform one or more of these steps, depending on your needs.

Fat Suction. This is usually done first, if at all. The surgeon makes a small incision (usually around your navel) and pushes the long, hollow metal suction tube through to make a tunnel under your skin. This does not sound delicate, and it isn't. Liposuction is a physically strenuous surgical procedure for your surgeon. The tube is drawn forcefully back and forth in that tunnel about ten times. Then the procedure is repeated in adjacent areas until all excess fat has been sucked out (see Suction Lipectomy). Depending on where the excess abdominal fat lies, the suction may be done through an incision above your pubic mound instead of, or in addition to, the incision at the navel.

Removal of Excess Skin. The skin above the pubic mound is incised for 6 to 8 inches *or* whatever length is needed to remove the fold of excess skin. (For people who have lost 50 pounds or so, the excess skin fold may go from hip to hip.) A person who has lost a great deal of weight may have a skin fold 3 or 4 inches wide and weighing 4 or more *pounds*. For a thin person whose skin has stretched from pregnancy, the excess skin will weigh *ounces*.

Tightening of the Muscles. After cutting through the skin, the surgeon separates the skin from the abdominal muscle beneath it and lifts the skin free up to the navel. The blood vessels that travel from the muscle to the skin must be cut and tied (ligated) or cauterized to stop the bleeding. The lower abdominal muscles are tightened by sewing the stretched muscle bundles close together; the muscles are not cut. Once the muscles have been tightened, the skin is pulled down over them and trimmed so that no excess skin is left behind. Since the navel is not moved, skin can only be pulled down a short distance or it may pull the navel out of shape. Finally, the skin is stitched together. Your abdomen is washed and bandages are put on.

"Mini-Tummy Tuck"

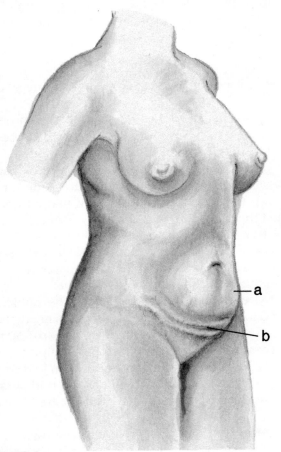

Figure 13-4.

This patient is a good candidate for a mini-tummy tuck. Only the lower abdomen (a) has loose muscle and some excess fat; the loose skin (b) is only on the lower part of the abdomen.

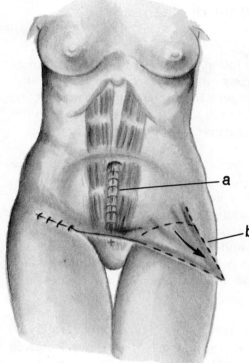

Figure 13-5.

The rectus muscle has been stitched in the lower part of the abdomen, below the navel, to tighten it (a). The excess central fat can be removed by suction. The excess skin (b) is being pulled down to be cut off.

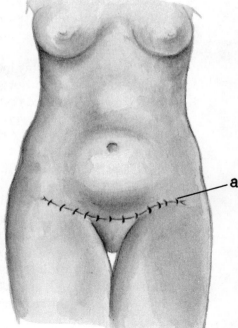

Figure 13-6.

The scar (a) is shorter than that needed for a *major* abdominal cosmetic operation, but it is not tiny. Notice that with a mini-tummy tuck, the navel is unchanged.

The Process of Recovery

What to Do About Pain

You will hurt after this operation, especially when you sit up or try to get out of bed, because of the pull on muscle and skin stitches. This pain is *not* agony, but most people need narcotic painkillers. These may be in pill form, but while you are in the hospital, you may need injections for the first 24 to 48 hours after surgery.

Some people have *no* pain after surgery—they tend to be people in peak physical condition. Smokers will have *more* pain than average, because they will tend to cough. The pain will *usually* be gone between 3 and 5 days after surgery. Then, you will have an intermittent aching that improves after a night's sleep and worsens at the end of a day. General anesthesia will be your biggest hurdle. You will be tired from the anesthesia for 2 weeks and will have continuing fatigue for up to 6 weeks.

The Healing Process

You can bathe or shower within 3 to 5 days after surgery. A shower is preferable, but if you take a tub bath, don't soak in the tub. You may be so sore that climbing in the tub puts you at risk for a fall.

You should *not* stay in bed. Most surgeons will want you up and walking the day of surgery, to decrease your risk of phlebitis. However, you will need rest. For the first week you'll spend much of the day resting and you will nap for 4 hours, or more, during the day. If you stay in the hospital after this surgery, you will go home after 1 or 2 days.

It will be hard to stand up straight at first. After 5 days, you can stand straight, but it takes a moment after you get up.

Your lower abdomen will be swollen. You may notice by the end of a day that the abdominal swelling is less, but your feet are puffy. You may not be bruised, but if you are it will show up first in your lower abdomen. After a week bruising will have moved to your groin. This does *not* mean that you have been bruised here; it means that gravity has pulled the bruising down. You will be too sore to sleep on your stomach for 3 to 4 weeks.

Bandages

You will have gauze over the stitches in the lower abdomen, held on with underpants or tape (the tape *hurts,* so avoid it if possible). You may also wear a girdle, body stocking, or binder. You will need gauze over the incision for 2 to 3 weeks, for comfort.

Your surgeon chooses what bandage to use. Until quite recently, the abdomen was wrapped with layers of elastic bandages, most of which rapidly came loose. These days your surgeon is more likely to ask you to buy a comfortable panty girdle or body stocking before surgery. This can be fitted on you as a bandage and kept in place for several days. Or your surgeon may order a special surgical girdle for you—these tend to be expensive. I prefer my patients to find a girdle that fits them, since shapes vary. Your surgeon may prefer to use a binder— an elastic wrap around your abdomen, usually held together with a Velcro strip. Male patients prefer this. It is easier to put on than the girdle, but it tends to need frequent adjusting to keep it in place.

Taking Care of Your Wound

You'll have little wound care to do, other than changing the gauze bandages once a day after you shower or bathe. Some surgeons will not let you bathe until your stitches are out—this may be *2 weeks.* I think it helps to leave your bandage on while you shower or bathe. It's easier to remove wet than dry.

Stitches

You will have internal stitches in your muscles, if these were repaired. The muscle stitches do not come out. You will have some absorbable stitches in the deep skin layers. You will probably also have a "pull-out" stitch—starting at one end of your incision and ending at the other end, running below your skin. This stitch does not leave cross-hatch scars, and it can stay in for 2 to 3 weeks. However, it is not as precise as the individual stitches ("interrupted sutures") that you see outside, across your skin. These will leave scars if they stay in for more than 5 to 7 days. They are removed within a week.

Scars

The scar goes across your abdomen, just above the pubic mound. It will be approximately 6 to 8 inches long. If you had fat suctioning, you will probably also have a scar near the navel, where the suction tube was inserted. This scar will not be noticeable. However, the scar near the pubis will probably be red, lumpy, and firm for 6 to 18 *months* after surgery. This is *not* a good scar area—its advantage is that it is not visible when you are dressed.

Tips

- Before you consider a mini-tuck, you should, ideally, be down to your normal weight, not be planning a pregnancy, and have tried spot exercising to tighten your stomach muscles.
- The surgery will dry your skin, because the trauma of surgery decreases the skin's oil production. Buy a large jar of body cream and rub it gently into the abdominal skin—staying away from stitches—once your bandages are off.
- Your abdomen will be sore and swollen. Wear loose clothes for up to 6 weeks after surgery.
- You can decrease the swelling in your abdomen with the pressure of an elastic body stocking or panty girdle (women) or an abdominal binder (men). A binder is like an extra-wide belt that spans the abdomen from hip to ribs and is worn under your clothes, fastened with Velcro or hooks. Many pharmacies carry them.

Back to Work

You can return to work after 2 weeks. Occasionally, a person returns as early as 10 days—but very tired. Even at 2 weeks, work will be a strain if you had general anesthesia—less if you had local with sedation. You can manage a desk job if you arrange nothing extra for the first 2 weeks back.

Back to Parties

You will be able to enjoy an early-evening dinner party 3 weeks after your operation. A cocktail party, a late evening, or dancing are out for 4 to 6 weeks after surgery.

Back to Sports

You can do easy stretches after one week—you should feel a pull, but not more. If you had local/sedation, after 2 weeks you can swim slowly for 15 minutes and do 15 minutes of exercises, again not going beyond a pulling sensation. You can also walk or work out with a bicycle. You will progress each week—and you'll be back in shape at 6 weeks.

If you had general anesthesia, you cannot make rapid progress. The anesthesia slows you down, and too much exercise will delay your recovery. Stretches and gentle swimming are fine for 2 to 4 weeks. After 4 to 6 weeks you can do most sports—but no contact sports until 6 weeks.

"Mini-Tummy Tuck": Recovery-at-a-Glance

This chart represents the *average* recovery times for this cosmetic operation.

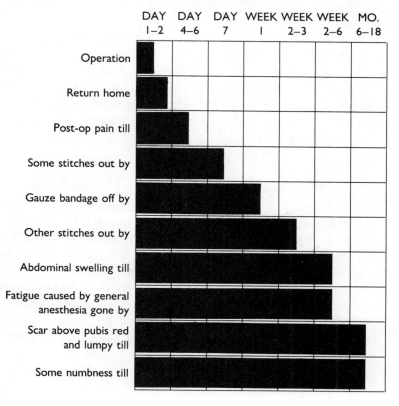

	DAY 1–2	DAY 4–6	DAY 7	WEEK 1	WEEK 2–3	WEEK 2–6	MO. 6–18
Operation	■						
Return home	■						
Post-op pain till	■■						
Some stitches out by	■■■						
Gauze bandage off by	■■■■						
Other stitches out by	■■■■■						
Abdominal swelling till	■■■■■■						
Fatigue caused by general anesthesia gone by	■■■■■■						
Scar above pubis red and lumpy till	■■■■■■■						
Some numbness till	■■■■■■■						

Back to Sex

For 2 weeks sex is out, because you may loosen an inside stitch or pull apart your incision. After that, sex is not harmful, but fatigue—especially if you go back to work early—may leave you without sexual desire for several weeks more.

How Much It Costs

Your surgeon's fee could be as low as $1000 to treat only excess skin—or as high as $3000 if muscle repair and fat suctioning are also needed.

Your hospital cost will range from about $1000 for local anesthesia with sedation if your tuck is done on an outpatient basis to $3000 for general anesthesia and several nights in the hospital.

Insurance Coverage

Insurance will not pay unless you can prove that the muscle weakness or skin excess is causing a medical problem such as skin crease infections or back pain. Since this operation is for lesser abdominal problems than those needing the full tummy tuck, your insurance company will not be easily persuaded that the operation is medically necessary. If your problem or your insurance company might be the exception, turn to the insurance section of Major Cosmetic Abdominal Surgery to know exactly how to handle insurance.

My Assessment of This Procedure

The mini-tuck has been developed over the past 10 years for people who need some abdominal improvement but for whom the major "tummy tuck" is too much surgery for too small a problem. About half the "tucks" I do are major; half are "mini." For some people, the decision is hard. A mini-tuck isn't enough but the major tuck seems like too much to go through.

An abdominal bulge may reflect not only skin, fat, and underlying muscle, but also your posture, spinal alignment, and the fat stored around your intestines. Therefore, the surgical results are at times unpredictable.

Side Effects and Complications

Side Effects

The side effects and complications of mini-tuck **surgery** are similar to those that develop from a major tuck, but since the "mini" surgery is less extensive, the risks are correspondingly less.

You will have a scar in the lower abdomen, which will be lumpy, firm, and red for 6 to 18 months. Your skin will be largely numb in the midabdomen, with diminished feeling at the sides. The feeling begins to return within weeks and may have returned in all but scattered patches within a few months.

However, **liposuction** has its own complications and problems. The area that is suctioned may develop ridges from the tunneling under the skin and from unevenness in the fat removal. The suctioning may irritate the skin, leaving patches of brownish discoloration that may be faintly visible—permanently. Also, the suctioning can cause a blister like accumulation called a seroma deep in the skin. This may absorb or it may need to be drawn off with a needle in the surgeon's office (don't panic—the numbness of your skin after surgery makes this *painless*).

The ridges from the suctioning are partly from swelling, which subsides in 6 to 12 months, but also from irregularities which may leave a permanent waviness in the skin. Studies show that about 10 percent of people after liposuction have—or would like to have, given the time and money—touch-up liposuction to smooth out such less-than-perfect areas. The newer smaller suction tubes may greatly lessen this problem.

Complications

Bleeding, infection, phlebitis, and poor healing are all possible, as they are after the major "tummy tuck," but with this less extensive surgery, complications are correspondingly rarer. Disappointment is probably the most common "complication"—a bad scar, distorted navel, waviness from liposuction, or residual protrusion in your lower abdomen; in other words, still dissatisfied that your stomach isn't "bikini perfect."

Rebecca: Still No Bikini

Rebecca was 38 and had lost 10 pounds in the past year. She had two children and was not planning to have more. Her lower abdomen bulged forward noticeably, giving her a "swaybacked" look. Her problem was in the lower abdomen and was not bad enough to justify a major tummy tuck, so I advised her to have a "mini." Rebecca's goal was to wear a bikini. I told her that surgery would improve her appearance but I could not predict if she would want to expose her abdomen.

At surgery, I did liposuction of the fatty deposits, repaired her stretched muscle, and removed excess skin. There was not much. She had little bruising and swelling, but her scars were lumpy and red. Also, although she now had a nice profile, she still didn't feel right in a bikini. Even though she knew surgery couldn't promise what she wanted, she was disappointed with her result.

Emory: No More "Jelly Roll"

Emory had been overweight for 10 years. He finally lost 75 pounds after marrying the woman of his dreams. She helped him diet—and told him that he should rid himself of the large "apron" of skin hanging over his groin after his diet.

Emory was in good physical shape—he and his wife swam every morning in their pool. His muscles were strong. His problem was the excess skin.

Emory had surgery as an outpatient with local plus sedation. I removed 12 pounds of excess skin and contoured the lower abdominal skin to lie as smooth as possible. He did not need a liposuction.

Emory was sore, which was inevitable. He wanted to work after one week, but his wife insisted that he not push himself. He was delighted to be without his "jelly roll," as he called his stretched skin.

Isabel: Leotard Perfect

Isabel was 30, slim, the mother of one child, and a devotée of body building when she came to see me for a mini-tuck. Her complaint was that her "line" in her leotard held her back from success in body building competition. The bulge was from weak muscles, damaged from a Cesarean section and Isabel wanted it surgically corrected.

Isabel had no excess fat. She had a little loose skin, but her chief problem was damaged muscle. I did a mini-tummy tuck with no liposuction and minimal *skin removal. The operation repaired muscle that had been stretched by pregnancy and scarred by the Cesarean incision from navel to pubis.*

Isabel had general anesthesia and spent one night in the hospital. She did body building exercises for her arms the day after surgery. She was tired but had no pain—a result of her excellent muscle condition. She went back to work as an aerobics instructor after 2 weeks, but she led her classes for the first week without actively demonstrating.

The operation did what she wanted—her now-flat abdomen looked perfect in a leotard except that her lumpy scars showed through, very faintly. She won her next competition.

What Other Patients Say

- **Actress, 41** (after weight loss): "It's marvelous except for my scar. And I'm too chubby. And I'm out of shape. But the *surgery* did what it was supposed to do. The rest is me."
- **Airport supervisor, 59** (after multiple operations for a bladder problem): "I had an infection, which I'm prone to get. I was out of work a full month. I used to *feel* my lower belly when I sat down. That's gone. Haven't looked at the scars, so they must be fine. My wife gets a chuckle because she says I don't walk as though the bottom is falling out anymore. Easiest operation I've had."
- **Mother, 26** (after a pregnancy and losing 20 pounds): "My husband got worried when I had the surgery. He joked that it meant I was getting ready to leave him. He said he loved me, no matter how I looked. Pregnancy destroyed my figure, and I wasn't about to live with that—at any age. I'm good enough to wear baby doll pajamas again, and tight jeans, and that was all I asked."
- **Divorced socialite, 44** (after pregnancy): "I had a sloppy lower abdomen. Surgery tightened things up. That was all I asked."

Liposuction

What Surgeons Call It

The technical term for this procedure is suction lipectomy or suction assisted lipectomy.

What It Will Do

This procedure permanently removes fat deposits by sucking them out, making your body proportions permanently better.

What It Won't Do

Liposuction does *not* replace weight loss. If you are fat before, you will be fat afterwards. However, it gets rid of fat deposits like thigh or tummy bulges that won't go away except with extreme dieting that leaves you too thin.

How Long It Lasts

Liposuction is permanently effective because the suction removes the fat cells in which the fat in that body area was stored. However, fat cells elsewhere in your body will continue to store excess fat.

When to Have It

Suction lipectomy may work well for you if you have unsightly bulges anywhere on your body that dieting and exercise can't improve. If you are dieting, wait until after the diet to have suction lipectomy and let it smooth out the bulges that remain at your new weight.

Dieting and fat suctioning achieve the same result: both remove fat from under your skin. But, you can't control *where* you lose the weight on a diet. Before you rush to a cosmetic surgeon for a fat suction, though, get down to your best *realistic* weight. You *may* find that your "disproportionate" hips can be dieted away—dieting is safer and cheaper than fat suction!

Where to Have It

This operation is usually done on an outpatient basis in a doctor's office operating room *or* a surgery center operating room *or* a hospital operating room. You may need to stay in the hospital overnight if a large amount of fat is suctioned from your body.

Conditions That Increase Your Risk

Phlebitis can occur and has been fatal to a patient after suction lipectomy. If you have had phlebitis you are at an increased risk of having it recur.

Usual Anesthesia

Local anesthesia with sedation is used when small areas are suctioned—for instance, around the chin. General anesthesia is required for most liposuction of the hips, buttocks, and thighs.

How Long It Takes

This depends on how much will be suctioned. On average, 1 to 2 hours is needed, unless the treated area is small.

The Operation
(Figure 13-7)

The exact procedure your surgeon uses will vary according to what you are having done. However, most people have suction of the hips and buttocks, so that is what I'll describe here.

Before

You will arrive about an hour before your surgery, having had nothing to eat or drink since midnight the night before. If the suctioning is going to be extensive, you may have donated a unit of your own blood for use during your surgery, to avoid the risks from transfusions from a stranger. For general anesthesia, your blood and urine will be tested to be sure that you are not anemic and that your kidneys are working properly. This might be done the morning of surgery, or a day or two before.

You will change into a hospital gown. Your surgeon will see you and, with you standing, will mark the areas that he will suction. (He may have done this the day before.) An IV will be placed in your arm so that you can be given a solution of dextrose and/or saline to prevent dehydration during surgery. You will be given some sedation by mouth, injection, or IV after your anesthesiologist has seen you. You will then be taken to the operating room.

Once you are on the operating table, a safety strap will be fastened over you. Elastic stockings may be placed on your legs. Sticky pads will be put on your chest for the heart monitor, and a pad will be put on your hip as a ground for the electrical cautery device that is used to seal off bleeding vessels. You will be given an intravenous drug such as pentothal and you will go to sleep.

Once you are asleep, the areas to be suctioned will be washed with surgical soap. If both your buttocks and thighs are being suctioned, you will be turned over halfway through the surgery. Usually, the surgery will start with you on your stomach, because so much of the fat will be on your sides and back.

During

After sterile surgical drapes are put over your body, your surgeon will make a tiny (about an inch) incision in the first suction area. He will push the suction tube through the incision into the excess fat. Then he will move the tube back and forth repeatedly in the excess fat. (The large suction tubes require considerable physical strength. The new smaller ones make liposuction less strenuous for a surgeon.) The back-and-forth motion of the tube loosens the fat cells and vacuums them out of your body. The fat comes out first, then blood from small torn blood vessels. When more blood than fat is coming out, the suction is over.

Your surgeon then removes the suction tube and goes to the next area, making a tiny incision as before and inserting the suction tube. He may return to the first area at the end to do more until it matches the other side. When he has finished the areas within reach—for instance, suctioning your waistline, hips, and buttocks from the back—he will stitch each incision. Then you are turned onto your back, for suctioning of fat deposits on the front of your body.

During your surgery, you will be given lots of intravenous fluids to replace fluids being suctioned out of your body. The suctioned material is measured, and your surgeon may give you a transfusion of plasma protein or your own blood, if he suctions out more than about 1500 milliliters (several quarts). If your suction surgery is extensive (1000 milliliters or more), you may be given alcohol intravenously to decrease your risk of blood clots in your veins. Not all surgeons do this, but it appears to help in preventing clots from forming.

Minor Suctioning

For minor suctioning when you are awake, the routine is the same until you reach the operating room. Then, instead of being put to sleep you will be sedated until you relax. Your surgeon will then inject the fat deposit with local anesthetic and will make a tiny stab incision—you will feel pressure, but not pain. You will feel more pressure when the suction tube is inserted. During the suction, you will be aware of vibration or friction under your skin. You may feel some stinging pain near the end—when the

Liposuction

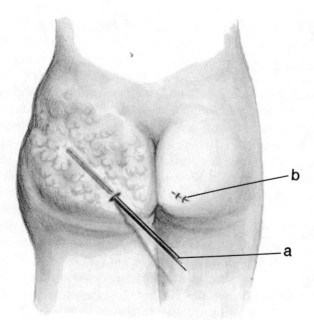

Figure 13-7.

This figure depicts the suction cannula (a) being inserted through a small incision in the buttock, and into the fat deposits of the hip. It will be moved back and forth 20 to 30 times in each of many similar positions to remove the fat. Note that the scar (b) intentionally lies above the buttock crease, so as not to show in sports clothes.

suction tube has removed the fat and suctions near the muscle beneath. Suctioning done with local anesthesia is usually brief and will rarely last over 30 minutes.

After

At the end of your surgery, the soap is washed off your skin and a Band-Aid or gauze is placed over each incision. Support bandages or a girdle are put on (see Bandages), and you are taken by stretcher to the recovery room. If you had over 2000 milliliters suctioned, you will almost certainly spend a night in hospital. If you had 750 to 1500 milliliters suctioned, you are likely to be allowed to go home that day. If you had only minimal suctioning—500 milliliters or less—you will almost certainly go home that day.

The Process of Recovery

What to Do About Pain

You will ache and be sore after liposuction surgery. If your hips and buttocks have been suctioned, you may be uncomfortable in virtually any position, sitting or lying down. You will be given prescriptions for pain, or you may take an acetaminophen (Tylenol) for mild pain. Do *not* take aspirin or any aspirin-containing product. The salicylate in the aspirin may make you bleed and will make your bruising much worse. By 2 days after surgery, you may feel stiff and sore, but you should not hurt.

The Healing Process

You will need to wear a snug support garment like a long-leg panty girdle for about 2 weeks, or until all your bruising is gone. The general anesthesia will leave you very tired for 10 to 14 days. You will be swollen at first, and swelling *may* obscure all or most of your improvement. The swelling will take about 2 weeks to resolve so that you can really see your new contour.

Bandages

- If your abdomen, thighs, or hips are being done, your surgeon may ask you to buy a long-leg panty girdle, or he may order one for you from a surgical supply company.

- If your chin is suctioned, you will have a support bandage, either an elastic wrap or a surgical chin support.
- If your lower legs or ankles are suctioned, you will wear knee-high support stockings.

You'll wear your support bandages until the bruising is gone, or, if on your face, for 5 days. Usually, for the first 2 to 5 days, you will not change the bandages. (The crotch of the panty girdle is cut out, to allow you to go to the bathroom.) After about 5 days, you can remove the bandages to bathe.

Taking Care of Your Wounds

Even when the liposuctioned areas are large, the *wounds* are small. Your wounds will need no special care. Your suctioned skin will be dry. Rub body cream into the dry skin once or twice a day until the dryness is gone.

Stitches

You will have a few stitches in each incision. These are removed 7 to 10 days after surgery.

Scars

You will have a small (1 inch or less) scar in each suctioned area. If your hips and thighs were suctioned, you will have six small incisions: one in each buttock crease, one at the top of each buttock, and one in the groin crease on each side, in front. These scars are usually a quarter-inch wide and pink or brown. The color fades in time but won't vanish. However, the scars are placed so that even most bikinis will cover them.

Tips

- Liposuction was developed in Germany and France and was introduced to the United States about 5 years ago. It does *not* make you thin. It cannot replace dieting . . . alas.
- Suction lipectomy *will* remove excess fat from areas that are fat out of proportion to the rest of your body.
- Cellulite is the popular name for the indented irregular appearance of the skin that is seen over the hips and thighs and buttocks of some overweight women. Liposuction removes *underlying fat*—it does *not* change the skin texture!

- Wear loose clothes. You will be stiff and will want to get into clothes easily.
- Ice will not help the large suctioned areas when they ache. You may find that sitting is uncomfortable, but a soft down pillow may make it tolerable.

Back to Work

The anesthesia will leave you tired. You will not be able to work for 7 to 14 days. Besides, when your hips, thighs, and buttocks are suctioned, it will be about a week before you can walk and sit comfortably enough to think about work.

Back to Parties

Wait 2 weeks, minimum, and preferably 3. The anesthesia leaves you tired, *but also* your legs will tire and swell easily. You won't want to dance, and standing will make your legs ache. An early-evening sit-down dinner party is reasonable at 2 weeks, but it will be too much if you are also returning to work.

Liposuction: Recovery-at-a-Glance

This chart represents the *average* recovery times for this cosmetic operation.

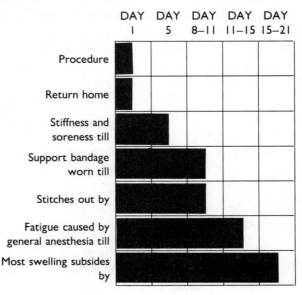

	DAY 1	DAY 5	DAY 8–11	DAY 11–15	DAY 15–21
Procedure					
Return home					
Stiffness and soreness till					
Support bandage worn till					
Stitches out by					
Fatigue caused by general anesthesia till					
Most swelling subsides by					

Back to Sports

You can do stretching and bending exercises between 10 and 14 days after suction lipectomy. You may be allowed to swim after 14 days—it stimulates your body to absorb residual swelling. Most sports involve vigorous leg work—tennis, aerobics, bicycling, dance, jogging. You can't do these for at least 3 weeks. If you start too early, your legs will ache and may swell.

Back to Sex

If you have no excess fluid or blood in the suctioned areas, you can resume sex after 1 week. However, the fatigue and numbness and swelling in your skin may make sex less pleasurable than usual. You will still be bruised, too. It's easier on *you* if you wait 10 to 14 days.

How Much It Costs

Costs will vary greatly, because a suction lipectomy can be for one small area or several large ones. Suction of a double chin, done in the office with local anesthesia, could cost as little as $500.

On the other hand, if your hips, thighs, and buttocks are suctioned at one time, your surgery requires general anesthesia and is much more extensive. You may pay $3000 to $5000 (or more) for your surgeon, and at least $1000 and up to $3000 for general anesthesia and a hospital stay.

Insurance Coverage

Insurance will *not* pay for liposuction except in unusual circumstances—for instance, if scarring from a car accident left extensive indentations that required contouring with suction lipectomy.

My Assessment of This Operation

This technique is still new. It is extremely good for a problem plaguing surgeons and patients for years—how to eliminate fat in the body. Newer techniques continue to be developed. For instance, the smaller suction tubes now available that probably cause less skin irritation, swelling, and bleeding. More advances will probably be made in the next several years.

Side Effects and Complications

Side Effects

One side effect which you cannot control is where your future fat will go. After liposuction, you may lose a pound or two that you don't regain. However, if you regain more weight, it has to go somewhere. Your body will store it in new areas. You could have your hips suctioned to perfection and find that your breasts, arms, or chin now get heavy when you gain weight. This of course can be reversed by dieting.

Fat suction is done "blind." Your surgeon feels the suction tube as it moves under your skin. The suctioned area quickly swells, making it more difficult for your surgeon to determine exactly where the excess fat lies. About 10 percent of patients will have minor areas that need resuctioning to get a good result. This is often a minor procedure done on an outpatient basis and under local anesthesia. Depending on your surgeon's policy, you may have to pay for this. The cost is almost always much less than the original surgery, but discuss cost with your surgeon ahead of time.

Some people have more skin color than others. Liposuction may irritate the skin and stimulate it to produce a blotchy brown color in the suctioned area. This may require skin bleaching cream and time (a year or more) to fade. (Most people know if their skin tends to discolor. If minor skin trauma leaves you with brown marks, you are more likely to get skin blotchiness after fat suctioning.)

Because the fat cells are pulled out of your body, the suctioned area will tend to ooze fluid into the suctioned space. You may develop a fluid collection (seroma) or a blood clot (hematoma) where you were suctioned. These can usually be treated by drawing the blood or fluid off in the office with a needle and syringe. In rare cases, re-operation to drain the fluid is needed.

Complications

Your most serious complication would be developing a blood clot in a leg vein (phlebitis). This itself is not so serious, but if one of the clots breaks loose and moves to your lungs, it can cause serious breathing difficulty. Fat suctioning often requires general anesthesia, which increases the risk of phlebitis. Also, surgery being done around the legs seems to irritate the leg veins. It's also possible that the fat suctioning may release chemicals—and fat—into your bloodstream.

Finally, the fat suctioning makes you less active than usual, and this also increases your risk of phlebitis. Your surgeon will use various ways to protect you. Elastic leg bandages, early walking, being physically fit, and intravenous alcohol all may be used. If you do get a leg blood clot, it may show up as leg swelling or pain. You will need leg and lung tests and will need to take blood-thinning medication for 3 to 6 months.

Jeannine: No Skimpy Tennis Togs

Jeannine was in her forties and loved to play tennis. She hated her heavy hips and thighs and had them suctioned. This definitely improved her shape, but her goal had been to wear skimpy tennis dresses. She hadn't worn them before her fat suction surgery, because her thighs looked too heavy. But she didn't wear such sports clothes afterwards, either. The fat suction left her hips splotched with brown and the swelling gave her skin a roughened texture that lasted for over a year.

Rona: Some Residual Lumpiness

Rona was an attractive young woman writer who had heavy hips. Despite daily exercise and being slightly underweight her hips were far too heavy. Rona had her hips suctioned and was thrilled. One side was perfect. The other had a small residual lump but she felt that this, compared to what she had been, was totally insignificant.

Rupert: Hard to Please

Rupert was in his early thirties and worked as a design engineer. He was slightly overweight, and always had been. He was a little out of shape, but he exercised on occasion. He had a bulge around his waist at the back, just above his buttocks (sometimes called a "love handle"). He wanted it gone. Rupert had fat suctioning in this area. The fat suctioning smoothed out the love handles, and the two scars (one on each side, high on the buttock) were not noticeable. Still, Rupert wasn't completely pleased. He felt that with the fat gone, his skin now was looser and that bothered him. He had known that the liposuction would loosen the skin, but there was no way to remove the loose skin without leaving a scar across his lower back. He was pleased with the fat suction, but not with his body.

Clarissa: Thrilled

Clarissa had lost 30 pounds. She was in her twenties and very physically active. Fortunately she had not damaged her skin elasticity, but she knew she would never be thin, and her buttocks, hips, thighs, and abdomen all had bulges she wished were gone. Clarissa had extensive suction lipectomy—on every bulging area. Most of the suctioning was on her hips and the least was done on her inner thighs (an area that can be oversuctioned because the fat is so delicate here). Clarissa had 2000 milliliters of fat suctioned out of her body and had a blood transfusion (of her own blood). She spent a night in the hospital. She was bruised from her waist down for several weeks, and she was out of work for 10 days—but she was thrilled. In profile and in front view she had lost the fat deposits that had made her body bulgy. She kept her weight off and preserved her new profile(s).

What Other Patients Say

- **Housewife, 40**: "I wanted a 25-inch waist back. I didn't get it. I went from a 29 to a 28. Still, I like the difference."
- **Woman jogger, 29**: "I'm a perfectionist and my buttocks were the last part I needed to fix up. Running didn't get it off. The suction did."
- **Female secretary, 35**: "I sit all day and every fat cell sank down. It made a world of difference to how I feel about myself. I don't cringe in front of the mirror anymore."
- **Male college student, 21**: "I had a double chin. And I wasn't fat but my chin made me look fat. Now it's gone. It was neat."
- **Businessman, 45**: "I knew it wouldn't do wonders. I'm fat. I'll always be fat. It got rid of a bulge I couldn't stand any longer."

Arm Lift

What Surgeons Call It

This operation is known technically as a brachioplasty or resection of lipocutaneous excess of arms.

What It Will Do

Cosmetic arm tightening aims to remove excess skin and underlying fat from your arms so that you don't have loose skin hanging from them.

What It Won't Do

The operation will not necessarily make you feel comfortable exposing your arms if you now cover them with clothes. It *may*, depending on how you scar.

How Long It Will Last

This operation is permanent, because it removes the stretched skin from your arms. In time, this skin may loosen to a slight degree, but it would take years before more surgery was needed. An exception would be if you gained a lot of weight (50 pounds) and lost it again. That would stretch your skin and *might* stretch it enough to need more skin removed.

When to Have It

Loose skin tends to develop on your arms in middle age, when some of the muscle bulk in the arms decreases. Working out with weights may fill out the loose skin, so it is worth a try for minor looseness. However, if you have been overweight and have lost weight, your skin may be flabby—at any age. If the skin is stretched beyond what exercise will reasonably fill in, surgery is your next step.

Where to Have It

Unless it is done in combination with other procedures so that general anesthesia is necessary, this procedure is usually done on an outpatient basis in a doctor's office operating room *or* an outpatient surgery center *or* a hospital operating room.

Conditions That Increase Your Risk

If you have a known tendency to form **lumpy scars** that take a long time to fade, you might consider whether your improvement will be worth the scars. The surgery may make your arms swell temporarily. If you have any underlying condition that affects your arms, you will be at higher risk from this operation. A woman who has had a **mastectomy** should probably *not* have this operation. The mastectomy will have injured the lymph glands on the side of the mastectomy. An arm lift may cause permanent severe arm swelling.

Usual Anesthesia

An arm lift is usually done with local anesthesia and sedation. However, if it is done with other body contouring operations, the local anesthetic may exceed a safe dose for you. Thus, general anesthesia may be required.

How Long It Takes

Duration depends partly on how much excess skin is on your arms. In general the surgery will take 2 hours to do.

The Operation
(Figure 13-8)

Before

You will arrive about an hour before your surgery, having had nothing to eat or drink since midnight the night before. After changing into a hospital gown, you will go to a preoperative area or directly to the operating room. An IV will be placed in your arm so that you can be given a solution of dextrose and/or saline to prevent dehydration during surgery. Your surgeon will see you to mark the surgical area with purple surgical ink. You will need to sit up, with your arms out in the air.

Once you are strapped on the operating table, sticky pads will be placed on your chest to monitor your heart. Also, a sticky pad will be placed on your thigh under your gown to serve as a ground to make the surgical cautery safe to use. (The cautery means using an electrical instrument to seal off bleeding vessels.) Your arms will be strapped to support boards at your side or supported with straps to a bar over your head. They will be washed with surgical soap. Sterile drapes will be placed under and around your arms and over your body in such a way that you cannot see the surgery.

You will be given sedation through your IV, and your surgeon will inject local anesthetic into one side. (He may inject both sides at once if the skin to be removed is less than usual. The injections are most often done in two stages, to avoid too much local anesthetic in your body at one time.)

During

Your surgeon will cut into the skin where he has marked the excess. The nurse will hold your arm and move it so that the surgeon can work. Once the skin is cut, he will cut into the fat.

Arm Lift

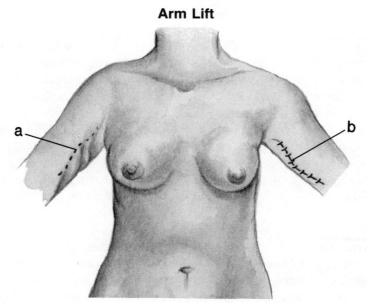

Figure 13-8.

Loose arm skin can be tightened. As you can see, the incision, indicated by the dotted line (a), is made on the *inner* surface of the arm. After the surgery, the skin is pulled tight. The scar (b) goes up to the axilla (armpit) and may go as low as the elbow.

Nerves, veins, and lymphatics lie deep in the fatty tissue. Your surgeon will leave the deeper layers of fat to avoid injury to these structures. Once the skin and fat have been removed, your surgeon adjusts the armpit skin to lie flat. Then the cautery will be used to seal off blood vessels. The surgeon will then put in the stitches to sew the skin together again. When one side is done, he will operate on the other side. Then your arms are washed free of soap, and the bandages are put on.

After

After the surgery, you go to the recovery room for about an hour. You can then be taken home to go to bed to rest.

The Process of Recovery

What to Do About Pain

Your arms will ache and feel sore. You will want to keep them propped up on several pillows, but that may put pressure on the incision lines. You may end up with no position that is really comfortable. (Supporting your *elbows* will work better—it takes pressure off the incisions *and* supports your arms.) You may need narcotic pain medication for a day or two. After that for most people acetaminophen (for example, Tylenol) is all that is needed except perhaps at night, when incisions tend to hurt. Do *not* take aspirin, because it will increase bruising and the risk of bleeding.

The Healing Process/Bandages

You will be bandaged for about 5 days. The first bandage will be several layers of gauze on the inside of your arm, with padding around the arm, all held on with one or two elastic wraps. This is bulky. (Wear loose-sleeved clothes to the operating room, or be prepared to have to cut the sleeves to accommodate your bandage.) After 5 days, your surgeon will remove the bandages but will keep your arms wrapped with an elastic bandage. You will feel comfortable with this support. After yet another 5 days, you will probably need no bandage other than tape strips across the incisions. These can be removed after another week.

Your arms will be visibly bruised and swollen for 2 weeks. Residual swelling may persist for weeks—noticeable when you put on tight-sleeved clothes.

Taking Care of Your Wound

With the lighter bandage after 5 days, you will be allowed to unwrap the bandage to bathe or shower. Pat or air dry the surgical areas. Put hand cream on your skin wherever there are no stitches. (The bandage will make your skin dry and itchy.) Then put on a layer of gauze and wrap on the elastic bandages again.

Arm Lift: Recovery-at-a-Glance

This chart represents the *average* recovery times for this cosmetic operation.

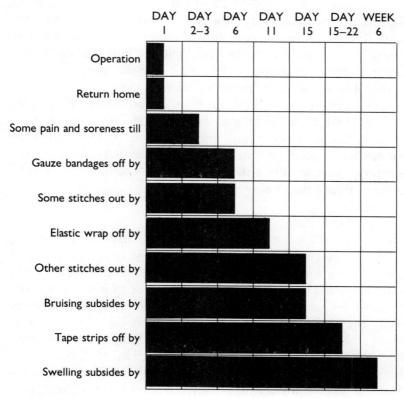

	DAY 1	DAY 2–3	DAY 6	DAY 11	DAY 15	DAY 15–22	WEEK 6
Operation	■						
Return home	■						
Some pain and soreness till		■					
Gauze bandages off by		■					
Some stitches out by		■					
Elastic wrap off by			■				
Other stitches out by				■			
Bruising subsides by					■		
Tape strips off by						■	
Swelling subsides by							■

If any elastic bandage feels too tight—loosen it. If your hands are puffy and swollen, you aren't keeping your arms up enough, the bandages are too tight, or both. Call your surgeon to let him know.

When you no longer need any bandage, keep the skin lubricated with lots of cream. Once the tape strips are off the scar you can rub cream into the scar as well to soften it.

Stitches

You will probably have several layers of stitches. The deepest layer of absorbable stitches will support your skin during healing. These don't always absorb completely. If tiny white dots appear in your scar, it is usually from an "absorbable" stitch that has not been absorbed and is working its way out. Your surgeon can remove it at the office.

The next layer of stitch will probably be a long, strong stitch extending from one end of the incision to the other under the skin. The stitch ends come out at either end of the incision. These "running subcuticular" or "pull-out" stitches are pulled out from the skin about 14 days after surgery. Their advantage is that they leave no stitch marks on your skin.

The last kind of stitch will be the traditional "interrupted suture," tied across your skin and secured with a knot. These stitches line your skin up as finely as possible. They can leave marks in your skin, so they are removed about 5 days after your surgery. However, the arm may heal slowly, and some of these stitches may have to stay in longer.

Scars

An arm lift will leave a long straight or S-shaped scar running down the inside of each arm from under your armpit to above the inner side of your elbow. This area does not tend to heal with fine white scars. You must assume that your scar will widen to about a quarter-inch or more. In time (6 to 18 months) these scars may blend in with your surrounding skin, but they may always be clearly visible. If your surgical goal is to have arms good enough to go sleeveless, balance that goal against the scars which may keep you from going sleeveless. However, the scars lie on the inner arm—the least conspicuous place. And, surgery is the only way to tighten loose, flabby skin here.

Tips

- An arm lift will leave a scar on the inside of your arm. If you are addicted to *sleeveless* dresses, invest in a few with sleeves to cover your arms to your elbows while you heal.
- Weight loss and being out of shape decreases the muscle bulk of your upper arms. If you are planning an exercise or weight *gain* program, postpone surgery until after you've achieved these goals.

Back to Work

As long as clothes conceal your bandage, you can work as early as 5 to 7 days after the surgery, unless the sedation has left you too tired. Your arms will ache at the end of a working day, and you should not be lifting or carrying. If yours is a "telephone" job, or if you direct others, work may be reasonable. For other jobs, 7 to 10 days is better than overusing your arms before they heal.

Back to Parties

You can go to a party after 5 days, if your clothes conceal the surgery. However, you will lack the energy to enjoy a late party, and your arms will ache by the end of the evening. They may also swell. Thus, it is best to avoid a party for 10 to 14 days. If you plan to dance, allow yourself 3 weeks.

Back to Sex

The tightening of your arm muscles during sexual stimulation can be enough to loosen or tear out a stitch. Also, you may fling your arms, forgetting for the moment to protect them. Although you can probably "get away with" having sex as early as a week after surgery, you should wait 2 weeks if you don't want the risk of pulling apart a segment of the incision, which would give you a wide scar in that area.

Back to Sports

You can limber up your legs and body after a week, but not your arms. You can take long walks and bicycle. After 10 days, you can swim, using a kickboard to rest your arms. You can play tennis after about 2 weeks—but no hard hitting for 3 weeks. Rowing, working out with arm weights, and any ball sport where you might get hit should wait for 3 to 4 weeks. If you play contact sports, you had best wait 4 weeks or more, depending on how roughly you play.

How Much It Costs

Your arm lift will cost about $1500 to $2500 for your surgeon's fee and about $1000 for the cost of the operating room.

Insurance Coverage

Insurance will rarely if ever pay for this operation. The flabby arm skin, although unappealing to you, does not cause skin rashes or irritation (unlike excess skin around the groin) except in unusual cases. Unless your case is unusual, insurance will not reimburse you.

My Assessment of This Procedure

An arm lift only removes excess skin and fat and the recovery is fairly easy. It is the only way to improve the contour of your arms if stretched skin hangs from them. Your major preoperative consideration should be the scars that the surgery will leave.

Side Effects and Complications

Side Effects

The most important side effect of an arm lift is the scar. The scar should lie on the inside of the arm, but it is likely to be wide. It may be lumpy for many months, or, it may be slightly sunken compared to your surrounding skin. Makeup of course can be used to camouflage the scar. A concealer stick can cover up the pink color of the scar while it heals.

If too much skin is removed, your skin may form transverse indentations where the stitches pull the skin together. In 3 to 6 months, these will flatten, as your arm skin readjusts. If too little skin is removed, your arm may still be flabby—you may need further surgery to remove the remaining excess, about 6 months after surgery.

The swelling in your arms may make the skin numb, temporarily. Also, some nerves to the skin are cut during surgery. You may have patchy areas of permanent numbness after the operation. This is not likely to bother you, since feeling in the arm is not as important as feeling in the face, hands, and feet.

Complications

The least common but most serious complication is **lymphedema**: swelling of the arm from cutting the lymphatics, which return tissue fluid in the arm to the blood. This condition may occur if your surgeon made a circular incision around your arm rather than a vertical one, or if he has taken out much fat deep in the arm. If lymphedema develops, you may need to wear an elastic support bandage on your arm for months to stop the swelling—and perhaps need to wear it at night, or during the day, for a long time, or permanently. (If your surgeon plans a circle incision around your upper arm, tell him "*Stop."* This problem occurred more often in the early days of arm lifting but is less likely to occur now.)

Joe: "The Flab Is Gone!"

Joe had been a professional athlete in his younger days. Then he "turned to fat." At 50 he had saggy arms that he could not abide. Working out with weights only helped a bit. Joe had an arm lift done under local anesthesia with sedation. He was an active man and had a hard time resting after surgery. As a result, his arms seemed to hurt him more than most people. At 2 weeks, although his scar was very red, Joe was delighted. The flab was gone. He didn't care about the rest.

Laura: A Major Weight Loss

Laura was in her twenties. After losing 50 pounds, she embarked on a program to rid herself of the skin that hung from her arms and elsewhere. She started with her arms, because they showed. The stretched skin on her breasts and abdomen was hidden by clothes. Laura had her surgery under general anesthesia—she was terrified of being awake. After surgery, she threw up, but then felt good enough to go home. Laura had very little pain after her surgery. She returned to work after a week, despite feeling tired from the general anesthetic. Her skin formed some cross-lines where too much skin was removed, but these flattened within 2 months. Laura was pleased with the surgery.

What Other Patients Say

- **Grandmother of eight, 68**: "I did my face and didn't look old except for my wrinkled arms. My mother had the same thing. My scar tanned right away and doesn't show."
- **Journalist, 51**: "Enough wasn't taken the first time. I wanted it done right, so we did it again. And the scar was just as wide the second time. There's no way I'd show off my arms. I don't want someone asking me how I got the scars."
- **Saleswoman, 63**: "It was quite easy for me. I lost only a few days from work, less than a week. I'm thrilled with not having that flab anymore. I also got engaged 3 months after surgery, so I'm thrilled with life in general."

Lifting of Hips, Thighs, and Buttocks

What Surgeons Call It

The technical term for this operation is resection of lipocutaneous excess of hips/thighs/buttocks or body contouring of hips/thighs/buttocks.

What It Will Do

The operation tightens loose skin from sagging buttocks, hips, or thighs so that loose skin does not hang from your body.

What It Won't Do

The thigh lift only tightens the skin of the upper thigh. Many women are bothered by loose skin or wrinkles around the knee. A thigh lift won't help.

How Long It Will Last

This is a permanent operation: the excess skin and the fat beneath are gone. However, if you gain weight after surgery, you can re-stretch the skin and scar—and require further surgery.

When to Have It

If weight changes caused your problem, be sure that your weight is now stable—so that you won't re-gain that weight.

Where to Have It

The surgery requires general anesthesia and one or more nights in the hospital. Thus, it is generally done in a hospital operating room.

Conditions That Increase Your Risk

If you have had phlebitis (blood clots from vein inflammation) in one or both legs in the past, you risk developing phlebitis again. This condition makes your legs hurt and swell. More dangerously, blood clots formed in your legs may loosen and move to your lungs, causing serious trouble with breathing. If you have phlebitis now, surgery must be postponed. Your risk of renewed phlebitis can be reduced by leg exercises before and after surgery and surgical support stockings. Be sure to tell your surgeon if you have had phlebitis in the past.

Usual Anesthesia

These operations require general anesthesia, because the local anesthetic needed to numb the area would exceed a safe dose.

How Long It Takes

Lifting the skin of the hips, thighs, or buttocks will usually take about 2 to 3 hours.

The Operation
(Figures 13-9 and 13-10)

Before

You will be brought to the operating room about an hour before your surgery, having had nothing to eat or drink since midnight the night before. If your surgeon has not already done your surgical markings, he will do them in the preoperative area. He needs to do these while you are standing. Also in the preoperative area, an IV will be placed in your arm so that you can be given a solution of saline and/or dextrose to prevent dehydration during surgery. An anesthetist will examine you, and you will be given some sedation and probably a dose of antibiotic through your IV.

You will next go to the operating room, where a safety strap will be put on. Sticky pads will be placed on your chest to monitor your heart. A sticky pad will be placed on your thigh under your gown to make the surgical cautery safe to use. (Surgical cautery means using an electrical heat device to seal off bleeding vessels.) Next you will be given an intravenous anesthetic such as pentothal and you will go to sleep. A tube will be put down your throat so the anesthetist can keep you asleep by giving you anesthetic gases mixed with oxygen. Once you are asleep, the surgical area is washed with surgical soap, and sterile drapes are placed over your body and around the surgical area. (If you

Thigh Lift

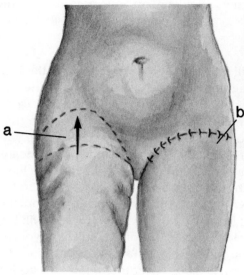

Figure 13-9.

The "before" view shows the upper thigh skin is loose. The dotted lines (a) indicate the amount of excess skin to be lifted and removed. In the "after" view, the final scar (b) lies in the crease of the groin. This surgery can lift the upper thighs but will *not* tighten loose skin around the knees.

Buttock Lift

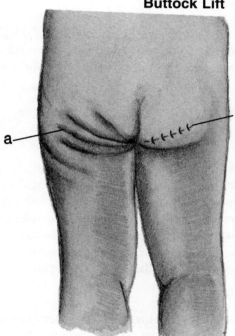

Figure 13-10.

The "before" view shows the skin of the buttock is loose and sagging (a). In the "after" view, the excess skin has been removed, as has the fat just below the skin. Note that the scar (b) is placed *above* the buttock crease. In time, the scar may shift downward. Thus a scar placed in the crease might shift further down, being too easily visible.

are having a buttock lift or a hip lift, you will be turned on your stomach for the surgery. You stay on your back for the thigh lift operation.)

During

Next the surgeon will inject dilute epinephrine into the incisions to diminish the bleeding. Then, following the marks, he will remove the excess skin down to the muscle, taking with it the thick layer of fat beneath the skin. If you are having a thigh lift, he will lift the skin to shift as much skin as possible up your leg. This is done to a lesser extent in buttock or hip lifts because the skin looseness does not extend down the back of the leg. Once the skin is cut out, the stitches are placed. You may need a drain (a plastic tube) under the incision if there has been much bleeding or fluid draining from the wound. Your surgeon will then operate on the other side. At the end of the surgery, your skin is washed to remove the surgical soap. Tape strips are placed across the incisions and gauze is placed over them. Finally, elastic wraps or a surgical girdle is placed on you.

After

From the operating room you go to the recovery room for about an hour. From there you will be taken to your hospital room.

The Process of Recovery

What to Do About Pain

The incisions are likely to hurt for several days, especially when you move or sit, which pulls on the stitches. When you are not moving, the incision area will ache and throb. For the first few days you will need narcotic painkillers by mouth, or by injection, given to you by the nurses while you are in hospital. By the end of a week, you will be stiff and ache at the end of the day, but should not need painkillers other than acetaminophen.

The Healing Process

You will need to see your surgeon a few days after leaving the hospital, and about a week after that. Your legs will tend to swell after the surgery, and you will need to wear knee-high support stockings for several weeks. The general anesthesia leaves most people very tired for at least 2 weeks—especially if the surgery lasted over 2 hours.

Bandages

You will have gauze bandages over your incisions—held on with tape, an elastic bandage, or a surgical support garment for 10 to 14 days.

Taking Care of Your Wound

You will be able to remove your bandages and to shower after a few days. Afterwards, pat the incision dry—or blow it dry with a cool hair dryer. Then cover the stitches with fresh gauze.

Stitches

You will probably have deep stitches that will absorb. There will be some stitches in the skin that will be removed after 5 to 7 days. You may also have stitches that stay in *longer*—2 or 3 weeks. These long-staying stitches are called pull-out stitches; they run under the skin exiting at either end. Thus they won't leave marks in your skin, even when they are in for a long time.

Scars

Your scars are the biggest drawback of these operations. The scar from a buttock lift lies in or above the buttock crease. The scar from the thigh lift lies in the crease of the leg, going from the groin in front around the inner thigh to the buttock in the back. These scars are moderately well hidden, although if they widen after surgery (and they often do) they may be visible in sports clothes. The hip lift will leave a long scar from your buttock out to the side of the leg. Today, with suction lipectomy available to reduce the fat deposits in this area, the hip lift is less popular, because of the scars.

Tips

- Elastic support hose after surgery will support your legs during the healing. Wear support hose for 6 weeks.
- Your skin will be dry after the surgery, so rub body lotion into the skin well away from the stitch line. When you bathe, use little soap—it will dry your skin even more.

- Skirts, not slacks, will be most comfortable for the first 2 weeks—they won't chafe surgical incisions.
- These operations remove excess skin and the fat underneath that skin. They are best done when you are in shape and have lost weight, if that is necessary.
- These operations *may* become necessary if you have had suction lipectomy of your hips, thighs, and buttocks and the skin is now loose. They are not usually done at the same time as the fat suction. Unlike fat suction, these operations leave long scars.

Back to Work

Realistically, you should allow yourself 2 weeks of recovery, and more if you can get it. There is the surgery and soreness to recover from, plus the fatigue of the general anesthesia. You will be too tired to work before 2 weeks are up.

Back to Parties

If you return to work after 2 weeks, avoid all parties for another week because you will be too tired to enjoy them. Apart from slow dancing, you should not dance until 3 to 4 weeks after surgery, when all the soreness is gone. Otherwise dancing won't be fun—you'll just hurt afterwards.

Back to Sports

You can go for a long walk or swim a few laps in a pool after 2 weeks, although you may not have the energy for sports if you go back to work at this time. After 3 weeks, you can begin more vigorous workouts and sports such as tennis or jogging. Rough contact sports are out for at least a month—they will be too much for your body and your incisions will ache afterwards.

Back to Sex

The incisions from these operations are slow to heal and lie close to the groin. You should avoid sex for about 3 weeks to allow the incisions to get strong—so that they won't inadvertently be pulled or injured during sex. You want to avoid causing them to bleed or hurt or damaging them so that your scars do not widen more than necessary.

Hip/Thigh/Buttock Lift: Recovery-at-a-Glance

This chart represents the *average* recovery times for this cosmetic operation.

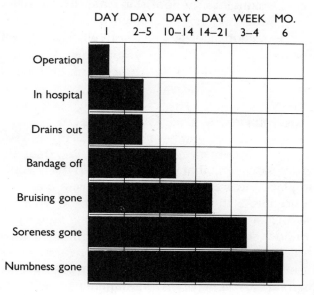

	DAY 1	DAY 2–5	DAY 10–14	DAY 14–21	WEEK 3–4	MO. 6
Operation						
In hospital						
Drains out						
Bandage off						
Bruising gone						
Soreness gone						
Numbness gone						

How Much It Costs

Your surgeon's fee will be approximately $2500 to $5000 for a lift of the hips, buttocks, and/or thighs. You will also have to pay approximately $2500 to $3000 or more for the operating room and several nights in the hospital.

Insurance Coverage

It is rarely worth the trouble to try to collect insurance. Most of these procedures are cosmetic. However, a few patients need the surgery because of extreme weight loss or a medical problem, such as adrenal malfunction, that led to sudden weight gain and then weight loss. If this applies to you, insurance may pay. Get the insurance company's *written* approval for the *dollar amount* that they will pay before your surgery. If you wait until after the surgery, they are much more likely to view it as "merely" cosmetic.

My Assessment of This Procedure

These operations are wonderful for people who have really loose skin from age, weight loss, or poor skin elasticity. However, the scars are long, wide, and may be sunken. These operations are not ideal for perfectionists who don't want any scar showing in a skimpy swim suit.

Side Effects and Complications

Side Effects

Scars are the major side effect that you must bear in mind. Although the surgeon can place the scars in the best possible area, the scars may become noticeable if they widen or shift, as they may after a buttock or hip lift. Most patients are happy with this surgery, but if you tend to form poor scars, think carefully before you go ahead.

Your skin will be numb after surgery, because many nerves to the skin are cut and because pulling on the skin makes the nerves malfunction temporarily. You may have permanent patches of numbness, but more commonly the numbness gradually fades over many months.

A blood clot (hematoma) or fluid collection (seroma) may develop under your incision after the surgery. This will delay your healing and may require drainage with a needle or through re-opening a small part of the incision. These cause a temporary wound-healing delay, and you heal rapidly once the problem is treated.

Complications

Infection can occur after these operations. Although it occurs only rarely, it can be temporarily disabling. The groin area has a very high bacterial count, so these operations are more infection prone than, for instance, breast or face surgery. If you develop a severe infection, you may need further surgery to drain the infection, antibiotics, and a longer stay in the hospital. Your scars will be worse—wide, red, swollen—for a long time—perhaps a year or permanently. Time and coverup cream will help to hide an unsatisfactory scar.

Infection can also seriously diminish the blood flow in the skin in these areas. This may cause scabbing of large areas around the scar, delaying healing for a month, or longer, or even making further surgery necessary to seal the wound.

Marjorie: Infection Left Scars

Marjorie had very loose thigh skin which she did not like. Her goal was to be able to wear a swim suit—to show off her legs. She was widowed and her children were in college. She thought it was time to do something for herself. Marjorie understood about the scars and had accepted them—she thought. Her recovery was complicated by a very rare infection. She required an additional week in the hospital, another week of convalescence at home, and daily office visits for another week. When Marjorie healed, her scars were lumpy and thick from the infection. Although she could see the improvement from the surgery, she felt disappointed because with the scars, she felt she would still not want to show off her legs.

George: An Adrenal Problem Led to Surgery

George was 18 when he developed an adrenal gland problem. In addition to gaining almost 40 pounds, he required major adrenal surgery. When he finally recovered—and lost the weight—a year later, his thighs had loose skin hanging down. He hated to think this was permanent. George decided to have a thigh lift under general anesthesia in the summer before college. He was very pleased to be rid of the hanging skin. The scars widened to almost an inch on his inner leg, but they were flat and not lumpy. They didn't bother him at all. He felt good about himself for the first time since he had become sick from his adrenal malfunction.

Lynn: No More "Awful" Buttocks

Lynn was in her late thirties. She was recently married and an avid sports enthusiast. No matter what she did, she felt her buttocks just looked "awful." They sagged like "an old cow." She wanted them fixed. Lynn had a buttock lift under general anesthesia. Her surgery was early in the morning. She was fit and had no bleeding, so she was able to go home after one night in the hospital. Lynn had no trouble with the surgery except that the antibiotics brought on a vaginal yeast infection (a complication of any antibiotic treatment). Even though she was too sore to sit for over a week and couldn't do sports, she felt that the brief yeast infection was the only real problem.

What Other Patients Say

- **Accountant, 27**: "I had a gastric bypass for obesity and really lost weight. If it weren't for being able to lift everything after I lost the weight, I'd just gain the weight back. I looked like a balloon that deflated."
- **Professional golfer, 49**: "I had a hip lift. My scars indented. I hate them. The indentation shows in tight sports clothes. There's no way to get rid of them. I can't say I'm pleased."
- **Mother of four, 37**: "I could *feel* the pulling of the scars for months after the surgery, but they look fine. I had my thighs lifted and my buttocks after my last baby. I like it."
- **Department store buyer, 60+**: "At my age—and I'm not telling—if you're thin, you sag. I sagged. My whole family sags. I had my legs and my rump lifted. I love it. The hips didn't need it. My breasts are next."

Index